THE NUTRITION NAVIGATOR

RESEARCHERS' EDITION

M.SC. HENRY S. GRANT

AMERICAN
DIET
PUBLISHING

KOBLENZ and WILMINGTON

ADP American Diet Publishing GmbH

Library of Congress Control Number 2014957226
ISBN 978-1-941978-24-5
Front cover design by Mahmood Ali
Interior design by Rose Hristova
E-Mail of the author: Grant@AmericanDietPublishing.com

ADP American Diet Publishing GmbH

Johannes Mueller-Strasse 12
56068 Koblenz
Germany

913 N Market Street
Wilmington, DE, 19801
United States of America

The data set for the algorithmic ordained statements concerning fructose, lactose and sugar alcohols is from the University of Minnesota Nutrition Coordination Center 2014 Food and Nutrient Database. The database license has been acquired for this book due to its high quality and scope based on international research. Statements regarding fructans and galactans have been drawn from four cited international studies. Those regarding fructans and galactans have been drawn from six different sources that are indicated in the tables. Nevertheless, the contents of the book bear no guarantee. Neither the author, publisher, any cited scientist nor the University of Minnesota is liable for personal injuries or physical or financial damage. Please note that the quantities of critical ingredients in the mentioned products, which are the foundation for the stated portion sizes, are relative and in part based on derivations. Portion sizes the reader is expected to tolerate are based on approximations of various details. The precise tolerable portion size of any product varies depending on its processing, country-specific composition, degree of maturity and cultivation.

ACKNOWLEDGMENTS

Special thanks to M. Thor and the nutritional research team of the University of Minnesota, J. S. Barrett, J. R. Biesiekierski, P. R. Gibson, K. Liels, J. G. Muir, S. J. Shepherd, R. Rose and O. Rosella as well as the rest of the gastroenterology research team of the Monash University, all other cited scientists for their research, B. Hartmann of the Bundesministerium für Ernährung, Landwirtschaft und Verbraucherschutz, G.-W. von Rymon Lipinski of the Goethe Universität, and H. Zorn of the Justus Liebig-Universität, for copyediting L. Gomes Domingues, F. Lang, C. R. Mundy, L. Popielinski and M. Vastolo, as well as my mother, sister and friends, especially C. Schlick and all other contributors who enabled me to write this book in first place.

To my daughter—Paula Anna

CONTENTS

Preface

This book shows you ways to find relief from abdominal discomfort due to any of the covered intolerances or from irritable bowel syndrome. With this book you will be able to identify those ingredients that lead to symptoms, enabling you to control your intake for a healthier and more worry-free life!

The book's information is drawn from intensive research and interviews with professors. The portions indicated in the food lists are based on results of laboratory research. An analysis of the US database has allowed us to produce practical recommendations regarding the portion sizes that your stomach can handle. Moreover, you will learn about the background and consequences of the ailments discussed. This book provides you with a broad spectrum of insights: removable key facts lists for your purchases, strategies to determine the amounts of critical foods you can stomach and even a discussion on the topic of stress management.

Nevertheless, only your doctor is qualified to make any mandatory nutritional recommendations. All those made in the book are non-binding. It is not possible to guarantee recovery, and there are other triggers of abdominal symptoms that may be relevant (see Chapter 2.2.6). This book should not be the sole basis for any decisions you make. Talk about any diet with your doctor before you begin in order to limit discomfort. You are responsible for your personal health, including how you choose to interpret data and specialists' advice.

As a long time sufferer, I know about the need for clarity and practical advice. The focuses of the strategy discussed in this book are quality and suitability for daily use. I wholeheartedly wish you ongoing success on your way to greater abdominal comfort!

Your author,

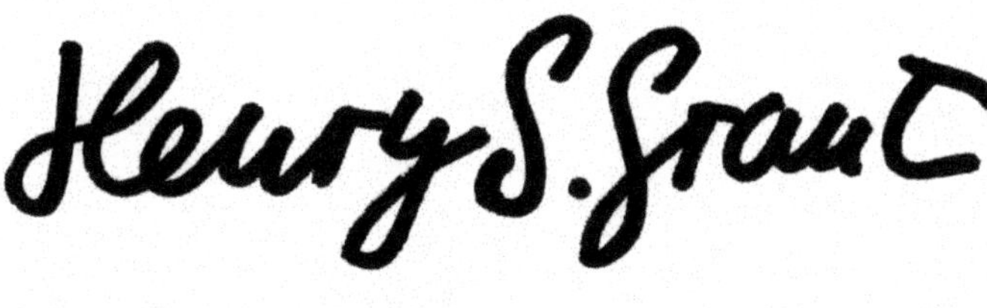

Henry S. Grant

1

INFORMATION

1.1 Why you deserve this book

You have courage. You took the initiative. By buying this book you have shown your will to overcome your discomfort. Many suffer due to such discomfort, yet only a few act, and you are one of them! You know that you and those around you will gain more from your life if you regain comfort in your belly. Hence, I welcome you to the mission of developing a successful nutritional routine.

If you bought the book so you could learn to adapt to those in your life suffering from intolerances, you will learn how in Chapter 2.5. This shows a consideration for others that would make anyone glad to be a guest at your table. Furthermore, you will find generally useful hints regarding healthy nutrition in Chapter 2.1.4, and in Chapter 2.6 you will learn to reduce stress in your everyday life and improve your decision-making skills.

If your employer or educational institution has given you this book as a gift, it is an expression of their appreciation of you and trust in your willingness to take action. The book has been written with the intention of enabling you to live more of a free life, by improving your digestive well-being. It will help you to change your life so you can stop losing happiness due to abdominal discomfort.

Before we begin, realize that starting soon after your birth, your mother ensured your adequate nutrition by giving you only baby food. Unlike creatures in the wild, we usually do not face natural restrictions concerning what we eat when. You, as an adult, choose what you want to eat. That being so, is it any wonder that finding a nutritional plan that fits your needs is a factor in your health? With this book, you benefit from a comprehensible description of current scientific research and probably the most useable food table on the market for countering food intolerance.

In this first part of the book you will find out which diagnostic procedures you should go through with your doctor before changing your diet. Moreover, the causes and effects of irritable bowel syndrome [IBS] will be explained, and you will discover the elements of foods that can cause abdominal discomfort. These are easily fermentable carbohydrates. We will call these comprehensive *bricks*, as a brick sits heavily in one's stomach. Some of these, like fructose and lactose, may already be familiar to you. Others are less well known and form one reason as to why discomfort persists for those who live on a "brick diet." Whether you have an intolerance or IBS, knowing about these triggers will help you improve your dietary health. After the triggers are discussed, the second part of the book will acquaint you with the nutrition navigator strategy. You can find out which bricks you can stomach well and how much you can eat of those that are problematic for you. Furthermore, you will read about the basic principles of a healthy diet. What's more, you learn how to stick to the diet in your everyday life, along with how you can reduce stress, which is also a factor that can upset your stomach. These are the aims of the nutrition navigator:

You **improve** your **quality of life** by gaining back **comfort** in your **stomach** while **maintaining** a **healthy diet**.

In order to help you achieve a healthy diet, the book guides you to choose portion sizes you are able to stomach with regard to fructose, lactose, sugar alcohols and other bricks in athletic products, beverages, cold and warm dishes, fast food chain products, fruits and vegetables and many other products and ingredients. The food table contains numerous brand-name products and enables you to reduce limitations on your choices as much as possible. If your doctor has made a diagnosis based upon nutrition diaries, he or she might choose to retest you after considering the data from this book. For example, the amount of sugar alcohols in some fruits and vegetables or the amount of free fructose in cereals is hard to discern from the currently available literature. Your doctor may thus be able to finally discover and accurately diagnose a specific intolerance. Additionally, you get two practical lists for your wallet, to make it easier for you to make smart purchases for yourself.
Only if you know which bricks you are able to stomach, along with the portion sizes of products that contain problematic ingredients, will you be able to

eat in a way that suits your profile and helps you avoid losing quality of life. Your mission is a challenging one. Bricks can hide everywhere—even in oral hygiene products and medicine. Please read this book's recommendations carefully and act accordingly. The consequences of being negligent about having an intolerance are harsh, as you will learn later. An unknown malabsorbtion of an ingredient can lead to depression and much more unpleasantness.[1] The "brick-eating dragons" presented in the following chapter are a fictive symbol of potential discomfort, while the "interception shield" is a symbol of the body's usual metabolism. The effects described, however, are real.

---

[1]Varea et al., 2005; Ledochowski, Sperner-Unterweger, Widner & Fuchs, 2000 & 1998a; Ledochowski, Sperner-Unterweger, & Fuchs, 1998b.

1.2 Prehistoric monsters take vengeance...

How do brick-eating dragons steal drive, fun and lust from you? Dragons were believed to have been stamped out in the Middle Ages—but some small ones persevered, and now they are back and are seeking revenge. Yet, we did not do them any harm. People had good reasons for hunting them in the Middle Ages for their extreme aggression. These so-called brick dragons are carrying out their vendetta by making themselves invisible and smuggling themselves into bellies. Even women and children are targeted. Anyone can be affected. They are called brick dragons here because they can only do harm if we eat too many of certain bricks. These bricks exist naturally in some foods and are usually used by our bodies to provide us with energy. However, as a brick dragon enters our stomach, it damages our stomach's engine or "brick interception shield," letting more bricks enter the dragon's lair, the bowel. There are different types of bricks. The penetrability of the interception shield can only be determined via tests that will be introduced later. Remember for now that for the dragons any means will do—revenge at any price—even if they themselves have to put themselves into a very uncomfortable place for their attacks. Some people may show no symptoms but still test positive for intolerance. They have an intolerance without having irritable bowel symptoms, suggesting that their shield is damaged for reasons other than a brick dragon.

How brick-eating dragons irritate us:

Some dragons build walls, and this leads to constipation. Others try to burn the bricks. The body is forced to extinguish the fire, leading to diarrhoea. Still others eat the bricks, and when they have collected enough energy, they blow up the stomach, resulting in flatulence and bloating.

Attack of the brick-eating dragons! Losses are suffered by…

↓ **Lust**

↓ **Health**

↓ **Fitness**

↓ **Vitality**

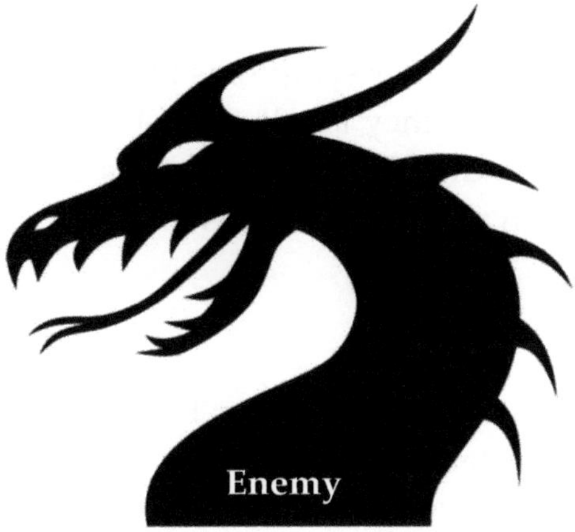

Brick-eating dragons are associated with extensive limitations to one's quality of life. Those who are affected are worse off with regard to their fitness, the frequency of their bodily pains, their vigilance, their vitality and their overall physical and mental health. Analogously, it is harder for them to discharge their social roles and enjoy emotional fulfilment.[2] As if that were not enough, those concerned are more likely to have sexual dysfunctions, such as reduced libido.[3]

It is not surprising that these symptoms leave their mark on absenteeism at work. A study in the USA[4] and one in the Netherlands[5] found that people with an untreated brick-eating dragon, i.e., an irritable bowel, miss school or work about twice as often as the general population. On average, this amounts to over five sick days per year. Increasing discomfort leads to a noticeable worsening of work efficiency, physical fitness, ability to fulfil social obligations, vitality, mental fitness and general health; sick days stack up.[6] Up to a certain point, the body is able to intercept bricks before they can reach the dragon. Those that are intercepted are used as usual to generate energy. When consumed in tolerable amounts bricks are good for the energy supply and gut flora and thus one's well-being.[7] If you eat more than your body can handle,

[2] Gralnek, Hays, Kilbourne, Naliboff, & Mayer, 2000.

[3] Fass, Fullerton, Naliboff, Hirsh, & Mayer, 1998.

[4] Drossman, et al., 1993.

[5] Donker, Foets, & Spreeuwenberg, 1999.

[6] Hahn, Kirchdoerfer, Fullerton, & Mayer, 1997.

[7] Muir et al., 2009.

however, your brick dragon rejoices and may affect your social and professional success as well as your love life. Luckily, you can and should fight back. Comprehensive studies show that the majority of those affected can substantially reduce their symptoms by adopting an appropriately low-brick diet. With such a diet, they ideally only target those bricks that their shield cannot effectively handle.[8] This is the book's aim. Still, before we get into strategy, you will learn about the diagnostic check.

Summary

Bricks are parts of foods. Your bowel has an interception shield. This shield can catch a certain amount of bricks and transform them into energy. This amount will be determined below. If you take in more bricks than your shield can intercept, however, then the result is discomfort, if you have an irritable bowel. By eating consciously, you can make sure that you take in only as many bricks as your shield can handle.

---

[8] Wilder-Smith, Materna, Wermelinger, & Schuler, 2013; Gibson & Shepherd, 2010; Goldstein, Braverman, & Stankiewicz 2000.

1.3 Diagnostic check

If you suffer from abdominal pains, bloating, constipation, flatulence or diarrhoea, do not accept your discomfort any longer; be the person who acts.[9] You can expect the whole procedure to take about half a year, but it will pay off: you are likely going to get your symptoms under control and minimize the limitations you face in your diet. The first step—before the book's actual diagnostic procedure begins—is to ask your doctor to refer you to a gastroenterologist in order to **avoid false diagnosis**.

The diagnosis will include a stool analysis, an ultrasonic check and some camera shots inside your stomach in order to reject other causes.[10] These tests will allow the specialist to check whether there is an abnormal bacterial colonization of the small intestine. This may lead to false positives in uncovering an intolerance to a brick type.[11] The next test looks for intolerance to gluten, an ingredient in grains, an intolerance to which is called celiac disease. In people who have untreated celiac disease the tolerance test for the brick sorbitol is often positive, even if they are able to stomach it.[12] Following this, a genetic test regarding hereditary fructose intolerance should be administered. Hereditary fructose intolerance is rare, but it is serious: the fructose test itself can be lethal to those with this disease.[13]

After other diseases have been ruled out, what follows are checks regarding three of the mentioned brick types. For the breath test, you will take a high dose containing fructose, lactose or sorbitol on different days. If bricks pass your shield and arrive at a brick-eating dragon, gases emerge from your intestine. These can and will then be measured in your breath. If the breath test is negative for fructose and sorbitol separately, please ask whether you can also do a combined test of fructose and sorbitol. The combined test is only comparable if the added amount of sorbitol is deducted from the amount of fructose. That is, if 5g of sorbitol is added to the fructose dilution, and the dilution of the previous fructose breath test contained 25g of fructose, then it should now contain only 20g of fructose in addition to the 5g of sorbitol.[14]

---

[9] Hahn et al., 1997.

[10] Raithel et al., 2013.

[11] Nucera et al., 2005.

[12] Corazza, Strocchi, Rossi, Sirola, & Fasbarrini, 1988.

[13] Ali, Rellos, & Cox, 1998.

[14] Gaby, 2005.

When the amount of gas in your breath reaches a certain level, the diagnosis is an intolerance towards the respective brick. Having an intolerance means that your shield's ability to intercept that brick is currently small, and bricks of that kind will be able to easily pass through to arrive at the brick dragon.[15]

The threshold for a positive diagnosis for a fructose dilution (typically containing 25–50g) is usually 20ppm (parts per million, a concentration measure). This threshold also applies for lactose and sorbitol.[16]

The recommended breath test, however, is not available everywhere. In Chapter 2.2.3 you will learn about a substitute test, in case you have no access to the breath test. In general, do not accept a diagnosis without a test. If none of the tests comes to a conclusive result, your irritable bowel syndrome is at least—for now—undefined.

For some people the breath test will give a positive result even if none of the usual symptoms are exhibited.[17] The general diagnosis for people who do suffer from symptoms is a functional gastrointestinal disorder. Irritable bowel syndrome belongs in this category. Irritable means that your stomach reacts sensitively to stimuli like air in the stomach—more on that in the next chapter. The bowel is the final segment of your alimentary canal and the dragon's lair.

In a study regarding the intensity of symptoms and intolerance to bricks, no differences were found between people diagnosed with "functional disorder of the bowel (by an intolerance)" and those diagnosed with irritable bowel syndrome. Thus, to simplify matters, remember that people who do suffer from the mentioned symptoms suffer from irritable bowel discomfort.[18] It makes sense to differentiate between a defined irritable bowel syndrome, for which it is clear what bricks one is intolerant towards, and an undefined irritable bowel syndrome, where either no intolerance exists towards one of the three bricks or no test has been conducted yet. Having an intolerance without this leading to discomfort is thus defined as having an intolerance without having an irritable bowel. Nevertheless, your doctor will tell you whether you have an intolerance or whether you have an—in this case undefined—irritable bowel syndrome.

Irritable bowel symptoms are similar regardless of whether the irritable bowel syndrome is defined or not because most of the bricks' effects are inde-

---

[15] Montalto et al., 2006.

[16] Raithel et al., 2013; Goldstein et al., 2000; D. Mishkin, Sablauskas, Yalovsky, & S. Mishkin, 1997; Truswell & Thorburn, 1988.

[17] Wilder-Smith et al., 2013; Corazza et al., 1988.

[18] Longstreth et al., 2006; Goldstein et al., 2000.

pendent of the type of brick, as they result from osmotic effects and fermentation and each brick can induce these. Bricks that pass your interception shield, i.e. are not metabolized by your body, lead to an accumulation of water and fermentation.[19] Incidentally, for up to 90% of patients with an irritable bowel, the syndrome can be defined in terms of an intolerance to one or more of the three bricks.[20]

If you suffer from irritable bowel symptoms, you are not alone: **20–30**% of Europeans have an intolerance, i.e., their bowel shield is too weak for one or more of the three bricks for which a breath test is usually conducted.[21] Worldwide, 10–15% of all people suffer from undefined abdominal discomfort.[22] About 20% of Americans, 9% of the Dutch, 22% of the English, 25% of the Japanese and 44% of West Africans are affected.[23]

Summary

If you regularly suffer from abdominal discomfort, visit a specialist. Checks can take up to half a year. Many others share your fate, but you are holding in your hands the key to fighting the symptoms!

---

19 Gibson & Shepherd, 2009.

20 Goldstein et al., 2000.

21 Raithel et al., 2013.

22 Quigley et al., 2009.

23 Wells, Hahn, & Whorwell, 1997.

1.4 Background of the disease

Irritable bowel syndrome is a common disease. The symptoms can usually be clearly differentiated from those caused by an allergic reaction by using approved methods such as the breath test diagnostic procedure. The symptoms exhibit themselves as an oversensitivity—not in the strength of your character, but related to your intestine. The exact causes are unknown. In some cases, infections and emotions may be an issue. The influence on emotions results from the close connection between the brain and the gut. On the one hand, a bad mood can cause your belly to grumble; on the other hand, a grumbling belly can adversely affect your mood. This link is useful to know to save us from foods we do not stomach well and to find a potential cause when we're having trouble with stress (see Chapter 2.6). You can imagine the diagnosis as a signal disturbance between head and stomach. The bad news is that this sensitivity appears in about 70% of those affected over the long term. The good news is that it does not cause cancer, and the ramifications can be reduced considerably in most cases. Due to the chronic nature of the disease, adjusting your diet as appropriate to your needs can supersede medical treatment. Most medicine has side effects, and a diet is often cheaper.[24]

Summary

An irritable bowel usually accompanies you for a long time. It is an oversensitivity of the digestive system. Anxiety coincides with grumbling in the belly. An irritable bowel is not a cause of cancer. By following an appropriate diet most affected people are able to overcome most of their symptoms. An effective diet can be better than medical treatment. A sensitive bowel is not a sign of weakness of character, but failing to adapt one's lifestyle to it may be interpreted as such!

[24] Quigley, Hunt, Emmanuel, & Hungin, 2013.

1.5 The bricks and how your belly is fighting

Bricks are carbohydrates that can either be absorbed by your body to be changed into energy or pass by your shield, in which case you have a dragon behind your barriers, gobbling bricks and breeding symptoms. Your body's brick interception shield works similarly to the toddler game in which the child pushes differently shaped blocks through openings in a box. If a brick fits through, it is intercepted and metabolized. What is tricky is that each human can stomach different amounts of the different bricks (has a different kind of shield). Some of the bricks cannot be efficiently intercepted by anyone's shield, but this is not an issue for people who do not have a brick-eating dragon. The following drawing illustrates that some bricks cannot be intercepted by the shield by the no entry-sign on the shield's round brick.

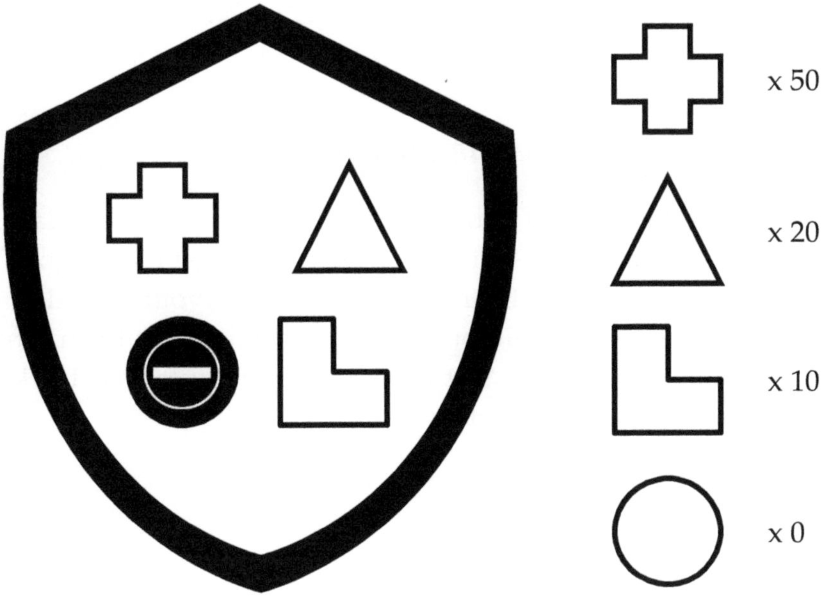

The depicted bowel shield can absorb cross-bricks very well with a capacity of over 50 pieces. Unfortunately, however, it offers no protection against round bricks. A round brick passes directly by to the affected person's dragon, which then reacts, e.g., by blowing up her belly or trying to spit fire. In such a case, the stomach reacts in the same way a dry sponge reacts when you put it in water. It sucks itself full and expands—the quenched water accumulates. Air and/or water lead to discomfort.[25] Therefore, if bricks enter the intestine it means:

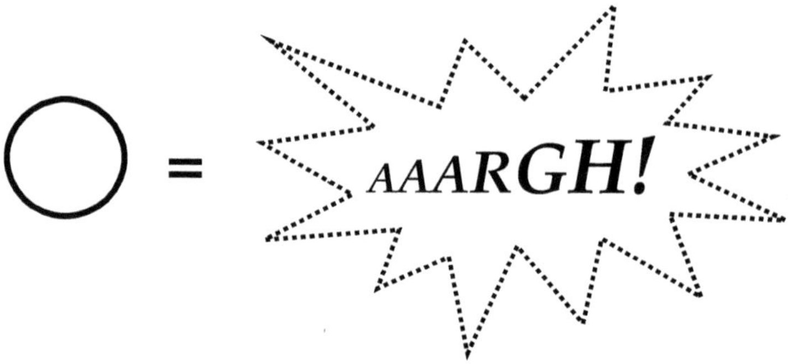

It depends on your shield

Did your breath test show that your shield's capacity for fructose, lactose and/or sorbitol is great? That is one-to-nothing for you against the dragon. You can continue eating those products that contain bricks your shield intercepts well—i.e., that you tolerate—without having to think about them. The others you have to avoid, more or less. But what are these mysterious bricks? In the following, you will find their profiles.

[25] Gibson & Shepherd, 2009; Lifschitz, 2000.

1.5.1 Brick number one: Lactose

In brief

Lactose is primarily contained in milk and other dairy products and is therefore also known as milk sugar. All toddlers need lactose and are able to stomach it. A lactose intolerance evolves after the fifth birthday at the earliest.[26] About 5–17% of the light-skinned and 50–100% of the remaining world population have a lactose intolerance. Even so, not all of those with lactose intolerance also have an irritable bowel.[27] What is more, those who are affected are usually able to stomach—that is to intercept—small amounts of lactose.[28]

Basic tolerance level (BTL): 1.5g per meal (as defined in the glossary).

There are four tolerance levels ranging from zero to three. These tolerance levels [TL] are used to determine one's tolerable portion sizes in the third part of this book. Applying the basic tolerance level [BTL], i.e. TL 0, you will be able to determine the portion sizes with which you can avoid symptoms induced by the respective bricks independent of your shield strength. The BTL portion sizes are the lowest for the respective brick. In order to find your TL, you will conduct a level test, as per Chapter 2.2.4. Observe the BTL during the implementation diet, unless your breath test shows that you tolerate the respective brick. You can find the portion tables in Chapter 3.

In one study, the symptoms appeared for those affected at 1.5g (though a 3g dose was not given for contrast). The authors were surprised that symptoms also appeared from lactose-free milk used for comparison.[29] The reason for this may be the prevalence of other easily fermentable carbohydrates that were contained in the test milk. These have a positive effect on the gut flora but can also trigger discomforts depending on the amount consumed.[30] The ingredients to which these symptoms can be attributed are galactans, which will be discussed later.[31] The amount of galactans in milk depends on the breed,

---

26 Raithel et al., 2013.

27 Lomer, Parkes, & Sanderson, 2008.

28 Suarez, Savalano, & Levitt, 1995; Barrett et al., 2010.

29 Vesa, Korpela, & Sahi, 1996.

30 German, Freeman, Lebrilla, & Mills, 2008; Gibson & Shepherd, 2010; Boehm & Stahl, 2007.

31 Kuhn & Gauhe, 1965.

race and lactation month of dairy cattle. The highest average amounts are to be found in cow milk with 0.137g/100ml,[32] followed by goat milk with 0.117g/100ml.[33] As 100mL of milk contains about 5g lactose and 0.137g galactans, about 0.03g will be added to the galactans for each gram of lactose. The BTL of galactans is thus crossed at 350mL of milk. In combination with other foods such as cereals, however, it can play a role regarding discomfort.

The tolerance threshold of pure lactose in cases of intolerance is likely to be 10g per day and thus about 3g per meal.[34] Thus you should be able to stomach the amount of lactose that is used in some medicine you take orally, as long as you avoid other products that contain lactose during the days of your treatment.[35] The BTL has been chosen as half of the recommended 3g per meal, as some affected nevertheless either completely avoid lactose or still feel that their tolerance threshold is lower.

Influence of fructans

For most people suffering from a lactose intolerance combined with an irritable bowel, simply reducing the consumed amount of lactose only partially leads to the symptoms' disappearance. Even though this may already be enough, it indicates that intolerances regarding other bricks play a role and may be worth considering in the nutrition plan.[36] Some lactose intolerant people suffer irritation from the brick fructans, which will be introduced in Chapter 1.5.3, more than by lactose.[37]

---

[32] Balasubramanya, Sarwar, & Narayanan, 1993; Jensen, Blanc, & Patton, 1995.
[33] Meyrand et al., 2013; Newburg & Neubauer, 1995.
[34] EFSA, 2007; Suarez et al., 1995. Milk acid bacteria, which are being used to produce cheese, are able to break down these galactans. For that reason their share in cheese is perhaps lower Makras, Van Acker, & De Vuyst, 2005. However, more specific data is not available yet.
[35] Raithel et al., 2013.
[36] Vernia, Ricciardi, Frandina, Bilotta, & Frieri, 1995.
[37] Teuri, Vapaatalo, & Korpela, 1999.

Calcium

When you reduce the amount of dairy products you consume, it is important to increase your supply of calcium from other sources. An adult under 50 years of age should take in about 1,000mg (1,300mg for teenagers), and a woman over 50 (or a man over 60) should take in 1,200mg.[38] You can take in calcium through some lactose-free milk (replacement) products, some protein powders (1,200mg/100g), cheddar cheese (721mg/100g), almonds (236mg/100g), salmon and sardines (240mg/100g), spinach (210mg/100g) and figs (162mg/100g)[39] or by taking calcium tablets. Please only choose tablets that do not contain (critical amounts of) other bricks that are problematic for you, if possible.[40]

Depression

In a study of randomly chosen participants who were suffering from depressed moods, a breath test showed that over 70% of them had a brick intolerance, while the average percentage among people from the same region suffering from a brick intolerance was only 15%. This does not indicate that many who have an intolerance are depressed but that many people with depression have an intolerance. Thus, in further research, tests were conducted to work out how many randomly selected people with an intolerance showed signs of depression. For 28.5% of the test group—a number significantly greater than the general population—the scores denoted depression.

Serotonin, a neurotransmitter that elevates one's mood is produced by the body from tryptophan, which is contained in food. Presumably at least some of the bricks that pass the interception shield merge with tryptophan to form a non-absorbable substance. This reaction reduces the amount of available tryptophan and causes the body to produce less serotonin. Hence, the bricks that arrive at the dragon's lair hinder the body's ability to let positive feelings emerge.[41] In an experiment in which fructose and sorbitol consumption was reduced, depression scores normalized for most participants. Keeping within the tolerance levels that apply to you when choosing your portion sizes can therefore improve your mood (your serotonin metabolism) because fewer bricks arrive at the dragon's lair. Extra discipline is required to maintain the

---

38 Ross et al., 2011.

39 U. S. Department of Agriculture [USDA], 2013.

40 McCoubrey, Parkes, Sanderson, & Lomer 2008.

41 Varea et al., 2005; Belitz, Grosch, & Schieberle, 2008.

portion thresholds in cases of depression, however: a lack of high spirits (tryptophan) can foster a hunger for sweets. Now, sweets often contain bricks. If an intolerance is present, the intake of the respective bricks further lowers one's mood, creating a vicious circle.[42] You can find the amount of bricks contained in sweets in the lists in Part 3. Even if you are not depressed, please remember that in the presence of a dysfunctional metabolism, depression can result from consuming too much of foods that contain problematic bricks. Affected people should always seek help rather than trying to counter these effects through sheer willpower.

Enzyme capsules

Assuming your body can metabolize 3g lactose by itself, taking enzyme capsules pays off once you are past the 3g tolerance level number 1 with your meal. Please make sure the enzyme capsules are free of other bricks that are problematic for you; for example, some contain sorbitol and mannitol. In order to be effective, the lactose enzymes not only have to arrive at the small intestine without being destroyed by acid before they get there, but they need to do so at the same time as the lactose. For this purpose, stomach acid-resistant capsules seem most appropriate. One study found that the most effective capsule was only able to break down 2.7g of lactose. At least four capsules would thus be required to take in a 250mL glass of lactose-free milk, which makes up for 12.5g of lactose after subtracting the 3g from that amount.[43] You can find the required amount of capsules in the K-column of the food tables contained in the third part of the book.

---

[42] Ledochowski, Sperner-Unterweger, Widner & Fuchs, 2000 & 1998a; Ledochowski, Sperner-Unterweger, & Fuchs, 1998b.

[43] O'Connell & Walsh, 2006.

Which foods contain this brick?

All (mammal) milk products contain milk sugar, as do many processed foods and consumable products such as breads, bologna, sauces and medicine (although the amount in medicine is often unproblematic if no additional products containing lactose are consumed). Raw milk tends to contain the highest amount of lactose, while some sorts of dry cheese, like cheddar, are nearly free of it. Luckily, you can intercept and metabolize at least some limited amounts of lactose, and there are enzyme capsules as well as numerous milk replacement and lactose-free products available, including rice milk. But be mindful that soymilk contains other bricks, fructans and galactans, while rice milk is free of them.[44]

[44] Biesiekierski et al., 2011.

1.5.2 Brick number two: Fructose

In brief

Fruit naturally contains fructose, and it is therefore known as fruit sugar. For 39% of those affected by unexplained regular abdominal discomfort, symptoms arise after the consumption of 15g fructose; for 70%, they appear after a dose of 30g.[45] People around the globe consume between 11 and 54g per day, or 4–18g per meal.[46] Accordingly, fructose triggers discomforts for many people who have an irritable bowel. As with the other bricks, the tolerable amount varies individually. If you do not have a fructose intolerance, there is no need to watch your fructose intake;[47] the fructose TLs only apply to those with a fructose intolerance or a currently undefined irritable bowel syndrome.

BTL: (Glucose balanced fructose 5g per 100g)[48]
Glucose-free fructose 0.5g per meal[49]

If you are restricted in your ability to stomach fructose, please get acquainted with the following factors that affect your body's fructose assimilation:

Influence of glucose

Imagine your interception shield (see Chapter 1.5) is being carried by a giant guard. Fructose is like a brick with the characteristics of a fly, and catching it is usually a challenge for the guard, especially when numerous fructose units appear at once. It is another game when glucose, a drop of sugar juice with the reaction time of a slug, enters the stage. Like any fly, fructose loves to come to rest on glucose, so the guard will have no trouble intercepting it. At times, however, sorbitol appears on the scene, as well, like a buzzing mosquito. Sorbitol is especially hard to catch and distracts the guard from the fructose.

---

[45] Choi, Johlin, Summers, Jackson, Rao, 2003.
[46] Gibson, Newnham, Barrett, Shepherd, & Muir, 2006; Park, & Yetley, 1993; Virtanen, Räsänen, Mäenpää, & Åkerblom, 1987.
[47] Gibson & Shepherd, 2009.
[48] The food contains fructose and glucose in equal amounts. Thereby, fructose is absorbed much better.
[49] Shepherd & Gibson, 2006. The amount of fructose that exceeds the amount of glucose in the food.

Hence, when sorbitol is present, more of the brick fructose gets through to arrive at the dragon.

This means that when quantities of glucose equal or exceed those of fructose, fructose interception is strongly improved.[50] Therefore, let us differentiate between glucose-balanced and glucose-free—or just "free" fructose. You can stomach much more fructose if it is balanced with glucose. According to the amount of gas measured during breath tests, glucose-balanced fructose is intercepted ten times more easily than free fructose.[51] For foods where the relationship leans more towards fructose than glucose, you can create balance artificially by eating foods that contain a lot of excess glucose.[52] A note regarding the tolerance level (TL) of glucose-balanced fructose: different studies show that people who are intolerant towards fructose are nevertheless able to stomach up to 50g of glucose-balanced fructose.[53] The limitation for glucose-balanced fructose[54] has only been mentioned due to an ambiguous study result. Despite the apparently optimal assimilation rate in a balanced glucose relationship, at a dose of 17g per day, 0.4g arrived at the intestine.[55] When the test was repeated with 98g of balanced glucose, the amount was still just slightly higher at 0.56g; however, due to the study setup, bacterial decomposition prior to the analysis may have distorted the result. Balanced fructose is disregarded in the food list because of the dubiousness of the test results. You can, however, adjust your consumption according to the sugar amount per 100g as shown in the ingredients, if you want, because sugar consists of one part glucose and one part fructose. At the same time, you can determine your adequate portion size with regard to free fructose in this book's food tables. If you want to limit your sugar consumption, and a beverage contains too much of it, you can dilute it with a suitable amount of water. It is good to reduce sugar consumption in general (see Chapter 2.1.4).

---

[50] Riby, Fujisawa, & Kretchmer, 1993.

[51] Kneepkens, Vonk, & Fernandes, 1984.

[52] Raithel el al., 2013.

[53] Latulippe & Skoog, 2011.

[54] Shepherd & Gibson, 2006.

[55] Barret et al., 2010.

Influence of sorbitol

If you have a fructose intolerance, you should try to avoid sorbitol as much as possible. Sorbitol inhibits the assimilation of fructose and is itself poorly absorbed by many people; thus, it is the dragon's best friend.[56] Unfortunately, no hint for an adequate BTL could be found. Still, you can determine your own TL as part of the tolerance level strategy upon finishing the three-week introductory diet (see Chapter 2.2.4).

Hereditary fructose intolerance

If you have been diagnosed with a rare and unfortunately not yet curable hereditary fructose intolerance, consuming fructose can be lethal. Please seek your doctor's advice.[57] You can use the food table in this book to determine foods that are free of fructose.

Folic acid deficiency

A fructose intolerance often negatively affects folic acid absorption. As a folic acid deficiency increases risk of cardiovascular disease, it would be sensible to take suitable supplements.[58] Otherwise, folic acid is contained in Kellogg's® Corn flakes (323µg/100g), some protein powders (280µg/100g) and short-grain rice (225µg/100g), for example.[59] The recommended daily dose is 300µg for men, 250µg for most women and 400µg for expectant mothers.[60]

Depression

Please see page 15.

---

[56] Raithel et al., 2013; Latulippe & Skoog, 2011; Shepherd, Parker Muir, & Gibson, 2008.

[57] Ali et al., 1998.

[58] Ledochowski, Ueberall, Propst, & Fuchs, 1999; Verhoef et al., 1996.

[59] USDA, 2013.

[60] Scientific Community on Food, 2000.

Enzyme capsules

Xylose isomerase is available on the market. The author is aware of only one study that aimed to prove its efficiency, and it showed symptoms improving by about 41%.[61] Whether this justifies the current high sales price remains for you to decide.

Foods with excess glucose

Few foods have an excess of glucose while being free of other bricks. When you eat one of the following foods together with a food that is restricted due to its amount of free fructose, you may be able to multiply your TL-adjusted portion size of the restricted food by the factor that applies to your TL. If you are interested, just test it out for yourself. Your multiplier is shown in one of the last four columns of the next table.[62] You can also purchase pure glucose as a powder online, though high sugar consumption should be avoided due to potential health implications (see Chapter 2.1.4).

Foods	Portion weight	Free glucose	BTL x	TL 1 x	TL 2 x	TL 3 x
Avocado (Florida)	37.5g	0.72g	2.25	1.5	1.25	1.25
Maple syrup	30g	0.32g	1.5	1.25	1	1
Mozzarella	28g	0.16g	1.25	1	1	1
Sweet corn	82g	1.22g	3.25	2	1.75	1.5
Thin slice of pineapple	56.3g	0.68g	2.25	1.5	1.5	1.25

Which foods contain this brick?

Nowadays, fructose is the cause of the sweet taste of many foods. It is added in the form of honey, gelling sugars and corn syrup. In the absence of an intolerance, humans can smoothly break down fructose. The way you mainly take in fructose depends on your nutritional habits. In the USA, about two thirds are taken in as soft drinks and enriched convenience foods and about one third as fruit. In Finland, the relationship is reversed.[63]

---

[61] Komericki et al., 2012.

[62] USDA, 2013; Latulippe & Skoog, 2011.

[63] Gibson et al., 2006.

1.5.3 Brick number three: Fructans

In brief

Fructose evolves while fructans metabolize, hence the similarity of their names.[64] It has been discovered that during the exploitation (fermentation) of **short-chain**[65] fructans by brick-eating dragons (bacteria), gas emerges.[66] However, that is not all; our body barely uses fructans. Up to 89% of them—more than of any other brick—are dished up for the bacteria in the colon.[67] What makes matters worse is that other bricks like fructose are digested much less effectively when more fructans are consumed.[68] For some lactose intolerant people, the discomforts induced by fructans are worse than those triggered by lactose itself.[69] As with holds for the other bricks, people without an irritable bowel are hardly bothered by them. If symptoms persist and are not reduced satisfactorily by limiting consumption of fructose, lactose and/or sorbitol, try reducing the amount of fructans and galactans (to be presented later in the book) in your meals.[70]

BTL of the sum of fructans and galactans: 0.5g per meal.[71]

Which foods contain this brick?

We primarily take in fructans when eating the following (tolerable amounts for the BTL in parentheses): garlic (one clove), onions (15g), artichoke (17g), cereals (21–45g) and noodles (147g), as well as pastries like bread, cake, cookies and pizza. Grain products contain far fewer fructans than vegetables, but the quantities in which we eat them makes them a primary source of fructans. Onions hold second place.[72] There is no relation between fructans and gluten. Even gluten-free bread often contains fructans, albeit about one third less than

---

64 Falony et al., 2009.

65 Category: Inulin, kestose and nystose.

66 Rumessen, 1992.

67 Barret et al., 2010; Molis et al., 1996.

68 Knudsen & Hessov, 1995.

69 Teuri et al., 1999.

70 Biesiekieski et al., 2011.

71 Barrett et al., 2010; Shepherd & Gibson, 2006.

72 Moshfegh, Friday, Goldman, & Ahuja, 1999.

common bread. Rice bread is free from fructans as the dough is commonly made without wheat, in contrast to potato or cornbread. In addition, spelt bread is especially well tolerated (250g) compared to rye or wheat bread (one slice each). Fructans are also contained in some fruits. Limit yourself, for example, to three fourths of a banana, half a nectarine and two slices of pineapple. The high amount of fructans contained in chicory or in Jerusalem and regular artichokes calls for avoidance.[73]

In tolerable amounts, fructans have positive effects, so they are added to various foods as inulin. For example, some beverages, brands of butter, candies, cereals, chocolates, ice creams and yogurts contain inulin. The added amounts of inulin are not always certain, aside from the derivations mentioned in the food table of this book. And so, to be on the safe side, you can avoid products that list inulin in their ingredients, use similar products in the food table of this book as a reference for the consumable amount according to your fructan TL or make a single-product test using the amount you can tolerate as a guideline (see Chapter 2.2.6). Some people are also allergic to inulin.[74]

You can even meet the 0.5g-per-meal BTL for fructans with little adaptation to your diet. Fructan-containing products are often consumed with other foods. When reviewing the portion sizes in Part 3 of the book, consider that when you combine fructan-containing foods, the respective single portion sizes decrease. In order to combine a fructan-containing product with another product that contains fructans or galactans you can, for example, bisect both portion sizes.

Influence on the nutrient supply

A reduction in fructans can require you to plan your intake of proteins, short-chain fatty acids and fibre.[75] You can find compensation strategies from Chapter 2 onward.

---

73 Biesiekierski et al., 2011; Muir et al., 2009; Muir et al., 2007; van Loo, Coussement, De Leenheer, Hoebregs, & Smith, 1995.

74 Gay-Crosier, Schreiber, & Hauser, 2000.

75 Biesiekieski et al., 2011; Muir et al., 2009; Dukas, Willett, & Giovannucci, 2003; Cummings & Macfarlane, 1997.

1.5.4 Brick number four: Galactans

In brief

Short-chain galactans[76], like short-chain fructans, are poorly absorbed by the body and arrive at the intestine in large chunks.[77] As fructans and galactans are similar oligosaccharides, they share a BTL of 0.5g in sum.[78]

BTL of the sum of fructans and galactans: 0.5g per meal.[79]

Buy prebiotics?

The European Food Safety Authority (EFSA) has repeatedly disregarded the claim that prebiotics and probiotics have a positive effect on the gut due to lack of solid proof. It regards them as at best potentially helpful.[80] Prebiotics producers ascribe artificial galactans a contribution to improved gut flora. A study set up by in collaboration of an employee of a prebiotics producer suggested that 3.5g of a special kind of artificial galactans improved the gut flora and thereby led to an average improvement of 37% regarding symptoms like abdominal pain, bloating, constipation, diarrhoea and flatulence.[81] Health claims are also associated with short-chain fatty acids that emerge during the breakdown of galactans by bacteria. Some artificially produced galactans produce less gas when they are assimilated by bacteria than those that occur naturally. However, as stated before, the EFSA refuses to support prebiotics beyond their statement regarding their potential.[82] Over 80% of participants in a study who followed this book's approach and consistently limited their consumption of fructose and fructans according to the BTLs listed experienced relief from their symptoms by about 70%.[83] Moreover, reducing the amount of bricks that arrive at the colon might a have favorable effect on mood (see page 15). These findings support the principles underlying this diet.

---

[76] Category raffinose and stachyose.

[77] Gibson & Shepherd, 2010, Suarez et al., 1999.

[78] Shepherd & Gibson, 2006.

[79] Barrett et al., 2010; Shepherd & Gibson, 2006.

[80] EFSA, 2013; Binnendijk & Rijkers 2013; EFSA, 2012b.

[81] Silk et al., 2009.

[82] EFSA, 2013, McKenzie et al., 2012; Silk, Davis, Vulevic, Tzortzis, & Gibson, 2009; Rycroft et al., 2001.

[83] Shepherd & Gibson, 2006.

Enzyme capsules

There are special enzyme capsules available that may help you to avoid symptoms that may otherwise be induced by galactans, though their effectiveness is disputed. They contain the enzyme alpha-galactosidase and are made from the mildew aspergillus niger, though packages may not fully reflect this information; they also contain the brick mannitol, a sugar alcohol, prevalent in mushrooms, to which some people exhibit allergies. You should be careful with these enzyme capsules if you have a fructose intolerance, as the galactans are metabolized into fructose by the enzymes. Unless your body immediately intercepts the fructose, it arrives at the intestine. There, gas-producing bacteria rejoice, since you have done some of their work for them.[84] So, you actually gained nothing. These enzyme capsules can only be helpful if you tolerate fructose and sorbitol and do not have an allergy to aspergillus niger.

Which foods contain this brick?

Beans and bloating go hand in hand for some—critical amounts of galactans combined with fructans (BTL portion size in parentheses) can be found in beans (1 tbsp., 15g), peas (1 tbsp., 15g), chickpeas (9 tbsp., 135g) and soybeans (3 tbsp., 45g). Vegetarians should pay particular attention to these. Considerable amounts are also contained in oat flakes (5 tbsp., 75g), lentils (5 tbsp., 75g) and wheat or rye bread (one slice, 42g).[85] Moreover, short-chain galactans are also contained in milk.[86] Agar and carrageenan[87] also contain galactans, but those they contain are longer and are not fully broken down by gut bacteria.[88] At times people suffering from an irritable bowel are suspicious towards these. Due to a lack of solid evidence, these are not considered in this book.[89] Still, if you have doubts about them, you can explore their impact yourself by adopting an alternative diet (see Chapter 2.2.6).

---

[84] Falony et al., 2009.

[85] Biesiekierski et al., 2011; Muir et al., 2009.

[86] Boehm & Stahl, 2007; German et al. 2008.

[87] Michel, Nyval-Collen, Barbeyron, Czjzek, & Helbert, 2006.

[88] Chi, Chang, & Hong, 2012; Necas & Bartosikova, 2013.

[89] Watson, 2008.

1.5.5 Brick number five: Sorbitol and others

Some fruits and vegetables naturally contain sugar alcohols like sorbitol. Furthermore, they are used as sweeteners and as carriers for some medicines. Often sugar alcohols are only mentioned in code on packages. In Chapter 2.4 you will learn how to identify the relevant information on labels.

BTL for the nine sugar alcohols being considered, including sorbitol: 0g.

Foods containing sorbitol often trigger abdominal discomforts.[90] Sorbitol is unproblematic if a breath test or substitute test indicates you can tolerate it, and that you can tolerate fructose as well. If you only have a fructose intolerance but not a sorbitol intolerance, you can use the sorbitol-adjusted portion sizes for fructose as indicated in the tables of Part 3 of this book. If you have a sorbitol intolerance, it makes sense to determine your personal TL (see Chapter 2.2.4) due to the radical BTL of 0g. There are three reasons in favor of this BTL:

1. The breath test for sorbitol shows an intolerance present at 5g in **58%** of those experiencing abdominal discomfort due to an irritable bowel and **53%** of healthy participants (based on a combination of studies with a total of 564 participants).[91]
2. If you have a fructose intolerance, sorbitol will aggravate your symptoms. Fructose emerges when sorbitol gets broken down. Meanwhile, sorbitol hinders already-present fructose from being intercepted because fructose and sorbitol share a transportation mechanism where sorbitol is preferred.[92]
3. Sugar alcohols are incompletely absorbed by many and can sometimes even lead to a water aggregation in the small intestine, reducing the intestine's ability to metabolize nutrients. On average, 25–40% of consumed sugar alcohols arrive at the colon.[93] Even small amounts of sorbitol can trigger discomforts.[94]

---

[90] Raithel et al., 2013; Gibson & Shepherd, 2010; Barrett et al., 2010; Ledochowski et al., 2000.

[91] D. Mishkin et al., 1997; Fernández-Bañares et al., 1993; Hyams, 1983.

[92] Gaby, 2005; Raithel et al., 2013.

[93] Langkilde, Andersson, Schweizer, & Würsch, 1994; Barrett et al., 2010.

[94] Rumessen & Gudmand-Høyer, 1987.

Influence on symptoms

In a Dutch study in 1993 high amounts of glucose were added to apple juice, reducing symptoms caused by apple juice by 80%.[95] However, the added glucose also bound the released fructose from sorbitol degradation.[96] Assuming that one third of symptoms caused by sorbitol arise due to non-degraded sorbitol, another third by the free fructose emerging from sorbitol that has been broken down and the remaining third due to fructose whose interception was hindered by sorbitol, sorbitol causes 30% of the discomfort resulting from apple juice. Considering the average amount of sorbitol contained in an apple (about 0.56g sorbitol and 4g of free fructose), 1g of sorbitol combined with free fructose causes about three times as many symptoms as 1g of free fructose alone, and 1g of sorbitol alone causes about twice as many symptoms as 1g of free fructose.[97] This relationship is taken into account in the amount recommended for foods that contain both fructose and sorbitol.

Which foods contain this brick?

Sugar alcohols occur naturally in different fruits and vegetables (fresh as well as dried). Moreover, they are added as sugar replacements in a large number of products, including beverages, candies, convenience foods, diabetic products like jelly (up to 57g/100g) and chocolate (up to 40g/100g), breaded fish and meat, ice cream, juices, medicine, oral hygiene products, sauces, sugar-free chewing gum (up to 2.5g/piece), sugar-free mints (up to 2g/piece) and even sausage.[98] As you can see, some diabetic products contain more than 20g of sorbitol. In one study, 84% of the 39 healthy participants had a sorbitol malabsorption for a 20g dose. Consumption of these products therefore deserves caution.[99]

---

95 Hoekstra, van Kempen, & Kneepkens, 1993.

96 Gaby, 2005.

97 Kneepkens, Jakobs, & Douwes, 1989.

98 Corazza et al., 1988.

99 Ladas, Grammenos, Tassios, & Raptis, 2000; Hyams, 1983.

1.5.6 Abdominal discomfort in children

Children ages 14 to 58 months were administered 250mL of apple juice in a study. Afterward, all children who suffered from chronic diarrhoea, as well as 65.5% of the healthy children, tested positive for malabsorption. Avoiding apple juice led to recovery for **all** of the children.[100] This result corresponds with other research that shows that many children suffer from diarrhoea and abdominal pain if they drink too much fruit juice. Juices that contain high levels of sorbitol have commonly been identified as triggers.[101] Generally speaking, you should give your child a maximum of 10mL juice per kilogram of body weight.[102] Moreover, you should avoid giving them fruit juices that contain sorbitol or high amounts of free fructose, like apple or peach juice.

---

[100] Kneepkens et al., 1989.

[101] Hyams, Etienne, Leichtner, & Theuer, 1988.

[102] Lifschitz, 2000.

1.6 Summary of Part 1

Your stomach is able to intercept some bricks and metabolize them into energy. However, the capacity for doing so differs from human to human. Lactose is primarily contained in milk products. Sufferers of an intolerance can usually tolerate small amounts well. When reducing the amount of lactose one consumes, it is important to make up for the simultaneous reduction in calcium intake. Fructose is most common in fruits, soft drinks and cereals. Combined with sorbitol, it is absorbed more poorly; combined with glucose, it is absorbed better. The most common dietary sources of fructans include grain products like bread, cereals and noodles, as well as garlic and onions, and they are not broken down well by the body. Galactans, which are predominantly found in beans, lentils and grains, are similarly poorly absorbed. The strictest BTL is associated with sorbitol, which should be avoided for the most part. Sorbitol is mainly found in many diabetic and light products, some fruits and vegetables and sauces and breadings. Stevia, by the way, is free of sorbitol.

Basic tolerance levels (BTLs)

The following table contains all of the BTLs previously introduced. Use it as a guide to the bricks you are intolerant to, at least during the three weeks of the introductory diet, and partially afterward during the level tests. Whether it is for the next wedding, project presentation or sailing trip, there are occasions when you especially want everything to run smoothly regarding your digestion. You can feel more secure on days like these if you manage your meals according to the BTLs for those bricks that you have an intolerance to. The BTLs are:

Glucose-free fructose	0.5g/meal
Glucose-balanced fructose	5g/100g
Lactose	1.5g/meal
Sorbitol and other sugar alcohols	0g/meal
Sum of fructans and galactans	0.5g/meal

As you adjust your diet according to the BTLs that are relevant for you, you can avoid those carbohydrates that cause discomfort as best as is practicable.

This page has been intentionally left blank.

2

STRATEGY

2.1 Mission planning

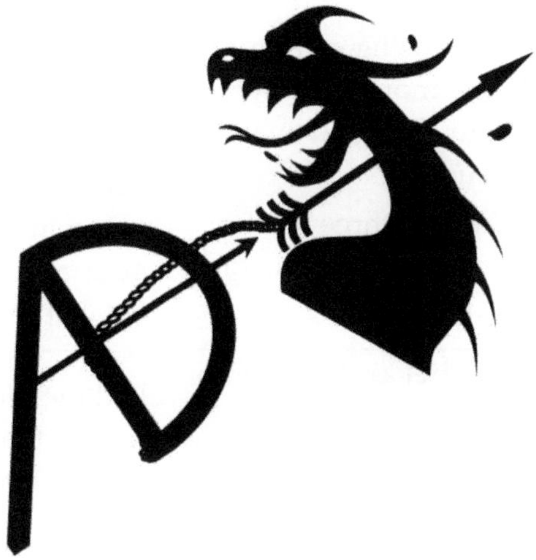

Stop letting brick-eating dragons attack and tempt you. Get ready for the dragon hunt. With positivity and discipline, chances are that we will chain your dragon. As the dragon is invisible, the best strategy is to feed it as few bricks as possible. Meanwhile, if you stay on your guard and wield your interception shield by eating portions close to the recommended maximum for your TL, the dragon will have a tough time. You can thereby reduce to tolerable amounts the consumption of those bricks that induce your symptoms to tolerable amounts. In order not to restrict yourself unnecessarily by avoiding foods that you love, you can **determine your personal tolerance thresholds for the bricks by taking a level test (Chapter 2.2.4).** See a qualified doctor to authorize this process, especially if the person with the intolerance is a child.

2.1.1 Roadmap

In the following strategy table, you will find the five major steps, their urgency, their titles, their durations and their purposes.

1)	Required	**Symptom test (sheet)** Duration: four days	Determining your status quo: Which symptoms do you have, and how severe are they?
	Optional	**Breath test from a specialist** Duration: six days	Identifying the bricks you absorb with difficulty. The target is to reduce your effort in Step 3.
	"quick-exit option" after positive breath test	**Keep the BTL for those bricks towards which you have an intolerance.** Fill out the following symptom test sheet once more after two weeks for four days and evaluate your diet's success. Duration: At least three weeks, depending on your satisfaction; see column on the right.	A) You are satisfied. Do you want to reduce your limitations to the extent possible? Perform the level test (see Step 5). B) You are unsatisfied. First perform Step 3 and then at least the substitute test for fructans and galactans. If no improvement occurs, test the alternatives shown in Chapter 2.2.6.
3)	Required	**Introductory diet and symptom test (sheet)** during the last four days. Duration: three weeks	Did the diet according to the BTLs lead to the expected reduction of symptoms? If no, see Chapter 2.2.6.
4)	Optional: Instead of Step 2	**Substitute test (for the breath test)** Duration: five weeks for all bricks	Uncovering the discomfort triggers for which no breath test is offered. Moreover, reducing the effort for Step 5.
5)	Optional	**Level test** Duration: 1 brick ~½ month 2 bricks ~1½ months 3 bricks ~2½ months 4 bricks ~5 months	Enabling you a diet that is as varied as possible while taking your intolerance(s) into account by determining your TLs.

The broad strategy is to determine your shield's interception capacities. The first step is checking your status quo. To do so, note down your symptoms on the following test sheet. It is important to choose days on which neither drugs nor sickness nor stress might influence your symptoms. If you aren't sure if you have produced contaminated results on a given day due to any of these factors, cross out the day and fill out the next one you consider unaffected. **Important: This also holds true for all of the subsequent tests. If you are in doubt as to whether the day was "normal," on which no uncommon circumstances distorted the symptoms, repeat the test to get a more reliable result.**[103] On days where you track your symptoms, carry a copy of the symptom test sheet with you. Ideally, you should fill it out immediately after your main meals, e.g., at 7am, 1pm and 7pm. After the four days of your status quo check, you should also classify the type of stool you usually have. Depending on whether you have constipation, diarrhoea or a mix of both, you are type IBS-C, IBS-D or IBS-M. If you are spared constipation and diarrhoea, your IBS type is un**classified**. Take that information with you when you visit the doctor.

After tracking your symptoms for four days, you can take a breath test to determine malabsorbtions. To do so, please ask your doctor to refer you to a gastroenterology specialist. If this type of test is not offered in your area, you can take a substitute test after following the introductory diet (see Chapter 2.2.3). To follow the introductory diet, read on to Chapter 2.2.2. This also holds for the "quick-exit option." You can disregard those bricks towards which the breath or substitute test does not indicate malabsorbtion. **Even if malabsorbtion is detected, you may be able to stomach more than the BTL portions.** You can therefore determine your personal TL with a level test (see Chapter 2.2.4) if the introductory diet reduced your symptoms. This is to save you from unnecessarily harsh restrictions on foods you enjoy. For example, if you have a lactose intolerance and like cheese, you can determine the highest tolerable amount of cheese per meal in Step 5. Be prepared to spend at least half a month on the level test (see page 32). You can be sure afterward that you are neither straining your body too much nor excessively restraining your consumption of foods you enjoy. Only an individual level test can lead you to that result.

In the quick-exit option, you skip the introductory diet (at least at first) but try to determine whether adhering to the BTLs for those bricks you don't absorb well according to the breath test has enough of a positive effect for you to

---

[103] Vesa et al. 1996.

just consider those bricks. If your symptoms don't improve to your satisfaction, go back and follow the introductory diet and conduct at least a substitute test for fructans and galactans. If this does not lead to satisfying results, read Chapter 2.2.6.

During the introductory diet, you keep those BTLs that are relevant for you (see Chapter 2.2). Exception: If the breath test comes out negative for fructose, lactose and sorbitol, the BTLs apply to all bricks. If symptoms improve while you are on the diet, continue with the substitute test for fructans and galactans. To be on the safe side, you can also do the substitute test for the remaining bricks, in order to exclude potential interdependencies like between sorbitol and fructose, which can be found together in apple juice, for example, as a cause. Otherwise, you will find alternative strategies in Chapter 2.2.6. If you have not done the breath test, all BTLs apply.

After two weeks of the quick-exit option or after the introductory diet, make an efficiency check by filling out the symptom test sheet again for four days. To evaluate the effect, compare the status quo check symptom test sheet with the efficiency check symptom test sheet. If you have fewer symptoms at the end of the diet—that is, if your evaluations for the efficiency check are clearly lower than those for the status quo check—the diet was a success. You can learn how to mathematically determine the diet's success in Chapter 2.1.3. **Put your symptom test sheets into a folder.** The most important one is the final test of **your introductory diet,** as you can use it as a **reference for all of your further tests**.

Stool types after Bristol

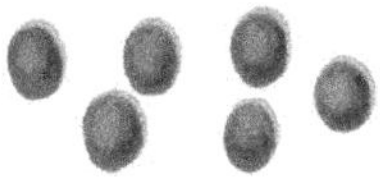	Separate hard lumps, like nuts (hard to pass)	**Type** A: Constipation **Value** 4
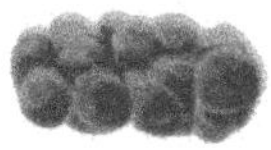	Sausage-shaped but lumpy	**Type** B: Constipation Value 2
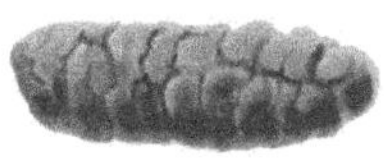	Like a sausage but with cracks on the surface	**Type** C: normal **Value** 1
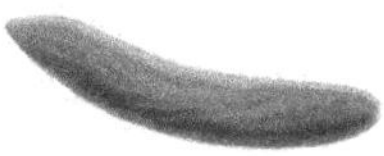	Like a sausage or snake, smooth and soft	**Type** D: normal **Value** 1
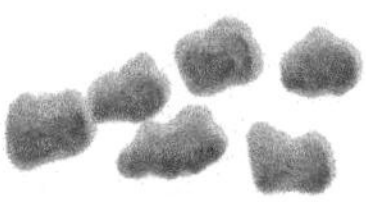	Soft blobs with clear-cut edges	**Type** E: Diarrhoea **Value** 2
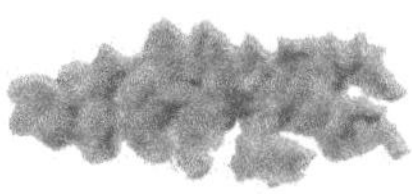	Fluffy pieces with ragged edges, a mushy stool	**Type** F: Diarrhoea **Value** 4
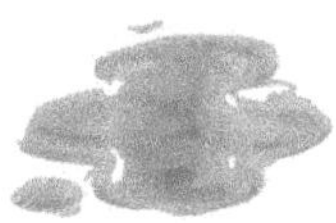	Watery, no solid pieces; **entirely liquid**	**Type** G: Diarrhoea **Value** 5

(Based on Lewis & Heaton, 1997; Thompson, 2006)

Types 3 and 4 are normal. The farther away your type is from these two, the worse your ailments.

2.1.2 Symptom test sheet

Test:______________________________ **End date:**____________

For each test, you need two copies of this page!

		Type/ Value		Defecation count		Stool grade	Bloating grade	Pain grade	
Day 1 prior	🐓		x		=				TEST DAY
	☀		x		=				
	☾		x		=				
				Total					
Day 2 prior	🐓		x		=				Day 1 after
	☀		x		=				
	☾		x		=				
				Total					
Day 3 prior	🐓		x		=				Day 2 after
	☀		x		=				
	☾		x		=				
				Total					
(Day 4 prior)	🐓		x		=				Day 3 after
	☀		x		=				
	☾		x		=				
				Total					

Note down your stool type in the morning 🐓, afternoon ☀ and evening ☾ and your stool value from 1 to 5 (see page 35) as well as the number of times you visited the toilet and multiply the stool value with the number of toilet uses to estimate the stool grade. In addition, evaluate bloating and pain from 1 to 5 according to the following scale:

1 No discomfort, like someone without symptoms
2 Hardly any discomfort relative to someone without symptoms
3 Medium discomfort relative to someone without symptoms
4 Severe discomfort relative to someone without symptoms
5 Very severe discomfort relative to someone without symptoms

2.1.3 Test result calculation table

You can probably trust your gut in evaluating your symptoms. If you prefer numbers, you can use the following two convenient procedures.[104] For the first application, you need the symptom test sheets from the status quo check[105] and the efficiency check.[106] You have the following two calculation options (please use a copy of the following table and a pencil); Option A is easier. With Option B, you save yourself calculation work for all the following tests and receive a statement regarding your tolerance.

A) Use the following table and calculate your results for all days up row B. A1 to A4 are the efficiency check days and A5 to A8 the status quo check days or, for the surrogate or level test, the test day and its three subsequent days. **A-grade calculation**: A1 = Stool total grade (grade in the morning plus grade in the afternoon plus grade in the evening) on Day 1. Note down the result in the cell with a cursive A1. Proceed likewise with all other A-numbers. Afterward, determine the **B-grades**: B1 = A1 plus total bloating grade on Day 1 plus total pain grade on Day 1. Then calculate B2 according to the Day 2 grades and so on. Now determine C2 and D2, i.e., the average of the status quo check days or, for the surrogate or level test, the average of the test and its three subsequent days. For the evaluation, compare D2 with the highest day grade from the efficiency check days. This is the largest grade of the grades B1 to B4. The further D2 is above the highest grade of that group, the more likely the introductory diet has worked or, if you took any other test, the more likely it is that you have an intolerance.

B) Calculate A1 to A8 as well as B1 to B8 with Option A. Then calculate C1 and D1 and proceed by calculating the further calculation steps in the table until L. To determine the efficiency of the introductory diet, also calculate C2 and D2. In an efficiency check of the introductory diet, compare D2 instead of L, the **l**id grade,[107] with K, the **K**.O. threshold grade,[108] for the interpretation. If D2 is greater than or equal to the K-grade, this points to an effective introductory diet. For the surrogate or level test, compare the K- with the L-grade, as explained in the following table.

Spare yourself time: Acquire the printer-friendly Excel version on www.Laxiba.co.uk/trc.

---

[104] From a statistical point of view the survey is slim and the result vague.

[105] Symptom test sheet filled out before starting the introductory diet.

[106] Symptom test sheet filled out at the end of the introductory diet.

[107] L = the day with the most severe symptoms following a live test.

[108] K = If the L-grade reaches this K. O. threshold, there is an intolerance.

	Efficiency check day					*Status quo check day* **day-after test**		
	1:	**2:**	**3:**	**4:**	*1:* **or Test day:**	*2:* / **1:**	*3:* / **2:**	*4:* / **3:**
A	*A1*	*A3*	*A3*	*A4*	*A5*	*A6*	*A7*	*A8*
B	*B1*	*B2*	*B3*	*B4*	*B5*	*B6*	*B7*	*B8*
C	*C1*	*C1 = B1 + B2 + B3 + B4* Add up the results of the cells B1 to B4. *C2 = B5 + B6 + B7 + B8* Add up the results of the cells B5 to B8.						*C2*
D	*D1*	*D1 = C1 ÷ 4* Divide your result in cell C1 by 4. *D2 = C2 ÷ 4* Divide your result in cell C2 by 4.						*D2*
E	*E1*	*E2*	*E3*	*E4*	*E1 = B1 - D1, E2 = B2 - D1* and so on. To calculate E1, subtract D1 from B1. Negative results are allowed.			
F	*F1*	*F2*	*F3*	*F4*	*F1 = E1* x *E1, F2 = E2* x *E2* and so on. To calculate F1, multiply E1 with itself. A negative times a negative equals a positive. Thus, each result must be positive.			
G	*G*	*G = F1 + F2 + F3 + F4* Add up the results of the cells F1 to F4.						
H	*H*	*H = G ÷ 4* Divide G by 4.						
I	*I*	*I* = Take the square root of your result in cell *H*. On your calculator, the symbol for square root is: √‾.						
J	*J*	*J = I* x 2 Multiply I by 2.						
K	*K*	*K = J + C1* Add the result in cell J to the result in cell C1. The **K**-grade is called **K**.O. threshold grade, as a D2 (used for checking the introductory diet's success) or L-grade that is greater than or equal to K suggests an intolerance.						
L	*L*	*L* = The biggest grade of the group B5, B6, B7 and B8. This group contains either the daily results of the status quo check (in that case D2 replaces L) or the results of the test day (B5) and its three subsequent days (B6 to B8). The L-grade is called **l**id grade, as it is used to evaluate the strength of the symptoms caused by an ongoing surrogate or level test. Analysis: *L* ≥ *K* indicates an intolerance, L< K a tolerance. An **L**-grade that is below the **K**-grade indicates a tolerance. A lid grade that is greater than or equal to the **K**.O.-threshold grade indicates an intolerance.						

2.1.4 Keeping your balance

Fundamental recommendations

1	Eat a rich variety of foods, i.e., something different each day and with lots of natural ingredients. Eat with a relaxed posture.	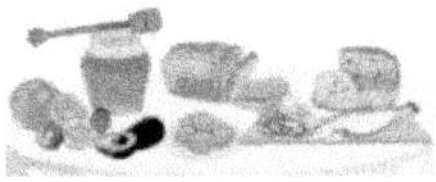
2	Take care of your supply of fiber, e.g., by eating potatoes, flaxseeds, lentils, nuts.	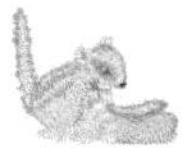
3	Ingest five portions of vegetables (ideally dark green, red or orange) and fruit.	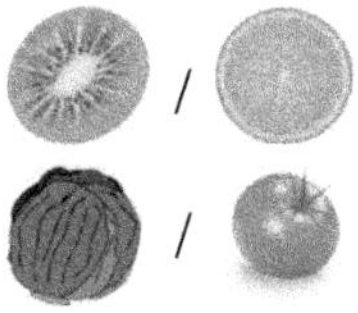 5/day
4	Have some reduced-fat milk products like reduced-fat milk, yogurt or cheese every day.	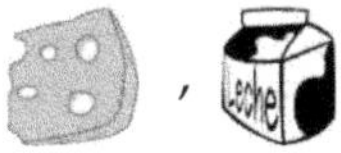
5	One or two times a week, eat fish and eggs, as well as 300–600g of low-fat meat, ideally poultry.	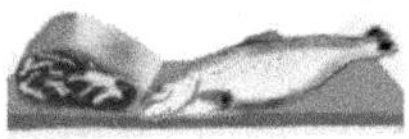
6	Use vegetable oils if possible, like canola oil, and fats.	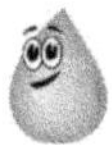
7	Reduce your consumption of salt and sugar.	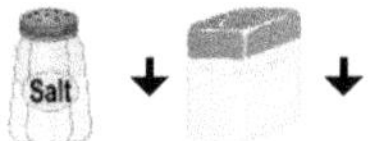
8	Drink at least 1.5 liters of non-alcoholic drinks per day. Best are unsweetened beverages and water. Drink alcohol minimally to moderately.	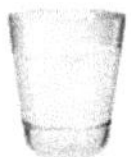
9	Preferably, cook fresh and at lower temperatures to reduce nutrient leaching.	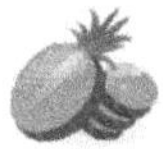
+	Stay fit: exercise regularly.	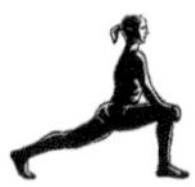

(DGE, 2013; Quigley et al., 2013; USDA and U. S. Department of Health and Human Services, 2010)

This page has been intentionally left blank.

2.1.4 Keeping your balance

Compensation needs due to your diet

If you reduce the fructans and galactans in your meals, you might have to compensate for the resulting loss of proteins, short-chain fatty acids and fibre. These three elements belong to a balanced diet. You usually ingest a large portion through fructan- and galactan-rich wheat products like bread, cereals and noodles, which you may be consuming less of. A regular intake of 20 to 38g of fibre, along with getting moderate exercise, can actually help to alleviate constipation.[109] As a guideline for your nutrition, find the recommended daily amounts in the following examples.

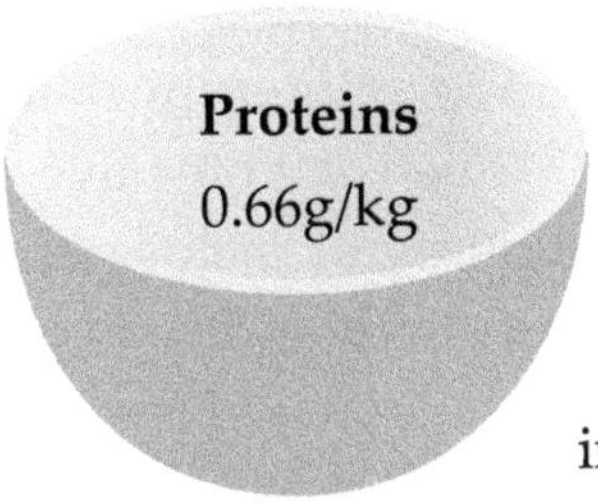

One needs 0.66g of protein per kilogram of body weight per day.[110] You can ensure your protein supply by consuming the following products. The rough amount of proteins per portion is shown in parentheses: 85g meat (28g protein), 85g fish (26g), 150mL instant coffee with or without caffeine (18g, but normal espresso contains only 0.3g), 200mL whole milk with added vitamin D (15g), 200mL whole milk or fat-free milk without additives (6g), 85g corn or wild rice (12g), 90g kidney beans (18g), 140g pasta (15g), 90g soy beans (14g), a medium-sized egg (7.5g), 90g lentils (8g), 110g potatoes (4g), 25g nuts, especially peanuts, peanut butter and almonds (5g), a slice of whole grain bread (5g), 25g cheese (4g), a slice of rice bread (3.5g), 30g cereal (3g), 24g rice bran (3g), 25g dark chocolate (2g) and 50g couscous (1.5g).[111] You may notice that maintaining a supply of protein is rather easy. Vegetarians, however, should plan their protein intake consciously.

---

109 Dukas, Willett, & Giovannucci, 2003; Quigley et al., 2013; USDA, 2013.

110 EFSA, 2012a.

111 USDA, 2013.

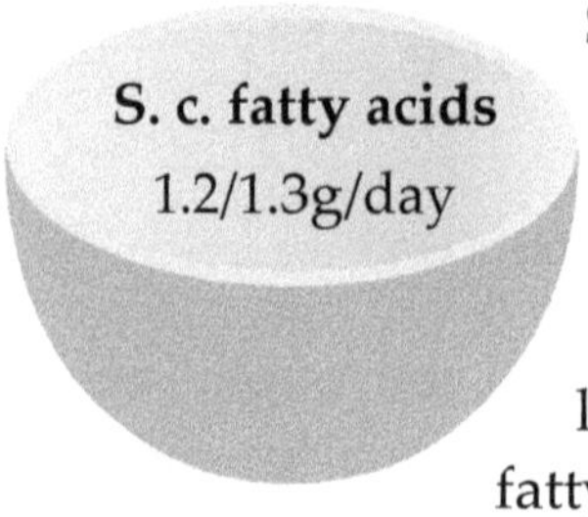

Short-chain fatty acids emerge as bacteria break down bricks, especially fructans. These are then partially absorbed by the intestine, as they are important sources of energy. They have a chain length of up to six carbon atoms, which is the basis for the following list.[112] Foods that are particularly rich in short-chain fatty acids include (fatty acids per portion without triglycerides in parentheses): 10g butter (0.5g), 25g goat's cheese (0.5g), 25g gouda, Swiss cheese, cheddar or Roquefort (0.4g), 50g mozzarella (0.3g), 47g M&M's® (0.3g), 25g blue cheese (0.25g), 20mL coconut oil (0.2g), 50g coconut meat (0.18g), 150g French fries (0.13g) or 20mL palm kernel oil (0.08g).[113] Even if your change in diet does not lead to a deficiency in short-chain fatty acids,[114] daily consumption of dairy products is recommended. As short-chain fatty acids ought to amount to 1/60 of the daily amount of consumed fats,[115] which ought to be 70g for women and 80g for men, the required minimum dairy intake is 1.2g per day for women and 1.3g for men.[116] Even if you have a lactose intolerance, you can usually consume small amounts of lactose and thus reach the target, for example, by eating three slices of cheddar. If you are a vegan, reaching the target is a challenge.

Omega 3 fatty acids

Another important food component is short-chain omega 3 fatty acids, although they are hardly affected by your diet. Women should take in 6.1g of the omega 3 fatty acid known as alpha-Linolenic acid, or ALA, while men should take in 7g.[117] Alternatively, maintaining a 2:1 proportion of omega 6 to omega 3 will lead to an intake of up to 9.6g per day for women and 11g for men. ALA fatty acids have a positive effect on your cardiovascular system.[118] The following foods contain high levels (rough ALA amount per portion in

---

[112] Mosby's medical dictionary, 2009; Falony et al., 2009; Campbell, Fahey, & Wolf, 1997; Cummings & MacFarlane, 1997; Ruppin, Bar-Meir, Soergel, Wood, & Schmitt, 1980.

[113] USDA, 2013.

[114] Cummings, 1981.

[115] FAO, 2008.

[116] CIAA, n. d..

[117] FAO, 2008; assumed energy of the fats is 20 %.

[118] Simopoulos, 1999; Connor, 2000; Mozaffarian & Wu, 2011.

parentheses): 200g fish (4g), 20mL linseed oil (10.5g) for which the consumed amount should be below 100mL per day (linseeds themselves contain 25% oil and thus 24g of linseeds, see page 56, at least 3g; however, during pregnancy you should avoid both),[119] 20mL canola oil (1.8g), 20mL mayonnaise (1g), 20mL soy oil (0.8g), 100g wheat crackers (0.8g), 70g French fries (0.3g), 16g peanut butter with omega 3 (0.5g), 25g walnuts (0.5g), 10g butter (0.3g) and 10g margarine (0.3g).[120] The data sheds a positive light on the fibre Strategy A as described in the following. You can reach the target amount of 7g for men just by consuming 1 tbsp. linseed oil per day. Alternatively, you can arrive at 6g, for example, by eating three portions of salad with 20mL of canola oil each and a slice of bread with omega 3 peanut butter. Apart from ALA, EPA (eicosapentaenoic acid) and DHA (docosahexaenoic acid) are also important. Your daily intake of EPA should be 250mg and of DHA, 500mg.[121] If you eat fish at any time during the week, you will usually have covered your need.[122] Krill or fish oil capsules containing these amounts are an alternative.

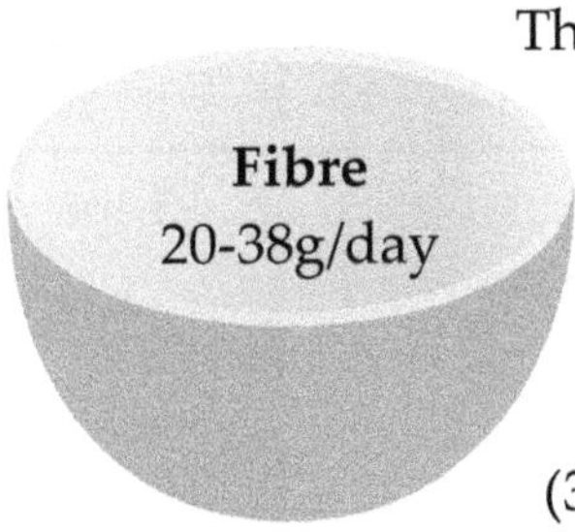

The following products are rich in fibre (fibre per portion in parentheses): 90g lentils (27.9g), 90g kidney beans (22.5g), 25g almonds (12g), 110g potatoes (8.7g), 30g bran cereals (up to 8.7g for Kellog's® All-Bran®), 24g linseeds (6.5g), 100g wild rice (6.2g), 24g rice bran (5g), one 42g slice of rye bread (5g), 30g wheat cereals (3.3g), 25g hazelnuts or pine nuts (2.7g), 25g dark chocolate (2.7g), 25g pistachio or pecans (2.5g), 60g (2.4g), 25g walnuts (1.7g), 25g chestnuts or butternuts (1g), 25g peanuts, coconuts or macadamia nuts (0.4g).[123] Fruits and vegetables contain about 1 to 5g per portion, e.g., avocado (1.7g), banana (3g), blackberries (4.4g), cauliflower (1.2g), salad (0.8g), olives (1.2g), orange (2.4g), spinach (7g), tomatoes (1.4g).[124] As fibre may be sort of a challenge, two different compensation strategies follow.

---

[119] Leinoel, n. d.; Tou, Chen, & Thompson, 1998.
[120] USDA e, 2013.
[121] EFSA, 2012c.
[122] USDA, 2013.
[123] USDA, 2013.
[124] Mount Sinai, n. d.

Strategy A: Linseeds

Linseeds contain a high amount of fibre and many omega 3 fatty acids. They are good at reducing constipation and can also help a little against pain and bloating. The downside of this all-around effect is that linseeds contain fructans and galactans. If you apply this book's strategy, the BTL portions you take in for fructans and galactans will be reduced to 28% (Level 1: 64%, 2 or 3: 86%) of their former quantity.[125] As you take in linseeds at three different times of the day, the amount per meal is 24g at most. This way the linseeds account for 6.5g of fibre at the highest daily stage. In order for your body to get acquainted with linseeds, start off in the first two weeks with one tablespoon combined with at least 75mL of water at breakfast. In the following weeks, you can then increase the intake amount according to the following table. The amount printed in normal type relates to the linseeds, and the amount in italics to the required minimum amount of water you should drink with it as a dilutor:

Week	**3–4**	**5–6**	**7–8**	**9–10**	**11–12**	**13–14**	**15–16**	**17f**
Breakfast	1 tsp *75 mL*	1 tsp *75 mL*	1 tbsp *150 mL*	1 tbsp *150 mL*	1 tbsp *150 mL*	1 tbsp 1 tsp *225 mL*	1 tbsp 1 tsp *225 mL*	1 tbsp 1 tsp *225 mL*
Lunch	1 tsp *75 mL*	1 tsp *75 mL*	1 tsp *75 mL*	1 tbsp *150 mL*	1 tbsp *150 mL*	1 tbsp *150 mL*	1 tbsp 1 tsp *225 mL*	1 tbsp 1 tsp *225 mL*
Dinner	-	1 tsp *75 mL*	1 tsp *75 mL*	1 tsp *75 mL*	1 tbsp *150 mL*	1 tbsp *150 mL*	1 tbsp *150 mL*	1 tbsp 1 tsp *150 mL*

(Blumenthal, 1998; McKenzie et al., 2012)

You can also accommodate linseeds in your meals. Whether the linseeds are whole or crushed should not make a difference. Make sure that you buy lin-

[125] J. Biesiekierski, personal communication, November 4, 2014; Biesiekierski et al., 2011.

seeds instead of psyllium as study results for suggest that psyllium is less effective.[126] Wheat bran as well has not been shown to lead to any improvement.[127] **Warning: Do not eat linseeds during pregnancy or lactation, as these can disturb your hormonal balance and cause premature birth.**[128] With 24g of linseeds you cover 7g of your fibre demand. One portion of fruits or vegetables contains 2.5g of fibre on average. You can reach your ideal daily fibre intake by eating five of them per day and adding wild rice to one of your meals together with the 17th week amount of linseeds as indicated in the last table.[129]

Strategy B: Brown rice/rice bran

This strategy focuses on rice bran, rather than on linseeds as in Strategy A (page 44). After all, rice bran contains 21g of fibre per 100g and thus accounts for 5g of the daily amount recommended for the plan's optimal stage. The advantage of using rice bran is that your TL of fructans and galactans remain unchanged. Furthermore, rice bran appears to be unproblematic during pregnancy. If for example you eat 30g cereal mixed with rice bran for your breakfast, 25g dark chocolate and 20g almonds, as well as two oranges in between; for lunch a portion of tomato salad with avocado and 45g of potatoes; and for your dinner, 45g rice as a side dish, you will have consumed about 28g of fibre in total. Hence, with a little bit of planning you can maximize your fibre intake and minimize your fructan and galactan intake, while avoiding fibre supplement capsules.

---

[126] Quigley et al., 2013; Tarpila, S., Tarpila, A., Grohn,
Silvennoinen, & Lindberg, 2004; Blumenthal, 1998; McKenzie et al., 2012.

[127] McKenzie et al., 2012.

[128] Tou et al., 1998.

[129] Mount Sinai, n. d.; Quigley et al., 2013.

Summary

Drink at least 1.5L of water per day and get moderate exercise. In order to keep your diet in balance you should focus on consuming the following:

Proteins: E.g., by eating fish, meat, eggs, rice or rice bran.

Short-chain fatty acids: E.g., by consuming dairy products. In case of a lactose intolerance, cheddar is suitable due to its low lactose content.

Omega 3: E.g., by using linseed oil or canola oil or eating fish or meat.

Fibre: E.g., by using linseeds or rice bran and eating five servings of fruit and vegetables per day, potatoes, rice, dark chocolate and a handful of nuts.

Please also make a point of enjoying a variety of foods. This especially applies to fruits and vegetables, to ensure that your body is adequately supplied with the vitamins that are important for your health.[130] What follows next is the first step of your LAXIBA strategy, a status quo check. This means you should fill out the symptom test sheet on page 36 for four days. Please also read Chapters 2.2 and 2.3 as you do so. Afterward, you will proceed according to the roadmap (see Chapter 2.1.1).

---

[130] Kennedy, 2004.

2.2 Your individual strategy

This chapter describes your introductory diet plan depending on your diagnosis. The diet has been well-tried.[131] However, should your symptoms not improve after three weeks of adhering to this diet, you should cease or, better, check whether bricks have been entering your meals after all.[132] One way to determine this is for you to keep a food diary and have a dietician or doctor check it.[133] If no critical bricks have been sneaking in, resign from the brick diet. In Chapter 2.2.6 you will find alternatives.

Diet code table

	FI [+] SI [+]	**FI [-] SI [+]**	**FI [+] SI [-]**	**FI [-] SI [-]**	**FI [?=+] SI [?=+]**
LI [+]	8	4	7	3	8
LI [-]	5	2	6	1	5
LI [?]	8	4	7	3	8

FI[+]=Fructose intolerance, FI[-]=No fructose intolerance,
LI[+]=Lactose intolerance, LI[-]=No lactose intolerance,
SI[+]=Sorbitol intolerance, SI[-]=No sorbitol intolerance.

Use the above table to determine your intolerance code. A [+] means that you have the respective intolerance and a [-], that you are untroubled by it. A [?] means that the diagnosis is uncertain. By using the assigned code, you can then find out for which bricks you should adhere to the basic tolerance levels (BTLs), up to a level test, in the "Diet code classification" table that follows:

---

131 Ong et al., 2010; Thomas, Nanda, & Shu, 2012; McKenzie et al., 2012; Goldstein et al., 2000.

132 McKenzie et al., 2012; Nanda, James, Smith, Dudley, & Jewell, 1989; Hawthorne, Lambert, D. Scott, & B. Scott, 1991; Parker, Naylor, Riordan, & Hunter, 1995.

133 Vesa et al., 1996.

Diet code classification

	FRUCTOSE	LACTOSE	SORBITOL	FRUCTANS & GALACTANS
1	☺	☺	☺	⮟
2	☺	☺	☠	⮟
3	☺	⮟	☺	⮟
4	☺	⮟	☠	⮟
5	⮟	☺	☠	⮟
6	⮟	☺	★	⮟
7	⮟	⮟	☺	⮟
8	⮟	⮟	☠	⮟

☺ = no restrictions, ⮟ = reduce consumption to your TL, ☠ = avoid consumption ★ = consumption of sorbitol is not a problem unless you consume it with fructose. It is recommended to use the sorbitol-adapted fructose column in the food tables.

A consumption limit for fructans and galactans generally holds for the introductory diet. Adhering to the BTL portions for all bricks is only required if the breath test was positive for all three bricks or if you did not take it. If the diet is successful, you should take the level test, described in Chapter 2.2.4, to reduce your restrictions as much as possible.

Procedure for the"quick-exit" option

Follow these steps if you have a lactose intolerance:

1) Reduce your consumption of lactose for three weeks according to the BTL portions and fill out the symptom test sheet at the end. If your symptoms improve to your satisfaction, continue this reduction in your lactose consumption. You may want to do the level test (Chapter 2.2.4). Otherwise, please continue with Step 2.
2) Follow the introductory diet according to your diet code as described earlier. If your diet is successful, do the substitute test for fructans and galactans afterward; it should come out positive. It will also make sense for you to take the level test (see Chapter 2.2.4), especially for lactose. If you remain unsatisfied, however, continue with Step 3.
3) Perhaps consuming less lactose has reduced your discomfort. Still, other foods could be affecting your symptoms as well. In Chapter 2.2.6 you will find suggestions as to which ones these could be and how you can test them.

2.2.1 It depends on the total load

You feel discomfort as soon as a threshold quantity of bricks arrive at the dragon. The more bricks arrive at your intestine the worse your symptoms are. In the food tables in the third part of the book, you will find the portion sizes that fit your TL. Yet, what do you do if you want to combine different foods, e.g., as you prepare to cook a recipe? The solution is to reduce the consumption for one or several of the affected foods far enough to reach your TL threshold. Let us say that you want to combine whole wheat bread and corn flakes, both of which contain fructans and galactans. To go below the BTL, restrict yourself to half a slice of the bread and three quarters of a corn flakes portion (22g). Don't worry if the reduced amounts aren't enough to fill you up: there are replacement products, low in or free of fructans and galactans (for example, rice bread, rice cereals, spelt and gluten free bread). Just look at the food table for similar products whose portions are less restricted.

2.2.2 Prevalence of the intolerance types

According to an extensive current study in Switzerland, 27% of people with abdominal discomfort were found to suffer from a fructose intolerance, 17% from a lactose intolerance and a further 33% from both.[134] However, the fructose dose of 35g that the study used is high for European conditions, if a Finnish study from 1987 still applies to contemporary diets,[135] and low for American conditions, wherein the average daily amount consumed is 54g.[136] Another research study using 25g fructose as its base level suggests a 49% average prevalence of fructose intolerance.[137] An analysis of several studies (see Chapter 1.5.5) shows that in general, 58% of those with irritable bowel symptoms have an intolerance of one kind or another. What is surprising is that lactose intolerance is only the second most prevalent intolerance in Europe, after sorbitol, yet the European market has adjusted itself better for those patients affected by lactose intolerance, especially with regard to food labelling. Those affected by a sorbitol intolerance, on the other hand, are forced to memorize technical terms to avoid eating sorbitol-containing products.

---

134 Wilder-Smith et al., 2013.

135 Virtanen et al., 1987.

136 Vos, Kimmons, Gillespie, Welsh, & Blanck, 2008.

137 D. Mishkin et al., 1997; Fernández-Bañares et al., 1993; Nelis, Vermeeren, & Jansen, 1990.

2.2.3 Substitute test

If no breath test is available but you want to find out which bricks you can stomach, then there is a substitute test. It determines the degree of an intolerance by gauging your symptoms after you have consumed the highest dose of the respective brick as is practical in your daily life. Of course, the test is only beneficial if your symptoms have improved through your consequent adherence to the BTL portion sizes for your problematic bricks.

As symptoms sometimes arise with a delay of up to three days, you have to schedule at least a week for the first brick that you want to test. Three days before the first test day, you must pay attention and always eat close (≤) to the BTL portion sizes of the bricks you are examining so that your pre-test meals do not affect your result. During the test day itself, keep all respective BTL portions, except for the brick that is being tested; on the three subsequent days all BTL portions hold once more. However, do not force yourself to eat more of the bricks than you did before starting the introductory diet, except for on the test day. On the test day, at the latest, as well as on the three subsequent days, fill out the symptom test sheet (see Chapter 2.1.2), unless you have already determined that you have an intolerance towards the tested brick. Use the symptom test sheet for the efficiency check days as a reference. If your symptoms do not worsen, then you are able to stomach the tested brick. If you want to test various bricks, you can spare yourself the three buffer days by testing the next brick on the fourth day after the last test day and proceed likewise with the other bricks you want to test.

Discuss the tests with your doctor beforehand so that he or she can consider the potential effects to and of your medical treatments and pre-existing conditions. For all the tests together, you need: a beaker, a 0.5L bottle, 100g of fructose and 20g of sorbitol, both which you can buy at your local pharmacy, scales and 1L of reduced-fat cow's milk without additives. In case of an intolerance you can use the remaining sugars for a level test later on. Now let us go through the test procedure:

Lactose test

At breakfast, drink half a liter of the milk, using the 0.5L bottle. Repeat at lunch unless your symptoms after the breakfast dose are so severe that you can already conclude that you have an intolerance. In addition to the milk, eat in accordance with your BTL portion sizes for the other relevant bricks.

Fructose test

Warning: before doing the test, confirm with your doctor that you do not have a hereditary fructose intolerance. For the test, add 25g (if you are in the USA or drink a lot of soft drinks use 35g) of fructose to a clean 0.5L bottle of water and shake it well. Then drink it completely on the morning of the test. In addition to the fructose, eat according to your BTLs on the test day and the next three days. You do not need a test for glucose-balanced fructose. If you want to pay attention to it, you can determine the amount you can tolerate by multiplying the TL amount of free fructose by ten.[138]

Sorbitol test

Proceed as for the fructose test, but replace the 25g of fructose with 5g of sorbitol.

Fructans and galactans test

Eat a generous portion of wheat cereal in the morning, beans with garlic and onions at lunch, brownies and crackers in between and a baguette or porridge dish in the evening.

As soon as you notice symptoms on the test day or the three subsequent days, which you can see mathematically if your **L**id **grade** is higher than your **K**.O.-threshold grade, you know you have an intolerance, and you can stop the test. In order to reduce your abdominal discomfort, drink still mineral water (usually up to three liters per day are salutary) and take a walk.

---

[138] Kneepkens, Vonk, & Fernandes, 1984.

2.2.4 Level test

Level test task list

# Tasks	Done when? ✔
1. You filled out the symptom test sheet for the status quo check.	
2. You asked your doctor to refer you to a specialist in order to do a breath test (if available).	
3. A) You decided to take the expedited ("quick-exit") option and found that your symptoms improved to your satisfaction.	
3. B) You performed the three-week introductory diet according to your diet code (page 47) and found improvement to your symptoms at the efficiency check (otherwise please proceed according to Chapter 2.2.6). If no breath test was available, you performed the substitute test.	
4. You decided which bricks you wanted to do the level test for (see page 56): the bricks that you have an intolerance towards as well as fructans and galactans.	
5. You estimated the time span for the level test: for one brick, it takes four weeks, for two bricks about eight weeks, for three bricks about 12 weeks and for four bricks about 16 weeks. However, the **acceleration option** lets you perform the tests right after one another (see page 56). You can thereby shorten the time span to 2½ weeks for one brick, 4½ weeks for two bricks, 6½ weeks for three bricks and 8½ weeks for four bricks.	
6. You convinced a partner to help you with your tests. They will mix your test liquids and interpret your symptom test sheets. You can count on their credibility and availability.	
7. You finished all of the tests, during which your testing partner adhered to the instructions on page 60, and you acted according to the flowchart on page 71.	
8. Finish: You talked your result over with your testing partner and entered your new combined or single TLs into the table on page 105.	

This page has been intentionally left blank.

Did your breath or substitute test demonstrate the presence of one or more brick intolerances? Then you should find out whether the BTLs fit for you. Each human differs in the amount he or she can stomach of each brick. Even in healthy humans the tolerated amount of fructose, for example, fluctuates between 5g and 50g.[139] Moreover, the amount consumed at once for the breath or substitute test is higher than what you would consume in a typical meal. The advantage of a high test dose is that you are unlikely to have symptoms from the respective brick in your everyday life if you are able to stomach it. However, in the case of an intolerance you should take a closer look, as the only thing that is yet certain is that you are in trouble when you consume an extreme amount. What is interesting is how much of a problematic brick you are able to stomach during normal nutritional consumption. For this purpose, you use the level test, where you increase the consumed amount in small steps, e.g., twice the BTL, to determine your tolerance threshold, while keeping the TLs for the remaining bricks. With every step, you then increase the tested consumption amount. The procedure is shown in the flowchart on page 71. The level test is finished last, after you have determined the levels that cause your symptoms for all tested bricks. If you use the mathematical Option B, this is the case when the lid grade is greater than or equal to the K.O. threshold grade. Take the test twice for each consumed amount to make sure your symptoms weren't caused by something else.

In order to make sure that you are also able to stomach your new single TL in combination with, if applicable, the new single TLs (that is, if your personal TL is above the BTL) of other tested bricks, next test all bricks with a new TL together. Note: there have to be at least three days between the two test days in order to avoid distorting the results.

Bricks to be tested

	Fructose	Lactose	Sorbitol	Fruc/Galactans
To be tested? Yes/No				
In which sequence (1, 2, …)				
(My calculated K.O. threshold grade is:)				

139 Rumessen & Gudmand-Høyer, 1986.

Now, choose the bricks that you want to determine your level for. Fructans and galactans are tested together. If you want to use the mathematical Option B, also enter your K-grade from the efficiency check. Important: disregard bricks that you can stomach and consume them as usual.

How a test week is run

<table>
<tr><th>Day 1–3 before the test day</th><th>On the test day</th><th>Day 1–3 after</th></tr>
<tr><td rowspan="2">Your brick consumption should surpass your current TLs by as narrow a margin as possible, but don't force yourself to eat more of anything than you want. Regulate only those TLs that have been confirmed by your partner so that you are uninfluenced on the test day, as symptoms can occur with three days' delay. If you do not feel as well on the test morning as you did at the end of the introductory diet, reschedule the test until you do.</td><td colspan="2">Fill out the symptom test sheet on the test day and its three subsequent days.</td></tr>
<tr><td>At breakfast, lunch and dinner consume only as much of the tested brick(s) as is part of the test dose and no more. For all other bricks, the current TLs hold as described on the left.</td><td>Keep your current TLs for your diet.</td></tr>
<tr><td colspan="3">Acceleration option: Perform the tests right after one another. Three days after the last test day, begin the next test day and thus save the three days described in the column on the left.</td></tr>
</table>

Start your test week three days before the test day, as symptoms may occur as many as three days after you consume the bricks that trigger them, and you want to start the test uninfluenced. On the days before the test, eat according to your current TLs. Your current TLs are those that you tolerated during the test and retest of the combination test described below. Initially, these are the BTLs (see page 105). After you have finished the first level test for all tested bricks, whether you perform a combination test and what it looks like depends on your results. It only makes sense if you do the test for at least two bricks and were able to stomach at least two bricks at the first tolerance level. For the combination test, test the respective bricks together at the higher tolerance level.

You do not have to fill out the symptom test sheet during the days leading up to the test (page 36), as you can use the efficiency check sheet as your reference, but from the day of the test to the third day after it, document your symptoms (unless you determine an intolerance earlier). Your testing partner prepares all test doses except for the fructans (F) and galactans (G). See the level table for F and G below to get a sense of the test quantities. For the test, eat the listed amounts of the following foods at the meals (M) breakfast, lunch and dinner. For the first test, these are the TL 1 amounts:

Level, amount/M	Portion size	Amount per day
Level 1 F: 0.5g, G: 0.5g	26g peas and 38g couscous	78g peas and 114g couscous
Level 2 F: 1g, G: 1g	53g peas and 77g couscous	159g peas and 231g couscous
Level 3 F: 1.5g, G: 1.5g	79g peas and 115g couscous	237g peas and 345g couscous

By consuming the listed amounts, you double the BTL at Level 1. In the following days, continue eating according to the BTLs. Then repeat the test at TL 1 to cover the result. Tell your testing partner whether your symptoms worsened at the test dose and give her or him the filled out test sheet. Afterward, proceed likewise with the next brick in order of precedence. When you have finished this with all bricks that are to be tested, you can perform a combined test of those bricks you were able to stomach at Level 1, perform a single level test or consider the level tests finished. If you want to test a level between two levels, you can calculate the dose as follows:

Lower dose + [(higher dose—lower dose) / 2]

If you can tolerate this dose, you should then adapt your multiplier for the food tables (see Chapter 3.1.1) by changing the word "dose" in the above formula with the multiplier. When your testing partner confirms you have an intolerance, the level test for that brick is over. Enter the highest TL for that brick in the table in Chapter 3.1.1. There you will find a differentiation between single TLs and combined TLs. At first, the combined TLs are the BTLs of all bricks you absorb badly. Later these may change if you can stomach a number of these bricks at a higher level when combined. You might also find that you are able to stomach two bricks while keeping the combined TLs of the other tested bricks but cannot tolerate both bricks together at the new level. In that case, enter the highest single level of these bricks into the single TL column. Note: if you determine an intolerance in a combined TL test concerning more than two bricks, it makes sense to repeat the test with only two of the bricks on the respective TL afterward. During this single-brick test, the TL that you were able to tolerate last holds for all other bricks. If you do tolerate one of these pairs at the new TL, note the tested TL as the combined TL for the two bricks. You can find the precise procedure in the flowchart in Section 2.2.5. A level test of balanced fructose is unnecessary; you will get the tolerated amount by just multiplying the level amount of tolerated fructose by 10 (see Chapter 3.1.1).[140]

For procedural reasons, wait until after you have repeated the test before trying to interpret the results. Please show your testing partner the table with the bricks for which you want to perform the level test (page 55). He or she can then adapt the test. Please also hand her or him the remaining sugars and measurement instruments from the substitute test (if taken).

How to handle symptoms

After noting test symptoms that were too severe to allow you to stomach the load, drink water (up to three liters per day) and take a walk to reduce your symptoms.

140 Kneepkens, Vonk, & Fernandes, 1984.

STOP: The following pages are for only your testing partner to read, as they contain information regarding procedural safety! Your partner's instructions will depend on results pertaining to your reactions; if you know how your partner is assessing you, you may alter your behavior and distort the results. Continue reading on page 71 to learn about the procedure resulting from your partner's tolerance statements. The three pages for your testing partner are preceded and followed by four empty pages. You should flick back from the end of the book to arrive at page 71 without reading them.

The **instructions** for your testing **partner** follow on page **60**. As the **reader** of the book you should leave them **unread**, to **produce** a **more accurate** test **result**. Hence, open a new page that is farther **ahead** and then **flick back** to page **71**.

The **instructions** for your testing **partner** follow on page **60**. As the **reader** of the book you should leave them **unread**, to **produce** a **more accurate** test **result**. Hence, open a new page that is much farther **ahead** and then **flick back** to page **71**.

The **instructions** for your testing **partner** follow on page **60**. As the **reader** of the book you should leave them **unread**, to **produce** a **more accurate** test **result**. Hence, open a new page that is much farther **ahead** and then **flick back** to page **71**.

The **instructions** for your testing **partner** follow on page **60**. As the **reader** of the book you should leave them **unread**, to **produce** a **more accurate** test **result**. Hence, open a new page that is much farther **ahead** and then **flick back** to page **71**.

Your friend wants to find out how much she or he can stomach of certain food ingredients. Unfortunately, a placebo effect is quite common in this test. Your role in this test is very important toward avoiding a false result. You are going to test each ingredient twice, each test taking about a week. On one of the two days, you are going to hand out a placebo mix instead of the real one. Your friend does not know about the placebo. Just say that the double test is required to get valid results, as you also have to keep track of certain behaviors she or he might exhibit. IMPORTANT: Keep quiet about the placebo until **all** tests are done (see page 72) and you have talked the results over. Waiting until the end of that final talk, is important as your friend may want more precise results. Between two test days are three monitoring days and three regeneration days.

Here is what you need: a beaker, a letter scale and three 0.5L bottles. Determine the ingredients to be tested on page 55 and for each of the following bricks being tested, prepare:

Fructose test: 0.5kg sugar, 100g fructose, vanilla extraxt and 1L of water.

Lactose test: 1L reduced-fat cow milk without additives, 1L of lactose free milk (please use cow milk that has been freed from lactose without a flavor or the label sugar free. Moreover, please do not use soy milk or rice milk for the test), vanilla extraxct.

Sorbitol test: 10g sorbitolm, vanilla extraxt and 1L of water.

If your friend has not given you the substances for the test solution, you can order them online or from a pharmacy. You can also ask your pharmacist to weigh the amounts you need.

From test to test, increase the level amounts according to the tables on the following pages. Begin with the TL 1 amounts of the highest ranked ingredient on page 55. Before repeating the test, note whether you first handed out the real or placebo mix and the result. Ideally you should ask for the symptom test sheet and write down L for reaL and A for plAcebo as well as the result. Then, keep all of the info sheets for the final discussion of all tests. If your friend has given you the K-grade, you can calculate the tolerance (see row L on page 37). If the L-grade is greater than or equal to K, this indicates an intolerance. There are three possible cases after each double test:

Case 1: Neither the placebo nor the real mix causes the symptoms to worsen, i.e., your friend is able to stomach the amounts of the ingredient, and it can be tested at the next level. Tell her/him that.

Case 2: Only the real mix causes the symptoms to worsen, i.e., your friend is intolerant for the amount. The test series for this ingredient is over, and your friend can be told. For a more precise level, you can proceed as per page 57.

Case 3: The placebo mix causes symptoms to worsen. Regardless of whether or not the real mix causes symptoms to worsen, as well, repeat the test with the same amount, starting with the placebo mix, but tell her that you reduced the amount to half of the dose. If your friend still reports an intolerance, abort the test and tell her/him (only until the final discussion) that s/he has an intolerance for the amount and the old levels remain current.[141]

After the test and retest of the first level of the ingredient with rank number 1, test the next ingredient in order (if applicable) also at the first level. After finishing all single tests for the stated ingredients at the first level, continue according to the level test flowchart on page 72. What follows may be a combination test:

Combination tests: For the lactose/fructose, lactose/sorbitol and lactose/sorbitol/fructose combination tests, use the cow milk and lactose freed cow milk together with vanilla extraxt according to the level amounts for lactose. For the fructose/sorbitol combination test alone, use 200mL of water. All ingredients to be tested are put into the liquids. For each one use the level amounts according to the single tables for the ingredients. After a tolerated combination test, the new combined tolerance levels hold for all further test days. Continue with another round of single tests for those bricks that were stomached well. This time, tell your friend that the new combined tolerance levels hold, and apply the Level 2 amounts for each test.

On the eve of one of the two test days, hand out three bottles with the real mix, and on the other one, three bottles with the placebo mix. At breakfast, lunch and dinner your friend drinks one bottle. Find the mixtures for each level in the following explanations and tables:

In the **left column** find the respective **level** and the **total amount** of substances per day, as it is easier to mix the **daily amount in one load** and **then divide** it among the **three bottles**. In the two columns on the right, find the amounts per bottle for the real/placebo substance.

Lactose: Required: 1L reduced-fat milk, 1L lactose free cow milk and vanilla extraxt. To hide taste differences between the normal and the laxtose free milk, please add a little bit of vanilla extraxt (**v.**) to both.

---

141 Latulippe & Skoog, 2011; Vesa et al., 1996.

Level and lactose amount, sum/day	Real (R) 3 × bottle with	Placebo (P) 3 × bottle with
Level 1 (3g/meal) per day 180mL milk and ½ tsp. of **v.**	4 tbsp. (60mL) milk 1 drop of **v.**	4 tbsp. lactose free milk 1 drop of **v.**
Level 2 (6g/meal) per day 360mL milk and ¾ tsp. of **v.**	120mL milk (100) 2 drops of **v.**	120mL lactose free milk 2 drops of **v.**
Level 3 (9g/meal) per day 540mL milk and 1 tsp. of **v.**	180mL milk 3 drops of **v.**	180mL lactose free milk 3 drops of **v.**

Fructose: Required: fructose and common sugar. Mix the following amounts with 200mL water (**w**) and add a little bit of vanilla extract (**v.**). Important: the bottles should not be diluted:

Level, real/placebo in g per day+600mL **w**	Real (R) 3 × 200mL **w** bottle with	Placebo (P) 3 × 200mL **w** bottle with
Level 1, 3 R/3.5 P, 1 tsp. v.	1g fructose 3 drops of **v.**	1.17g sugar 3 drops of **v.**
Level 2, 6 R/7 P, 1 tsp. v.	2g fructose 3 drops of **v.**	2.34g sugar 3 drops of **v.**
Level 3, 9 R/10.5 P, 1 tsp. v.	3g fructose 3 drops of **v.**	3.51g sugar 3 drops of **v.**

Sorbitol: Required: sorbitol and common sugar. Mix the amounts with 200mL of water (w) and add a little bit of vanilla extract (**v.**). Important: the bottles should not be diluted:

Level, real/placebo in g per day+600mL w	Real (R) 3 × 200mL **w** bottle with	Placebo (P) 3 × 200mL **w** bottle with
Level 1, 0.3 R/0.2 P, 1 tsp. v.	0.1g sorbitol 3 drops of **v.**	0.06g sugar 3 drops of **v.**
Level 2, 1.2 R/0.7 P, 1 tsp. v.	0.4g sorbitol 3 drops of **v.**	0.24g sugar 3 drops of **v.**
Level 3, 3 R/1.26 P, 1 tsp. v.	0.7g sorbitol 3 drops of **v.**	0.42g sugar 3 drops of **v.**

The **instructions** for your testing **partner** begin on page **60**. As the **reader** of the book you should leave them **unread**, to **produce** a **more accurate** test **result**. The book resumes on page 71.

The **instructions** for your testing **partner** begin on page **60**. As the **reader** of the book you should leave them **unread**, to **produce** a **more accurate** test **result**. The book resumes on page 71.

The **instructions** for your testing **partner** begin on page **60**. As the **reader** of the book you should leave them **unread**, to **produce** a **more accurate** test **result**. The book resumes on page 71.

The **instructions** for your testing **partner** begin on page **60**. As the **reader** of the book you should leave them **unread**, to **produce** a **more accurate** test **result**.

2.2.5 Symptom based test process

Procedural example with fictive bricks

In order to help you to remain impartial, the bricks are labelledhere after actual building materials: granite, wood and sandstone. Test the brick "granite" (having rank one in the example; see brick choice on page 55), "sandstone" (rank two) and "wood" (rank three). If, according to your testing partner, you could not tolerate "granite" during the first test at Level 1, then continue consuming that brick at the BTL amount. If you were able to tolerate "sandstone" at Level 1, however, that amount should now be considered your new TL for this brick if consumed on its own (not in combination with other bricks). Let's say, moreover, that you were able to stomach "wood" at the first level.

Next, perform a combined test of "sandstone" and "wood," as you were able to stomach the two bricks independently in the single tests. You can see this as you follow the [+] of the first diamond in the following flowchart. For this test, you will consume a mix of the two bricks in your test dilution bottles. While taking this test, eat according to the Level 0 portions for "granite," following the food tables in Part 3 of the book. If you are able to stomach that test load, enter Level 1 of "sandstone" and "wood" together with Level 0 of "granite," as a new combined TL in the table in Chapter 3.1.1.

Afterward, do another round of single level tests, as illustrated by the [+] of the second diamond in the line of the flowchart. Begin with the Level 2 test for "sandstone." The test dilution bottle then contains the Level 2 amount for "sandstone" and the Level 1 amount for "wood." On the test day, keep "granite" at Level 0. On the three days that follow, eat according to the Level 1 portion sizes of "sandstone" and "wood." If you tolerate the Level 2 amount of "sandstone" well, then do the Level 2 test of "wood" in which the test dilution contains the Level 1 amount of "sandstone" and the Level 2 amount of "wood." However, let's say you are intolerant towards that solution. If you follow the [-] at the third diamond in line (on the following page) and at the following diamond the [+], you find out that you would enter Level 2 for "sandstone" for the combined TL. Moreover, you learn that you can also do the Level 3 test for "sandstone." At this test again the Level 1 amount for "wood" is added. If you can stomach it, enter Level 3 for "sandstone" in the combined TL column.

Maybe you are interested in whether you can stomach more of the "wood" brick if you keep the BTLs for the other bricks. In this case, ask your testing partner to repeat the Level 2 test for "wood" with a mix that only contains the Level 2 amount of "wood" and none of the other bricks. During the test days, restrict yourself to the BTL portions of the other bricks. If you can stomach the Level 2 amount of "wood" now, enter Level 2 in the single TL column for wood and note down BTLs, as it only holds when you keep the BTLs of the other bricks.

Warning: you must not surpass any TL portion that holds during a level test, as it can distort the result. If this happens, you unfortunately have to repeat the test. Exception: you already finished the test after learning that you are intolerant towards that brick amount.

Level test flowchart

Starting with the rectangle in the upper right corner, read off the next step by following the arrows. A diamond means that the next step depends on the statement within the diamond being true [+] or false [-]. If the statement is true, follow the [+]-arrow, and if it is false, follow the [-]-arrow. In the rectangular fields, find a statement about what to do next. In fields that follow a field with a flag attached to it saying PATH 1 or PATH 2, you also find data in brackets or parentheses. These are only relevant if you were asked to follow the respective PATH at the end of the second page of the flowchart. The statements within the parentheses apply if you reach them via PATH 1, and those in square brackets if you were asked to follow PATH 2.

All instructions are based on the assumption that you want to take all level tests to the end, which you do not have to do. It might be enough for you to know that you are able to stomach the TL 1 portions. If this is true, just stop after the combined TL 1 test. The regular procedure ends as you reach a field with rounded corners. Enter the respective new levels into the table in Chapter 3.1.1.

What is the use of the combined test? The development of symptoms depends on how many bricks pass your belly's interception shield. Let's say you tolerate a higher level of various bricks in the single test. Exhausting the new portion sizes for these levels at the same time may still lead to symptoms due to interaction effects. Therefore, you want to check whether you are still able to tolerate the new portion sizes, when they are associated with the level advancements, at your shield's maximum combined exposure.

*Optional: Follow up level tests to find out the maximum single TLs of the bricks that were tolerated at the last level test.

**Optional: Follow up level test to find out the maximum new combined TL of the highest level brick(s). For non-tested bricks the current (new) combined TL portion sizes hold.

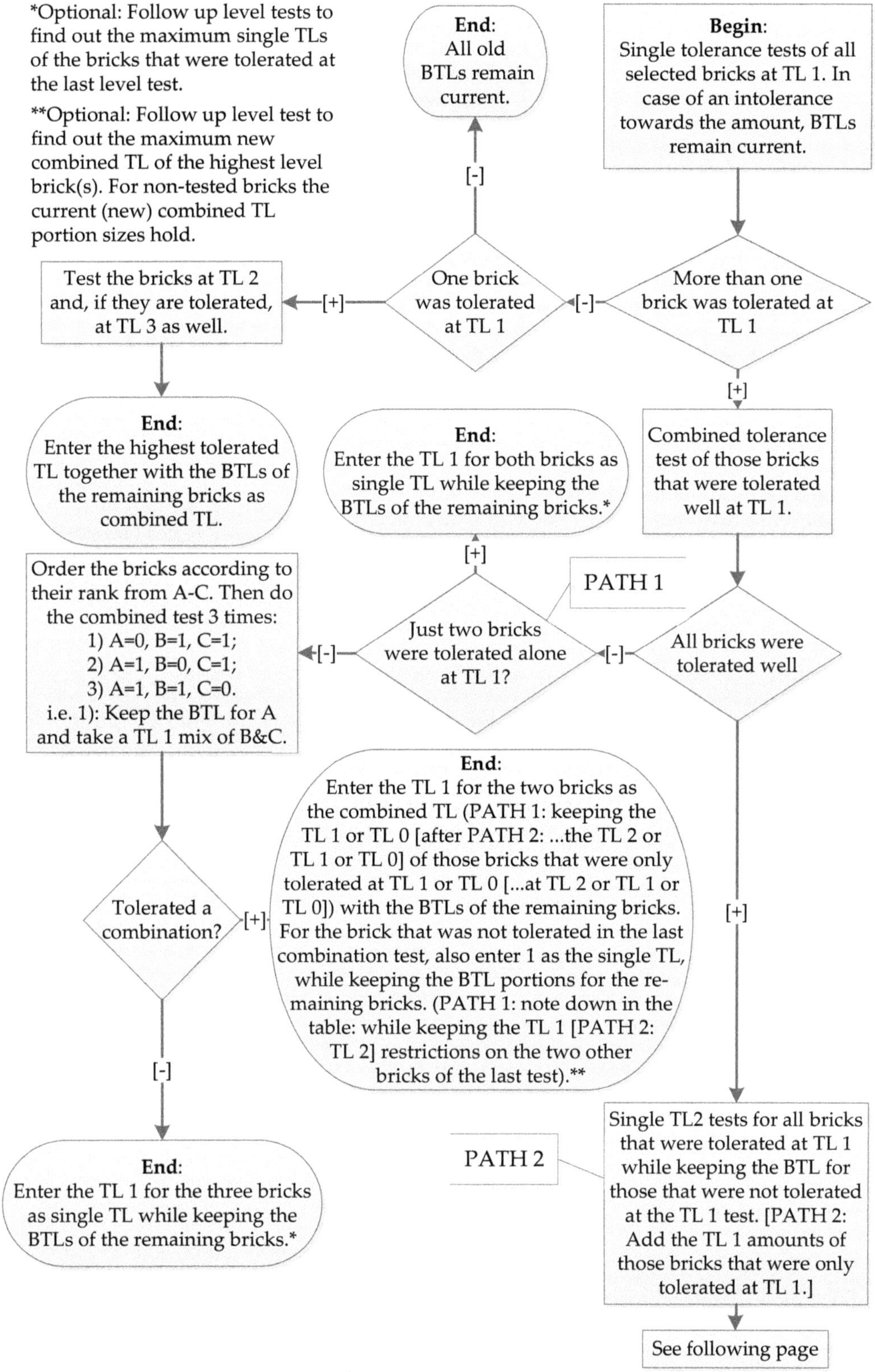

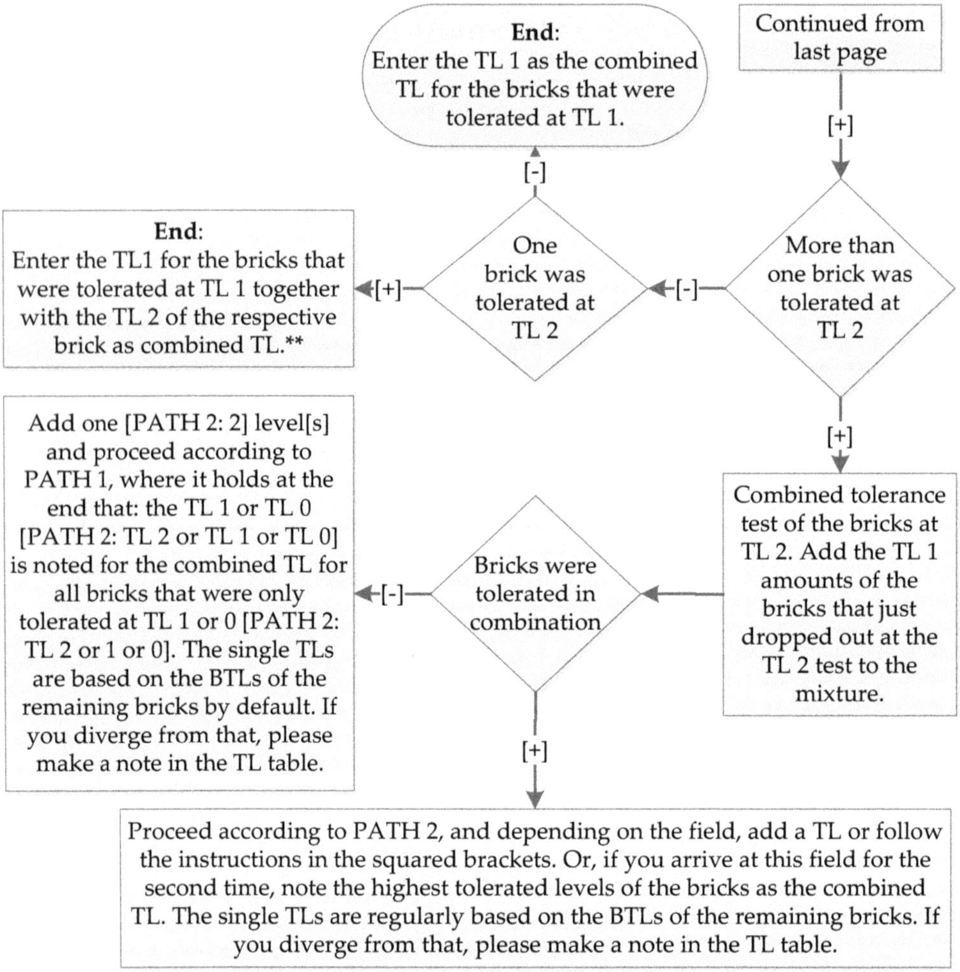
Continued from last page
[+]
More than one brick was tolerated at TL 2
[-]
One brick was tolerated at TL 2
[-]
End:
Enter the TL 1 as the combined TL for the bricks that were tolerated at TL 1.
[+]
End:
Enter the TL1 for the bricks that were tolerated at TL 1 together with the TL 2 of the respective brick as combined TL.**
[+]
Combined tolerance test of the bricks at TL 2. Add the TL 1 amounts of the bricks that just dropped out at the TL 2 test to the mixture.
Bricks were tolerated in combination
[-]
Add one [PATH 2: 2] level[s] and proceed according to PATH 1, where it holds at the end that: the TL 1 or TL 0 [PATH 2: TL 2 or TL 1 or TL 0] is noted for the combined TL for all bricks that were only tolerated at TL 1 or 0 [PATH 2: TL 2 or 1 or 0]. The single TLs are based on the BTLs of the remaining bricks by default. If you diverge from that, please make a note in the TL table.
[+]
Proceed according to PATH 2, and depending on the field, add a TL or follow the instructions in the squared brackets. Or, if you arrive at this field for the second time, note the highest tolerated levels of the bricks as the combined TL. The single TLs are regularly based on the BTLs of the remaining bricks. If you diverge from that, please make a note in the TL table.

2.2.6 Alternative strategies

General causes of abdominal discomfort

The following triggers have been found most often in an analysis of nutrition diaries. On a subjective scale from 1 (seldom) to 6 (very often): wheat 5, milk 5, coffee 5, eggs 5, potatoes 5, nuts 4, rye 2, barley 2, corn 2, oats 2, banana 2, onions 2, peas 2.[142] The malabsorbtions for all of these food products except for coffee, corn, eggs, nuts and potatoes can be explained by the scientific analysis of carbohydrates like fructose, lactose, fructans and galactans. The author was unable to find studies that analyzed the fructan and galactan content of eggs, coffee and nuts.[143]

Alternative diet strategy

Sometimes a product such as coffee causes discomfort or acts as a trigger for reasons other than the carbohydrates that are the focus of this book. In these cases try adopting an alternative introductory diet. In such a diet, you will abstain from coffee, corn, eggs, nuts and potatoes, as well as up to two to four other products or ingredients that you suspect might be causing you trouble. Before starting the diet take note of the greatest amount you are likely to consume of the affected foods at breakfast, lunch and dinner. You need that sheet later to find out which of the foods, if any, caused you symptoms. Then at the end of the three test weeks, use the symptom test sheet again to determine the efficiency of the diet by comparing it with your former status quo sheet. If you want, you can also employ the mentioned calculation methods, using the final sheet from your alternative diet as your efficiency check sheet. Before starting the diet, discuss potential personal risks with your doctor.

If the diet successfully relieved your symptoms, wait three days and then test the foods that you are abstaining from. Take a look at the notes you made regarding your usual portion sizes of the foods included in the test. Choose one of the foods, and on test day, eat the amounts that are typical for you at the times you usually eat them. On that day and the three that follow, fill out the symptom test sheet (see page 36) and, if you are using math Option B (see page 37), estimate your L-grade. During the test weeks, continue to avoid the

---

[142] Petitpierre Gumowski, & Girald, 1985; Nanda et al., 1989; Hawthorne et al., 1991; Parker et al., 1995; Stefanini et al., 1995.

[143] Biesiekierski et al. 2011; Muir et al. 2007, 2009.

foods you are testing as well as those you tested intolerant for. A negative test result indicates that you can safely consume the given food as you did before the alternative introductory diet. With a positive result, you have two options: either you can completely avoid the food or you can determine a tolerable portion size by performing a level test. For the level test, you divide your common portion by four. During the level test weeks, refrain from all symptom-inducing foods you found. On the test day, eat the to-be-tested portion size at the times you normally have your three main meals. Start with one fourth of your normal portion size. If your symptoms do not significantly worsen, repeat the test on the fourth day after your test day with half of your common portion size. If you can stomach this amount, repeat the test with three fourths of your normal portion. If you were not able to stomach one fourth of your normal portion size, you can choose to avoid the food or ingredient or test it further at a reduced test portion size. If symptoms arose at half your usual portion size, then consider your tolerable portion to be one fourth of a full portion; if they arose at three fourths, your tolerable portion is a half-portion. If you could not narrow your symptoms down to a critical food or ingredient, return to your usual diet. Low dosage antidepressants constitute one possible remaining alternative for addressing your symptoms, but consult your doctor to discuss this option further.[144]

[144] Quigley et al., 2013; McKenzie et al., 2012.

2.3 General diet hints

2.3.1 Good reasons for your persistence

Imagine that one of your best friends goes on a two-week vacation, leaving his beloved Labrador retriever in your care, along with some instructions about the dog's health needs as he has an intolerance towards an ingredient in some dog foods. You run out of dog food after the first week, and while you're on your way out of the house to get more, your partner stops you. "Hold on," s/he says, "There's still the dog food we give your aunt's dog in the pantry." You're tempted to give in and use it, rather than spend an hour driving to the store and back, but you read the ingredient list and know that one of the ingredients is harmful to the dog. Unlike the happy dog image on the package suggests, giving him this food causes him pain, flatulence and lethargy; catching a stick will be out of the question for this poor pooch, and you tell your partner so. "Don't be so worried," s/he argues. "The dogs we had growing up ate it all the time and never had a problem!" But you know that even if your partner's family did it all the time, it doesn't make it right for this dog. Hence, you give some thought about your friend's dog and his well-being is worth the investment of your money and time. The question that you now have to answer yourself is:

do you owe it to yourself, too?

In the end, I call upon you to take responsibility for your nutrition. Show respect to your body. Acquire the necessary courage and discipline. Your body is a part of you. Just as many vegetarians stand by their dietary choices for the duration of their lives, you should stand by your diet and your body. Be yourself. The key is not starting out perfect but starting at all and making small improvements every day. That is something you can do!

Your target should be to change your sustenance day by day, food by food, in such a way as to allow you to lead a largely symptom-free life. All beginnings are difficult, however, and as you leap the initial hurdles, you will find further motivation and discipline in discovering how much your nutritional changes are paying off for you.

The first step in that direction is to connect that goal with whatever is most important to you in your life. Independent of where your passions lie most strongly, you will improve on them by gaining more energy and improved wellbeing.

Thus, turn your attention and abilities towards eating in a way that will help you achieve your goals. Overcome any fears of change you might have by imagining that you have already done it. How? Cut out the following card and fold it as indicated. Then put it somewhere you can see it every day. Ideally, you can take a picture of yourself after a particularly successful milestone and put it on the drawing. Then let it encourage you to continue improving your nutrition each day.

Stephen William Hawking has never stopped producing outstanding scientific works despite suffering from amyosthenia.[145] Why? Because he is following his heart and because he has a positive attitude about life. Who seeks excuses when they're passionate about something? When it comes to passion, it is all about the how. It is about doing what is possible and thus it is always all about the solution. There are similar examples in sports. Melissa Stockwell achieves first class athletic performance despite having lost a leg. Her sport is her passion, and she finds ways to excel in it regardless of the circumstances life gave her.[146]

So what is your passion? Write it down. Then make it clear to yourself that a symptom-reducing diet will positively affect your passion. Then get on your way to making this nutrition a part of your life.

---

[145] Hawking, n. d..

[146] Stockwell, n. d..

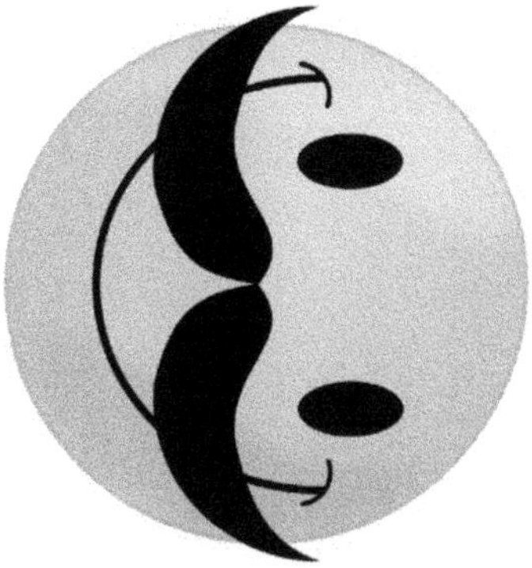

Eat ***smarter***
Live ***happier***
Laxiba.co.uk

Eat ***smarter***
Live ***happier***
Laxiba.co.uk

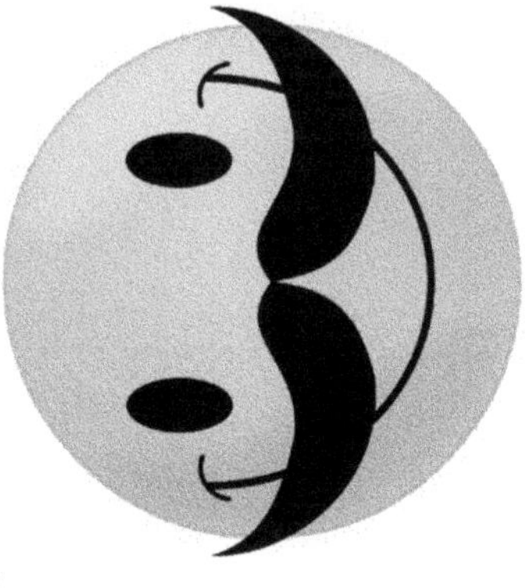

This page has been intentionally left blank.

2.3.2 Mealtimes

Even when and how often you eat can affect your digestion. Who are the greatest experts on that? People for whom a successful supply of energy is of the utmost importance—that is to say, athletes. An analysis shows that over 97% of elite Canadian athletes eat at least three times a day; 57% of them also take a snack in the morning, 71% in the afternoon and 58% in the evening.[147] Moreover, regular mealtimes have a positive effect on the cardiovascular system.[148] A study of more than 4,500 children showed that the risk of childhood obesity markedly decreases the more often children eat during the day.[149]

2.3.3 Reasons for using the bricks

What are bricks doing in medicine, sausage, and all manner of other things you consume on a daily basis? Some reasons bricks get added to products include savings in costs, as well as their use as a flavoring, a preservative, a thickener for meat products or a sugar substitute, e.g., for diabetic. In addition, lactose and sorbitol are used as medicinal carriers.[150] So far, there is no strong lobby against using bricks in foods or making them easier to avoid. Of course, these bricks also occur naturally, but that is not a valid reason to use them instead of the also naturally occurring Stevia in, for example, chewing gums.

2.3.4 Eating out

At home, restricting one's consumption of bricks is rather easy, but how about eating out? Some products that are usually safe include eggs, fish or meat without breading or sauce, kiwis, leafy salads dressed with oil, oregano, pepper and salt, oranges, pesto, potatoes, rice, tomatoes, tomato sauce and tortillas. Depending on your intolerances, you have to be careful with diabetics products and prepared sauces, as they often contain bricks like sorbitol. What about menus, however? Have you ever spent time at a restaurant considering

---

147 Erdman, Tunnicliffe, Lun, & Reimer, 2013.

148 Farshchi, Taylor, & Macdonald, 2004.

149 Toschke, Thorsteinsdottir, & von Kris, 2009.

150 Raithel et al., 2013.

what the ideal combination of menu items would be for you?[151] The good thing is that you can often ask for changes to be made to menu items without paying much extra, if you ask the server. You can likewise voice your needs to your hosts when you are invited to a meal. To make it easy, just hand out the out-of-home list (see Chapter 2.4.3). You can send it out with the following message, for example:

> *"Dear [name of the host],*
>
> *I was glad to receive your invitation to [occasion of the invitation], and I am happy to come. If it would not be an inconvenience for you to cook some of the foods that are included in the attached table separately from the other meals, then I would be pleased to take part in the meal, as well. Please tell me whether that will be possible so that I can plan accordingly.*
>
> *Thank you and see you soon!*
>
> *[Your name]"*

The out-of-home list also makes it easier for a restaurant kitchen to find a suitable meal for you. As fast food chains are not as readily equipped to adapt their menus, you will find many fast food chain products and the portion sizes you can stomach in the third part of this book. You can stay on the safe side by always having your book with you. However, it will hardly be always at hand, unlike a foldable list for your purse or wallet. In Chapter 2.4 you will find two such lists with the tolerable portion sizes of some common products. This list also includes information on brick names and brick-free products.

2.3.5 Convenience foods

Unfortunately, fructose, lactose and sorbitol are added to many convenience foods or are naturally contained in the ingredients. However, you will find exceptions, even when shopping on the cheap, including convenience foods that advertise the use of natural ingredients and those that contain tomato sauce. The leaflets (see Chapter 2.4) will inform you of which ingredients on a package are related to bricks.

---

151 Eisenführ, Weber, & Langer, 2010.

2.3.6 Medicine and oral hygiene

Everything you take into your mouth can cause symptoms if it contains a brick you cannot tolerate. Sorbitol in particular is found in many oral hygiene products. Examples of sorbitol-free toothpastes include Weleda® Calendula Toothpaste. Use dental floss without wax, and find a mouthwash such as TheraBreath® Fresh Breath Oral Rinse.

The search for sorbitol-free medicines may be especially hard, so ask your pharmacist for assistance. Many nasal sprays, eye drops and expectorants contain this additive. However, if you look hard enough, you will usually find alternatives for these as well.

Examples of sorbitol-free pharmaceuticals include: Allerest® PE Allergy & Sinus Relief – Tablets [CONTAINS LACTOSE] (frontal sinusitis), BecoAllergy® 10mg 7 Tablets (allergy) [CONTAINS LACTOSE], Imodium® Capsules classic (diarrhoea) [CONTAINS LACTOSE], Murine® Irritation & Redness Eye Drops (eye irritation), Otex Express® (eardrops), Teva® Loratadine 10mg 30 Tablets (hayfever) [CONTAINS LACTOSE], Venos® Chesty Coughs (expectorant) and Vicks® Sinex Micromist Nasal Spray (frontal sinusitis)

It is good to know that middle-sized capsules contain 0.58g at the most, and the largest, 1.6g per piece, while tablets are usually even a little lighter. For mixtures a teaspoon holds about 5mL/g and a tablespoon 5–15mL/g. Despite your best efforts at researching your own intolerances, you may find yourself unable to stomach a medicine for whatever reason. If you are having symptoms, search for alternatives. If in doubt, use the symptom test sheet. Write down your symptoms while using it and compare it with a record of your diet taken when you were not using the medicine, for example, on your efficiency check sheet. You can use any sheet where you recorded your symptoms after refraining from bricks that you are intolerant towards.

2.3.7 Nutritional supplements

If you take vitamin supplements, the following examples are brick-free:

UK: HealthAid® Vitamin B Complex Supreme Capsules, HealthAid® Vitamin B12 1000ug Tablets, Bioglan® Rest and Restore Night Multivitamin For Women Tablets, Bioglan® Rest and Restore Night Multivitamin For Men Capsules. The use of multivitamin supplements could not be shown in a long-term trial.[152] If you take them, make sure not to take too much of certain vitamins. Vitamins that can be unsafe in excess include B3 and B6, as well as A, D, E and K,[153] which can cause symptoms of poisoning if you overdose. It is thus recommended to discuss your intake with your doctor. One possible approach with these vitamins may be to take them in three-month cycles. That means taking them for three months and then taking the next three months off.

2.3.8 Positive aspects of the diet

While you restrict your intake of brick-containing foods, try to think more about what you eat and you will likely find better nutritional balance.

2.3.9 Testing yourself

Some of those affected by IBS reportedly struggle to absorb other ingredients like aspartame or maltodextrin. If you have reason to believe that this applies to you, follow the alternative introductory diet outlined in Chapter 2.2.6.

2.3.10 Protein shakes—nutrition for athletes

There is a questionable trend among athletes to take special supplements. If you are able to cover your protein demand with the products listed in Chapter 2.1.4, you have no need for protein shakes or the like.[154] Many energy bars and electrolyte products contain sorbitol due to their processed fruit content, but you can find sorbitol-free alternatives in pharmacies. These products have their own category in this book's food tables.

2.3.11 Sweeteners

Unlike many other sweeteners, such as those added to "light" products like sugar-free soft drinks, pure Stevia is sorbitol-free.

---

152 Briançon et al. 2011.
153 Webb & Whitney, 2008.
154 Test, 2008.

2.3.12 Fish and meat

Breaded fish and meat, processed (such as Bolognese, bratwurst or liverwurst) or with sauce, may contain bricks. Any bricks they contain should be included in the list of ingredients. In the following chapter, you will find leaflets to keep at hand listing bricks and their safe quantities.

2.3.13 These actions lead to lasting change

In order to achieve lasting success, it is important that you monitor your own nutrition. If you find yourself starting to ignore the recommended amounts, you should get back on track and restart your commitment as soon as possible. Write down your goal to adapt your nutrition to the stated food and drink portion sizes to reduce abdominal discomfort and improve your quality of life. Stay conscious of the negative consequences of eating "blindly" covered in the first part of this book. Why is it important to change your habits? Re-read your goal and then write down your five most important reasons for striving towards it. Moreover, answer this question for yourself: why it is important to act **now**?[155] Inform the people close to you about why changing your nutritional habits is important—ask them to support you. Short-term change is easy. The real challenge is continuing with your dietary commitments in the long run. One way to stay motivated is to write about the positive effects on your quality of life that come from keeping your diet (annotate a calendar or jot down your thoughts daily). It also helps to work with a partner. At our homepage, www.Laxiba.co.uk/coach, you can hire a coach who guides you through the steps in this book and the change process. Furthermore, you can find people in a similar situation to yours, exchange experiences with them and motivate each other at www.Laxiba.co.uk/team[156]

Imagine yourself living with few or no abdominal symptoms. You will have changed your diet in a way that significantly improves your wellbeing through determination and capability. The more vividly and multidimensionally you can picture what your life will be like after you have succeeded, the more likely you are to achieve that success.[157] If you lapse slightly, relax; refocus and sort yourself out for the next day. As you continually adapt your path

[155] Hillson, 2013; Michie, 2013.

[156] Stubbs, 2013.

[157] Fox, 2013.

(like you do when using a compass), you will reach your goal in the end. If you find that this strategy helps you, you can continue to follow it for the long run.[158]

2.4 The leaflets

Cut out the two leaflets on the following pages. Please fold them along the thick lines. Start with the dotted line. Then fold each leaflet again at the half-dashed line. You can now keep this important information at hand when you are out and about or shopping.

---

[158] Gilbert, 2013.

Front

Flyer for lactose, fructans & galactans

Non critical ingredients: lactose intolerance

Calcium lactate	Glucono delta-lactone	Sodium lactate
Lactate	Milk acid	Natriumlactat
Potassium lactate	(INS additive numbers: 575, 325-327)	

Critical ingredients: lactose intolerance

Lactose	Yoghurt	Whey
Cheese	Kefir, lassi	Milk(-powder)
Curd	(Concentrated) butter	Cream

Asian, Greek, Italian and Spanish meals rather contain little lactose. Asian rice meals also containing few fructans and galactans. Fish, other seafood, meat, black coffee, eggs and oils are also free from lactose. The same holds for fruits and vegetable although some of them contain fructans and galactans.

Back

Lactose is often contained in:

- cereals
- ice cream and sweets like chocolate
- coffee and milk, condensed milk
- dairy products
- breadings, sauces, puréed meat, Tzatziki
- sweet pastries like biscuits, cakes and tarts, cream

Fructans are primarily contained in:

artichokes, asparagus, banana, blueberries, bread, Brussels sprouts, cabbage,

cauliflower, cereals, chicory root, couscous, garlic, leeks, linseeds, nectarine, noodles, onions, pastries like biscuits and cake, pineapple,

pizza, products that inulin has been added to (like some cereals, chocolates and ice creams) raisins, semolina flour, shallots and sunchoke

Galactans are primarily contained in:

beans, lentils, linseeds, oat flakes, peas, soy products including tofu, sprouts, wheat and other grains

LAXIBA®

Interior left

Lactose, fructans & galactans free

Apple	Fish and	Oranges
Apricot	Meat	Parmesan
Carrots	Jelly babies	Pear
celery	Ice tea	Peppers
Chocolate sorbet	Ketchup	Potatoes
Coconut	Kiwi	Rice
Drinks without	Lettuce	Spelt flour
milk, yoghurt etc.	Oil & vinegar	Squash

Lactose poor for normal portion sizes

Butter ☺; 14g	Margarine 21¾P.; 9g	Swiss
Cheddar 33¼P.; 30g	Nutella ®32¼P.; 37g	cheese
Fondue sauce ☺; 53g	Parmesan ☺; 5g	☺; 30g

Per strong lactase capsule you take in, you can stomach about 75% more of each shown portion amount:

Portion unit shown as

Exemplar	Cup	Glas	Portion	Slice
E	C	G	P	S

☹=avoid; ☹²=1/4 unit at TL2; ☺=contains traces; ☻=is free of it

Calculation of the remaining TL-portions

Lactose (TL1)	L0 = ÷2	L2 = x2	L3 = x3
Fru-/Galactans (TL0)	L1 = x2	L2 = x4	L3 = x6

Interior right

High amount of lactose

Cacao ¼C.; 150g
Casserole ½P.; 238g
Cheese-sauce ¼P.; 66g
Condensed milk ½P ¼P.; 107g 200g
Creme-soup ½P.; 245g
Kefir ¼P.; 220g
Mashed-potatoe ½P.; 140g
Milk rice ¼P.; 107g 200g
Milk ¼G.; 200g
Mozzarella 9¾P.; 30g
Pan cake ½P.; 187g
Tart ½P.; 87,5g
Yoghurt ¼P.; 250g

F+G TL 0 portions

Apple strudel ¾ P., 64g
Asparagus ½P., 85g
Baguette 1¾S., 42g
Banana juice ½G., 200g
Granola bar ½P., 27g
Hamburger ½E., 100g
Hot dog ¼E., 199g
Kidney beans ¼P., 90g
Sandwich ☹
Shalot ¼E., 15g

Cake ¼P., 122g
Calzone ¼P., 168g
Cheese cake ☹P., 220g
Chop Suey ¼P., 166g
Cookie ½E., 45g
Corn Flakes 1½P., 30g
Couscous ¼P., 140g
Cracker ¼P., 30g
Crêpe ¾E., 55g
Crispbread ¼S., 42g
Danish pastry ¼E., 125g
Donut ½E., 105g
French toast ¼ P., 131g
Leeks ¼P., 89g
Lentils ¾P., 90g
Muesli ¼P., 55g
Muffin ¼E., 113g
Noodles 1P., 140g
Oat bran 1¼P., 55g
Onion Rings ¼P., 70g
Peas 1¼P., 15g
Pizza ½P., 209g
Plain dumplings ½P., 55g
Ravioli ¼P., 250g
Rye bread ¾S., 42g
Sandwich-cookie 3½E., 14,5g
Snow peas ¾P., 85g
Spring roll ¼P., 140g
Tofu ½P., 85g
Waffles ½P., 95g
White wholegrain wheat bread ¾S., 42g

Front

Flyer for fructose and sorbitol

Non problematic ingredients: sorbitol intolerance

Maltodextrin	Sorbic acid	Barley malt sirup
Sodium sorbate	Potassium sorbate	Calcium sorbate
Sorbitan...	Polyoxyethylene (20) -**sorbitan**-...	
(INS add. numbers: 200-203, 432-436, 491-495)		

Problematic ingredients: sorbitol intolerance

Sorbitol Lactitol	Mannitol (Ethyl-) Maltol	Xylitol Hexanhexol
Glucitol	Maltitol/-syrup	Inositol
Isomalt	Palatinit®	Sionon
Erythritol	Pinitol	
(INS add. numbers: 420-21, 636-37, 953, 965-7)		

Back

Find further tools at www.Laxiba.co.uk

Caution... free fructose is contained in:

- cereals with high fructose corn syrup (HFCS)
- many convenience foods
- jam sugar, honey and corn syrup
- some sweeteners
- many fruit, dry fruit and juices
- many soft drinks and alcoholic beverages

Sugar alcohols are often contained in:

- sausages, fish and meat that is puréed, pickled or has a breading
- convenience foods and readymade sauces
- chewing gums and mints, except for those that are only sweetened with Stevia. only traces of sorbitol are contained in: Wrigley's® Spearmint, Doublemint and Juicy Fruit®
- some sugar free, and isotonic beverages
- medicine and mouth hygiene products
- electrolyte products and energy bars
- bars, pralines, sweet pastries, tart, even readymade cream
- diabetic, dietary products

LAXIBA®

Interior left

Apple F:☹; S☹2;E 182g
Apricot F:D +¾ P; S¾;E 35g
Bals. vinegar F:D; S23;P 15,94g
Banana F:D +¼ P.; S9¼;E 118g
Beer F50; S10;G 200ml
Big Mac ®F5; S6½;E 215g
Bitter Lemon F☹; S:D;G 200ml
Blackberries F3¾; S:D;P 140g
Blueberry Muffin F:D;S:D;E113g
Broccoli F3; S:D;P 85g
Cauliflower F:D; S2½;P 85g

Cinnamon Toast Crunch ®F¼; S:D;P 30g
Coca Cola ®F½; S:D;G 200ml

Corn flakes F:D +1½ P.; S☺, 30g
Cranberries F:D +2¾ P.; S45¼;P 55g
Fiber One Original ®F41½; S:D;P 30g
Garden salad F8¼; S16¾;P85g
Ginger ale F☹; S:D;G 200ml
Lettuce F8¼; S16¾;P 85g
Oat bran F:D; S:D;P 55g
Pears F½; S¼;E 15g

Pickles F4¾; S1;E 85g
Pineapple F¾; S¾;P 140g
Strawberries F½; S¼;P 140g

Portion unit shown as

Exemplar	Cup	Glas	Portion	Slice
E	C	G	P	S

☹=avoid; ☹2=1/4 unit at TL2; ☺=contains traces; ☻=is free of it

Portion amounts for fructose (F) and sorbitol (S)

Fructose (TL 0)	L1 = x2	L2 = x4	L3 = x5
Sorbitol (TL 1)	L0 = x0	L2 = x4	L3 = x10

Interior right

7UP ®F☹; S:D;G 200ml
Black current F1; S:D;P 140g
Cabbage F:D +¾ P.; S58;P 85g
Champagne F31¼; S¾;G200ml
Cherries F10; S½;L 15g
Chicken, s.n's. F2½; S☺;L 15g
Chocolate F:D; S48; P 25g
Coffee F:D; S:D;T 150g
Granola bar F:D +4¼ P.; S71¼;E 35g

Grapes F¼; S½;P 140g
Honey Smacks ®F:D +12 P.; S83¼;P 30g

Honey F½; S1¾;L 15g
Ketchup F:D +¼ P.; S3¾;L 15g
Kiwi F1; S:D;E 86g
Lemon F:D; S:D;E 58g
Long island icetea F¾; S16½;G 200ml

M & M's ®F:D; S:D;P 40g
Mango F1; S4;L 15g
Mate-Tee F:D; S:D;G 200ml
Mayo F:D; S:D;P 15g
Melon F1; S14¼;P 140g
Milk F:D; S:D;G 200ml

Mushroom F:D +¼ P.; S¾;L 15g
Nectarine F8¼; S1;L 15g
Noodles F:D +¼ P.; S:D;P 140g
Oranges F2¼; S:D;E 140g
Peach F:D +½ P.; S¼;E 140g
Peppers F½; S:D;E 85g
Pepsi ®F½; S:D;J 200g
Pizza F:D +¾ P.; S¾;E 209g
Plums F:D +¼ P.; S¾;E 15g
Popsicle F:D +1¼ P.; S:D;P52g
Potatoes F:D; S45¼;P 110g
Raspberry F½; S1½;P 140g

Red Bull ®F:D +7¾P.;S:D;G200ml
Rice F:D; S:D;P 140g
Sauerkraut F:D; S¾;L 15g
Squash, bttrnt F:D; S:D;P 130g
Sugar free Chewinggums F¼; S☹2;E 2g
Sushi F:D; S1½;P 140g
Tomatoes F4½; S1;E 85g
Tonic Water ®F☹; S:D;G 200ml
Wheat bread F¾; S26¼;S 42g
Whopper ®F2¾; S1;E 315g
Winegum F:D+12 P; S:D;P30g
Wine F31¼; S¾;G 200ml

2.4.1 Fructose and sugar alcohols

If you have a fructose intolerance, be mindful of fructose and HFCS while reading through ingredient lists. To determine sorbitol-free products, however, you unfortunately have to navigate an unbelievable muddle of identifiers, despite the high prevalence of the condition:[159]

Noncritical ingredients for sorbitol intolerance[160]		
Maltodextrin	Sorbic acid	Barley malt syrup
Sodium sorbate	Potassium sorbate	Calcium sorbate
Sorbitan...	Polyoxyethylene (20) -sorbitan-...	

Critical ingredients for sorbitol intolerance[161]		
Sorbitol	Mannitol	Xylitol
Lactitol	(Ethyl-) Maltol	Hexanhexol
Glucitol	Maltitol/-syrup	Inositol
Isomalt	Palatinit®	Sionon
Erythritol	Pinitol	

[159] There is an immediate need for simplification here. The declaration "critical in case of a sorbitol intolerance" would spare many efforts.

[160] INS additive numbers: 200–203, 432–436, 491–495.

[161] INS additive numbers: 420–21, 636–37, 953, 965–67.

Caution...

Free fructose is contained in:

- Unknown quantities in cereals with high fructose corn syrup (HFCS) or isoglucose, glucose-fructose syrup, fructose-glucose syrup and high fructose maize syrup, unless listed in the food tables of this book
- Many convenience foods
- Preserving sugar
- Honey and corn syrup (fructose quantity is unclear)
- Some sweeteners
- Many fruits, dried fruits, juices and alcoholic drinks
- Many soft drinks

Sugar alcohols like sorbitol are also often contained in:

- Diabetic and dietary products
- Electrolyte products and energy bars
- Convenience foods and prepared sauces
- Chewing gums and mints, except those sweetened only with Stevia, for example. Traces of sorbitol are found in Wrigley's® Spearmint, Doublemint and Juicy Fruit
- Some "light," i.e., sugar free, and isotonic beverages
- Medicine and oral hygiene products
- Bars, pralines, sweet pastries, tarts, prepared cream
- Puréed, pickled or breaded sausages, fish and meat

Moreover, some fruits (like apples, apricots, bananas, cantaloupe, carambola, cherries, cranberries, grapes, guava, lowbush cranberries, mango, nectarine, peach, pear, pinapple, plum, pomegranate, raspberries, strawberries and watermelon) and vegetables (artichoke, asparagus, beets, cabbage, carrots, cauliflower, celeriac, celery, chestnuts, chicory, coleslaw, cucumber, eggplant, endive, fennel bulb, garbanzo beans (chickpeas), kale, kohlrabi, leeks, lettuce (boston), lettuce (green leaf), lettuce (iceberg), lettuce (red leaf), lettuce (romaine), mushrooms, olives, onions, pickled beets, radish, sauerkraut, sour pickles, soybean sprouts, spinach, tempeh, tomatoes and turnip), including juices contain sorbitol. Many alcoholic beverages do, as well, but brandy, gin, rum and whiskey for example, are often sorbitol-free.[162]

---

[162] Zorn, 2014.

2.4.2 Fructans, galactans and lactose[163]

Noncritical ingredients for lactose intolerance		
Calcium lactate	Glucono delta-lactone	Sodium lactate
Lactate	Lactic acid	Potassium lactate
Critical ingredients for lactose intolerance		
Lactose	Yogurt	Whey
Cheese	Kefir, lassi	Milk (-powder)
Curd	(Concentrated) butter	Cream

Asian, Greek, Italian and Spanish meals tend not to contain much lactose. Asian rice-based dishes are also low in fructans and galactans. Fish and seafood, meat, black coffee, eggs and oils are also lactose-free, as are fruits and vegetables, although some contain fructans and galactans.

Caution...:

Lactose is also contained in:

- Coffee with milk or condensed milk
- Cream
- Many cereals
- Many types of ice cream, chocolate and other candy
- Some breads and sauces
- Some sausages
- Sweet pastries like biscuits, cakes and tarts
- Tzatziki

[163] INS additive numbers: 575, 325-327.

High amounts of fructans are found in:

- Artichokes
- Asparagus
- Bananas
- Blueberries
- Brussels sprouts
- Cabbage
- Cauliflower
- Cereals
- Chicory root
- Couscous
- Linseeds
- Garlic
- Jerusalem artichokes
- Leeks
- Nectarines
- Noodles
- Onions
- Pastries and biscuits, breads and cakes
- Pineapple
- Pizza
- Products that inulin has been added to, such as some cereals, chocolate and ice cream
- Raisins
- Semolina flour
- Shallots

High amounts of galactans are found in:

- Beans
- Linseeds
- Lentils
- Oats
- Peas
- Soy products, including tofu
- Sprouts
- Wheat and other grains

2.4.3 The eating out list

Fruit	Vegetables	Warm dishes
Blackberries	Avocado, green	Brandy vinegar
Currants	Basil	Caviar
Dates, fresh	Chard	Chinese oyster sauce
Figs, fresh	Chives	Fish, meat, shrimp and shellfish*
Goji berries	Coriander	
Lemon zest	Green peppers	Kraft® Italian Dressing
Loganberry	Horseradish	
Papaya	Kelp	Kraft® Mayonnaise
Passion fruit	Oregano	Oils
Rhubarb	Parsnips	Kraft® Thousand Island Dressing®
	Peppermint, fresh	
	Rice	Pepper and salt
	Rosemary	Rice bread
	Rutabaga	Rice noodles
	Squash: Butternut, calabash, giant and spaghetti	Soy oil
	Thyme	Spelt flour
	Yam	Tabasco® sauce

*Non puréed and without breading and sauce.

Beverages	Others	
Black coffee	Baking powder	Pecan nuts
Brandy	Brazil nuts	Pine nuts
Gin	Brown sugar	Pistachios
Jasmine tea	Cashews	Pumpkin seeds
Maté tea	Coconut	Rice bread
Peppermint tea	Gelatin	Spelt
Rum	Ginkgo	Walnuts
Tequila	Liquorice	White sugar
Tonic Water	Macadamia nuts	
Vodka	Maple syrup	
Water	Peanut butter	
Whisky	Peanuts	

This page has been intentionally left blank.

2.5 For hosts

There will be someone in your circle of friends who has IBS or an intolerance towards one or more ingredients. Of course, as a host, you want to be considerate to your guests. In order to offer some suitable food options, ask whether anyone has an intolerance. This will give your guests a good impression, as you are demonstrating that their needs are important to you. Cut out the two leaflets from the preceding chapter. You can find therein the tolerable portions of a number of common foods. If one or more guests has a sorbitol intolerance, please ensure you cook sorbitol-containing ingredients separately.

Generally, you should be fine if you offer: black coffee, cheddar, corn flakes, eggs, fish and meat (non-breaded and without prepared sauce), French fries, kiwis, lettuce, lemons, margarine (not butter), nuts, oil with oregano, pepper and salt (as an alternative to sauce), oranges, peas, potatoes, rice, rice milk, salted popcorn, salted crisps, spinach, Stevia, sugar, tomatoes and water. Most herbs and spices, except for garlic and onions, are harmless. Adjusting to suit affected guests is actually quite straightforward. Just serve the tolerable foods separately from any sauces, garlic and onions, e.g., by using separate bowls for potatoes, butter, salad and dressing.

2.6 Stress management

Stress can affect your stomach and worsen irritable bowel symptoms. Hence, it is important to reduce it. Developing a solution-orientated way to manage your own worries can help you do so. How does that help? The more you stress over something, the more brain areas that are required for a reasonable decision are being set off. This happens, because in a certain way, our bodies are prepared for an earlier historical era. Dangerous situations like being attacked by a wolf pack left us with three options: fight, flight or playing dead. If we spent too much time thinking in such a situation, it was game over!

Now, completely different factors cause us to worry. In addition to such everyday concerns like air pollution, extreme temperatures and noise, many people worry about losing control over a situation. If you start to worry, fight and flight reactions are supported by the release of hormones that enable us to make quick, even if ill-conceived, decisions. Large parts of our brain are set aside for that purpose. You feel stress and tend to rather make impulsive then rational decisions. The third option your brain conceives in a dangerous situation, playing dead, somewhat corresponds to the extreme modern-day phenomena that is widely known as burnout.

You don't want to overreact or give up on your responsibilities and play dead like a hyena, so you need to maintain control of your body and mind. Appropriate actions in everyday life depend on rational thinking; this may require preventive measures. Once your body feels like it's in danger it is difficult to abruptly halt the rolling wheel of your body's emergency reactions. Yoga and progressive muscle relaxation before work are useful stress preventers. Using such techniques before going to work is sensible as it is seldom possible to take an hour off during the work day. Breaks and disruptions during your working hours are also **counterproductive** if you are dealing with complex tasks; they often lead to poor decisions, more stress and a short temper. Thus, try to avoid disruption when dealing with sophisticated tasks. However, interruptions of simple mental or physical labor lasting a few minutes, rather than seconds, are shown to offer slight positive effects. Taking breaks from hard physical labor, meanwhile, show even stronger benefits, lowering the risk of injuries and enhancing endurance.[164]

---

[164] Lombardi et al., 2014; Speier, Vessey, & Valacich, 2003; Zohar, 1999; Coraggio, 1990.

Still, relaxation alone might not be the solution. Often, you can identify the source of your fears; when you are in the habit of regularly acknowledging the deeper causes of your stress, you will be able to deal with them and develop appropriate solutions that allow you to manage risks and arrive at your goals.

By doing so, you can even use your fears—through the process of conquering them—to help you become more successful in your everyday life. Sit down at a quiet desk at the beginning or end of the day. Next, think about what you are worried about right now and which steps you need to take to prevent the feared outcomes.

It is helpful to create an Excel spreadsheet for doing so or to purchase the standardized and printer-optimized PaceAce-Version at a reasonable price at www.Laxiba.co.uk. If you want to create the table by yourself, call the first sheet "Worries" and the second one "Task List." Next, write down the following task headings in the first spreadsheet: "Current Worries," "Preventive measure A," "Preventive measure B" and "Preventive measure C." Then enter the following column titles in the second spreadsheet: "Task," "Priority," "Deadline," "Who does it?" and "Done."

You should write down your concerns in the first column of the first sheet. Then, think about what you'll need to do to prevent these worries from being realized. Think of three alternatives for each outcome. Enter these into the "Preventive measure A–C" fields next to each worry, A being the action you want to take first. Then, transfer "Preventive measure A" to the "Task List" sheet. Next, prioritize the tasks by employing an adapted version of the "Eisenhower method," an organization technique that takes importance and urgency into account, from A to E:

Task is important	Action now	Better done soon
Task is unimportant	Chance for completion after everything important has been done.	Dull moment task
Efface (don't do) task	**Task is urgent**	**Task can be postponed**

In the order from A to D, you then execute your tasks on a daily basis. Hence, you prevent worrying and free yourself from doubting whether you are doing the right thing at the moment. After assessing the tasks from A to D, you fill out the column "Deadline", where you enter the date at which you want to accomplish the task. Furthermore, you either note "I" or the name of the person that you want to delegate the task to in the column "Who does it?". Finally, you tick off the cell in the column „Done", when you have finished the task.[165]

Another important aspect is keeping your life balanced. This means that instead of delivering an over-the-top performance in one area but lousy results in all others, you want to do at least a satisfying job in all areas, in order to remain capable in the long run. Which of the family, spare time, relaxation and work quadrants are important is up to you, along with the results you're aiming for with them, such as spending time with those closest to you, taking daily walks, pursuing your hobbies and getting your work done properly. Furthermore, it is important to resist basing your success on external measures. You should nourish a healthy self-confidence and serenity in yourself. This also means knowing when the task you are doing has been done well enough. Some people get into time trouble because they over-deliver on some tasks and then have little time left to take care of other important tasks, which then causes stress.

Family: Spend time with those closest to you	**Relaxation:** Go out for a walk on a daily basis
Spare time: Pursue your hobbies regularly	**Work:** Get your work done properly

You can measure your progress with regard to the four quadrants on a monthly basis on a scale of 1 (very good) to 7 (very poor).[166] Always assign 7 points to the area that you're happiest with and other numbers to the remaining qua-

[165] Huether, 2014.

[166] Eisenführ et al., 2010; Berekoven et al., 2007; Farquhar & Keller, 1989; Winterfeldt & Edwards, 1986.

drants in relation to that one. Afterward, consider whether you want to make any changes to how you're approaching these areas of your life and how you can make those changes. You can also use the spreadsheet you created to manage your worries.

One final point on the topic of stress: be mindful of your mood, and try to stay positive! What you need to do that depends on you. Sometimes simply deciding to be in a good mood can do more than most people realize. Everyone has a load of problems to carry, and it's easier to carry it if you commit yourself to a positive outlook.

Do things that excite you as often as possible. Plan your activities around what is most important to you in your life. What that means is obviously personal to you! It is your treasure, per se, so you have to dig it out yourself. Abraham Lincoln had this to say, to send you on your way: "That some achieve great success is proof to all that others can achieve it as well."[167]

---

[167] Bowden, 2011.

2.7 General summary

1. What you are dealing with

Do you have an intolerance and/or symptoms? Then your bowel is easily irritated by certain substances in food called "bricks." Problems develop when your body doesn't intercept such bricks before they can cause symptoms. With a brick in your belly, you are carrying a burden. It is often a chronic condition, but it does not cause cancer. In most cases, the symptoms can be reduced to an acceptable level if you follow an appropriate diet.

2. Are you a special case?

According to the World Gastroenterology Organisation (WGO), up to one billion people worldwide are affected by a dietary intolerance.[168] In a way, you are lucky, as you can use this book to help you to reduce your symptoms.

3. Good reasons to follow this diet

An intolerance accompanies you for a long time, maybe even for the rest of your life. If the diet works, it is far cheaper than medical treatment and can sometimes be even more effective. Many medicines also have side effects. By examining different bricks one by one, you can find the one(s) that your body cannot tolerate. The level test will help you learn how to eat as freely as possible while continuing to gain nutritional benefits. You learn, as well, how to balance your diet despite reducing the consumption of certain foods. If the diet works for you, it will also lead to a general improvement in your well-being. You should find that you are ill less often, better able to concentrate, better at fulfiling social obligations, stronger at sports—your new diet can even positively affect your sex drive! Start today with the first LAXIBA® step: get the ball rolling by tracking your symptoms for four days using the symptom test sheet (page 53).

---

[168] Quigley et al., 2009.

4. This is why you want to take the level test

Tolerance thresholds are different for everyone. The more bricks you are able to eat, the fewer restrictions you will face in your everyday diet. You might save yourself effort and be able to enjoy a more varied selection of food.

5. What you should pay attention to for the diet

Two things: First, keep your TLs by restricting your portion sizes accordingly. This means that you only eat as much of the bricks as your stomach can handle. If you do not consume any bricks, you will lose your ability to handle your interception shield well (see Chapter 1.5), and you will be back at square one. Second, eat in a balanced way by consuming fats, fibre and proteins each day (see Chapter 2.1.4).

6. The last trump of the vexed brick dragon

It is important that you really want the changes this book can help you achieve. Your first step is thus to understand that applying a working solution is going to help you lead a better life. If you recognize how the improvements in your diet relate to attaining your heartfelt ambitions, you will be more motivated to keep going, even if you face setbacks. This is a strategic plan, not an overnight miracle cure!

It may help you to set a time each Sunday to fill out the symptom test sheet—independent of the other tests. This will remind you of your goal and let you break down the necessary steps towards it on a weekly basis. What is also important is that you become aware of the hurdles you will face. It will be hard to restrict yourself with regard to the consumption of some foods that you have come to love. Especially at the beginning, it will be unnerving to ask for dietary considerations as a dinner guest. Your nutrition plan will be new to others; you may feel criticized for your insistence on maintaining your new eating habits. Explain that you need to do it for the sake of your health. At the same time, express your appreciation for others' support. Moreover, try not give dietary advice unless you are asked for it—respect the eating habits of others. This makes them more likely to accept yours.

The brick-eating dragons are betting on one last card: the influence of your old habits. They usually creep in after you have kept your new diet for a few days. It happens when you have started to feel better and become less alert to the dangers! Use your suggested weekly check as a countermeasure. It reminds you of your plan. Keep to it and it will help ensure your brick dragon cannot further agonize you. Take it easy. If you keep realigning your nutritional habits with your goals, you will get closer and closer to achieving them in the long run.

7. Are there hints for general nutrition?

Drink at least 1.5L of water every day. Eat a variety of foods. Even if you are lactose intolerant, you can try to eat dry cheese (for example) in order to cover your need for short-chain fatty acids. If you are a vegan, you should plan your protein intake, and consider your fiber consumption, if you are restricting your fructan and galactan intake. In addition to following your TL portion sizes and taking in linseeds or rice bran and a handful of nuts, you might also like to eat beans, lentils, peas and so forth: it is ok to eat foods that contain bricks; they can even be good for you, as long as you keep within your TL restrictions. To do even more for your health, work out regularly.

What can you do if a fruit juice contains too many bricks to drink a regular glass full? By diluting it with water you can multiply your tolerable portion.

How can you save on cooking time? Cook larger portion sizes. This only takes a little longer than smaller portions, and warming the food up is quick. Rice and potatoes, for instance, can be kept in the fridge for days. Purchase lockable glass containers to store your food keeping it fresh longer.

If you are suffering **acute symptoms**, take a walk and drink up to three liters of drinking water per day.

8. The LAXIBA® quickie

Fructans & Galactans: Eat fewer beans, lentils, peas and grain products, such as pastries and noodles.

Fructose (& Sorbitol): Avoid apple and peach juices and drink orange juice instead, for example. Be careful with soft drinks.

Lactose: Reduce your consumption of milk or use replacement products such as rice milk. Dry cheese like cheddar contains only a little lactose.

Sorbitol: Be wary of diabetic, diet and light products, as well as dried fruit.

3

FOOD TABLES

3.1 Introduction to the tables

In the following section, you will learn about the tolerable portion sizes according to your TL for lactose, fructose, and the sum of nine sugar alcohols, fructans and galactans. The statements all relate to **one meal**, a-ssuming **three meals** per day, consumed at roughly 7am, 1pm and 7pm, i.e., each with a **gap** of about **six hours**. (However, this is mainly just a reference point to align your consumption amounts with. You do not have to change your meal times!)

First, you find the lists are ordered by category. Juices are found under fast beverages, for example. Alternatively, you can use the alphabetical keyword index, e.g., if you are solely interested in finding the tolerable portion size of an orange juice. The sizes are shown next to the foods in the tables. In the **category tables,** the portions are based on the following TLs, which have been chosen according to the brick amounts for each level: **lactose: TL 1; fructose (with or without sorbitol adjustment): TL 0 (BTL); sorbitol: TL 0 and 1; fructans and galactans: TL 0 and TL1.** In the **alphabetical keyword index**, which begins after the **category tables**, only the sorbitol-adjusted fructose is shown at TL 0 and TL 1. In the first row of each table, you will find the multipliers to determine the portion size for the other three levels.

3.1.1 Your personal tolerance levels

Cross out all bricks that you are able to stomach without restrictions in the table below. The first column lists the bricks. The following columns list the TLs (the higher your TL, the less sensitive you are despite your intolerance towardss products that contain the respective brick) and the respective threshold amounts per meal. In the last two columns you should enter, in pencil, the TL that applies to you—before having done the level test this is the BTL, i.e., TL 0. The table is pretty much self-explanatory. In the field "combined TL" you should enter the TL you are able to stomach in combination with other bricks. In the field "single TL" you should enter the highest TL for the brick as you keep the BTLs of the remaining bricks.

Brick	TL	g	Combined TL	Single TL
Free fructose g/meal	0	0.5		
	1	1		
	2	2		
	3	3		
Free sorbitol adjusted fructose g/meal	0	0.5		
	1	1		
	2	2		
	3	3		
Lactose g/meal	0	1.5		
	1	3		
	2	6		
	3	9		
Sorbitol and other sugar alcohols g/meal	0	0		
	1	0.1		
	2	0.4		
	3	0.7		
Fructans and galactans g/meal	0	0.5		
	1	1		
	2	2		
	3	3		

3.1.2 Explanation of the abbreviations

Overview

Here you can see an excerpt of a category table. The pattern for it is: "How many bananas/burgers/etc. can I eat per meal if I have an intolerance toward fructose/lactose/sorbitol (i.e. sugar alcohols) and/or fructans and galactans?"

Food category name[a]	Unit[b]	Lactose[c] + Unit/[c]	Fructose*[d] Fructose[d]	Sorbitol[e] Sorbitol[e]	Fruc/Galacta.[f] Fruc/Galacta.[f]	
Baguette, wheat	slice(s) 1.49oz/42g	☺	☺ ☺	☺ ☺	×1¾ ×3½	A
Grasshopper (drink)	glass(es) 8.4oz.fl/240mL	×1¼[g] + ×1 unit[g]	☺+ ×1¼ unit[h] ☺+ ×1½ unit[h]	☹[i] ×¾	×7 ×14	
Red wine vinegar	tablespoon(s) 0.5oz.fl/14.8mL	☺	☺[j] ☺[j]	☹ ×20	☺ ☺	

Level 0[k]: lactose measure ×½

Level 1[k]: fructose measure ×2

Level 2[k]: fructose-/sorbitol measure ×4. the rest ×2

Level 3[k]: sorbitol measure ×7. the rest ×3

: source of fruc/galactans data

+ Unit/: added tolerated amount of unit per strong lactase capsule

Fructose*: fructose, sorbitol adjusted

☺+ ×[Amount] unit: Per unit consumed you can additionally tolerate up to [amount] × fructose(*)-unit of another product.

☹: avoid; ☹[1]: ¼ at TL 1; ☹[2]: ¼ at TL 2; ☹[3]: ¼ at TL 3; ☺: only contains traces; ☺: is free from it

Explanation

a	Category of the foods that are listed below.
b	The measurement unit that the measures in the ingredient columns relate to. Below you find the gram amount of that measurement unit. The measure is the number with which you have to multiply the measurement unit in order to determine the respective portion size that applies to you.
c	Lactose = Here you can find the tolerable lactose measures at TL (tolerance level) 1. Your TL for lactose refers to your sensitivity toward lactose if you are lactose intolerant. Apart from the basic tolerance level (BTL), TL 0, the TLs 1 to 3 may apply. The higher your TL, the less sensitive you are towardss products containing lactose, despite your intolerance, and the higher portion sizes you can tolerate of such products. + unit/: Additionally tolerated measure per strong lactase capsule you take (only applicable to the restrictionts from the lactose content).

d	Fructose* = Measure for free fructose with adjustment for the effect of sorbitol on the fructose absorption at TL 0. Fructose = Free fructose without adjustment for sorbitol at TL 0.
e	Sorbitol = Amounts if you have a sugar alcohol (sorbitol) intolerance above ( ) at TL 0 and below ( ) at TL 1.
f	Fruc/Galacta. = Tolerable amounts in case of a fructan and galactan malabsorbtion. Above ( ) at TL 0 and below ( ) at TL 1. If there is a letter in the column to the right, then it identifies the source for the shown amount. Otherwise, the amount is estimated based on the amount of lactose contained in the food and therefore refers to the minimum quantity of fructans and galactans contained in the food.
g	1¼ = 250mL of the drink is tolerated even for a lactose intolerance at TL 0, as the statement is related to a 200mL glass (1.25 × 200mL = 250mL). + 1 unit/ = For each lactase capsule taken, one further 200mL glass can be stomached, as this is the measurement unit here.
h	☺+ ×[number] unit = More glucose than fructose is contained in the food. Hence, you can tolerate the product in case of fructose intolerance. What is more, due to the "neutralizing" effect of glucose on fructose (see Chapter 1.5.2), per consumed unit you will tolerate up to [number] times the TL 0 fructose amount of another food. For example, for a "grasshopper," 1¼× the fructose measure of another food can be additionally tolerated if the other food is consumed simultaneously. For safety you should halve the amount.
i	☹ = Avoid the food when keeping TL 0 for sugar alcohols.
j	☺ = You can stomach over 90 times the stated measurement unit. ☺ = The food is free of the respective brick.
k	Multipliers to calculate the portions, if a tolerance level other than the one named in the column header applies to you. If you want to determine the measure of lactose for a "grasshopper" for tolerance level (TL) 0, multiply the 1¼ with ½, which is about ½. Hence, you can tolerate half a glass, i.e., 100mL.

Note: Please always consider the ingredients stated on packages, as well, as the composition may vary, especially for non-brand name products. You can find a guide to portion sizes and lactose content in fish and meat products at the end of Chapter 3.5.3 under the heading "Lactose hideouts."

Table columns

Unit	Measurement unit for foods.
Lactose +unit/	In the upper section you will find the amount of a **unit** that you can stomach if you have a lactose intolerance at TL 1. In the lower section you will find the amount you will be able to additionally consume per strong (~12.000 FCC[169]) lactase capsule you take: +[number] unit, i.e., additional portion per capsule (this refers only to a lactose restriction).
Fructose*	Amount per **unit** that is tolerated in a fructose intolerance at TL 0, where the amount of sorbitol in the food is considered. In the keyword table, you will also find the **fructose*** amounts that apply for **fructose*** at TL 1. Here you partially find the special labeling "☺+ ×[amount] unit," which means that the food contains more glucose than fructose. Thus, in the case of **simultaneous consumption** of one **unit** of the "☺+ ×[amount] unit" food, up to the stated [number] times the respective measure of a food that is restricted due to fructose can be additionally tolerated at TL 0. If for ice cream the **fructose*** cell states "☺+ ×3 unit," for example, then that means that you are now able to tolerate ¼ plus 3 × ¼, thus, up to a whole portion of **unit** of grapes, whose normally tolerable **fructose*** portion is limited to ¼ of **unit**, if you eat them simultaneously with the ice cream (simultaneously means that you chew both foods at the same time in your mouth). For safety, halve the stated "☺+ ×[number] unit" amount. If a higher TL applies to you, you have to **divide** the + [number] unit" amount by the respective multiplier indicated in Chapter 3.1.3, as at a higher TL the **portions** are commensurably **larger**. For example, assume that your TL for **fructose*** is TL 2 and you read in the TL 1 row for **fructose*** in the Keyword Index that "☺+ ×3¾ unit" applies to one apricot. The TL 2 multiplier of **fructose*** is 2. When you divide 3¾ by the multiplier 2, this is roughly 1¾. At TL 2 you can stomach one portion of grapes. If you eat an apricot at the same time, you can then stomach 1 portion plus 1¾ × 1, hence, 2¾ portions of grapes.

169 Food Chemical Codex, measurement unit for enzymes.

Fructose	Amount per **unit in case of** fructose intolerance without consideration of the contained sorbitol for TL 0. Here you will also find the special labeling "☺+ ×[number] unit" explained above. Important: Fructose is only shown in the category tables and there at the bottom.
Sorbit	Amount per **unit** for a sorbitol (i.e., sugar alcohol) intolerance, above at TL 0 and below at TL 1.
Fruc/ Galactans	Amount per **unit** for a fructans and galactans malabsorption, above at TL 0 and below at TL 1.
🕮	Source upon which **fructans and galactans** calculations were based. If the field is **empty**, the indications are estimates based on the amount of lactose and are thus **less reliable**.

More elaborate explanation

In the **unit** column, beside the food name, you will find the portion measurement unit that applies to that food. The list of measurement units can be found at the top of this page. Below each measurement unit, you will also find the rough weight of a **unit.** In the columns to the right of **unit** you can find out how many **unit**s you can tolerate per meal dependent on which intolerance applies to you:

In the **Lactose** column you can find the tolerated amount of **unit** for tolerance level (TL) 1 and, below, the additionally consumable amount **unit** for each strong lactase capsule you take.

The **Fructose*/Fructose** column shows you the tolerable amount in case you are fructose intolerant. At the top you will find the maximum portion size when the amount of sorbitol contained in the food is taken into consideration (**Fructose*** shows the tolerable amount of **unit** due to the contained fructose and sorbitol in the product). Here, the amount of sorbitol is added to the amount of free fructose, and the portion is determined with regard to the TL of free fructose (see Chapter 1.5.2). In the category tables, the stated **Fructose*** amounts refer to TL 0. In the keyword lists you will also find the **Fructose*** TL 1 amounts below. In the category tables, however, below the **Fructose*** TL 0 amounts you will find the TL 0 amounts for free fructose (**Fructose**) without taking sorbitol into account.

The **Sorbitol** column contains the amount of **unit** that holds if you have an intolerance toward sorbitol. The statement is based on the sum of nine sugar alcohols contained in the food, including sorbitol.

The **Fruc/Galactans** column shows the tolerable amount of **unit** that results from the sum of fructans and galactans. At the top, you will see the amount that applies to TL 0 and at the bottom the one for TL 1. The column "🕮" refers to the source on which the calculation of the amount of **unit** for **fructan and galactan malabsorption** is based on, if any.[170] If **no source** is **listed**, the estimate is based on the amount of **lactose**[171] a food contains. In that case, concrete study results regarding the amount of fructans and galactans are not available for the respective food; the listed amount is less certain.

---

[170] A stands for Biesiekierski et al., 2011; B for Muir et al., 2009; C for Muir et al., 2007, D for Shepherd and Gibson, 2006, E for van Loo et al., 1995 and F for Muir et al., 2007, Van Loo et al., 1995, and G for Monash University, 2014.

[171] Balasubramanya, Sarwar, & Narayanan, 1993; Jensen, Blanc, & Patton, 1995.

Amount symbols used:

☺	Free consumption: the smiley shows you foods that are completely free of the given brick, such as fructose or sorbitol.
☺	Over 90 times **unit** can be tolerated.
¼, ½, ¾, 1, 1¼, 1½, 1¾, 2, etc.	The tolerated amount of **unit**, e.g., "cookie/piece/½" means half a cookie of the respective type can be tolerated per meal, and "soup/portion/1¾" means one and three fourths of a **unit** of the soup.
☹	The tolerated amount is below ¼ of **unit** for TL 3, so it's best to avoid it.
☹^{1}	You can stomach ¼ of **unit** if TL 1 applies to you; otherwise ☹ applies. If TL 2 (or 3) applies to you, you can tolerate ½ (or ¾) of **unit**. ☹^{1} is only shown in the category tables and is there only for **Fructose** and **Fructose***.
☹^{2}	You can tolerate ¼ of **unit** if TL 2 applies to you; otherwise ☹ applies. If TL 3 applies to you, the tolerable amount of **unit** increases to ½ for sugar alcohols only.
☹^{3}	You can stomach ¼ of **unit** if TL 3 applies to you; otherwise ☹ applies.
+ [number] unit	By taking a high-dosed lactase capsule, you can additionally tolerate the amount of **unit** with regard to lactose independent of your TL. If for example you consider drinking milk, and **unit** is one cup, +¼ unit in the bottom of the lactose row means that per lactase capsule you tolerate one fourth of a cup of milk more.
☺+ × [number] unit	The product contains more glucose than free fructose. The **simultaneous** intake of a portion measurement unit (**unit**) of the respective food can enable you to eat up to [number] times the TL 0 amount that is shown for other fructose(*) containing foods. To be on the safe side, divide the [number] by two, as glucose is already partially absorbed by the mouth, and sometimes the food is not chewed completely. For example, for a Kellogg's® Corn Flakes 30g portion, "☺+ ×1½ unit" is shown. If you divide the statement by two, it means that instead of the nor-

mal amount of 1½ tbsp. of apple sauce you are now able to stomach the 1½ tbsp. + 1½ tbsp. × (1½ unit ÷2 [in case you halve the amount for safety]), and thus about 2½ tbsp. in total. If a higher TL applies to you, **divide** the [amount] by the respective level multiplier (Chapter 3.1.3), as for higher levels the portions are higher as well. In the keyword list you will also find the TL 1 amounts for **Fructose***.

If you are keeping the BTL (TL 0) for sorbitol, avoid all products without a ☺-smiley in the upper part of the **Sorbitol** column. Please consider the gram numbers indicated when using the tables. Common portion sizes may be smaller than you think, e.g., 30g for corn flakes.

3.1.3 Level multipliers

The multipliers are there to help you determine the tolerable amounts of each unit scale if your TL deviates from the underlying TL, i.e. the TL that the amounts in the table hold for. In the category tables the multipliers are based on TL 0 for fructose and on TL 1 for all other bricks. In the keyword tables, all multipliers are based on TL 1. The increments have been chosen primarily for their tolerability. For fructose you will also find the deviating multipliers for the keyword table in the right column.

Lactose (Lactose), underlying TL: 1

TL 0 =Amounts ÷ 2
TL 2 =Amounts × 2
TL 3 =Amounts × 3

Sorbitol-adjusted free fructose (Fructose*) as well as **free fructose without considering sorbitol (Fructose)**, underlying TL: 0

TL 1 =Amounts × 2
TL 2 =Amounts × 4
TL 3 =Amounts × 6

Sorbitol-adjusted fructose (Fructose*), underlying TL: 1

TL 2 =Amounts × 2
TL 3 =Amounts × 3

Sugar alcohols (Sorbitol), underlying TL: 1

TL 2 =Amounts × 4
TL 3 =Amounts × 7

Fructans and galactans (Fruc/Galactans), underlying TL: 1

TL 2 =Amounts × 2
TL 3 =Amounts × 3

TABLES BY CATEGORY

3.2 Athletes

Athletes	Unit	Lactose + unit/	Fructose* Fructose	Sorbitol Sorbitol	FrucGalactans FrucGalactans
Clif Bar®,Chocolate Chip	piece 2.4oz/68g	9 +7½ unit	☺+ ×10 unit ☺+ ×10 unit	☹ 2¼	¾ 1½
Clif Bar®,Crunchy Peanut Butter	piece 2.4oz/68g	☺	☺+ ×10¼ unit ☺+ ×10¼ unit	☹ 2½	☺ ☺
Clif Bar®,Oatmeal Raisin Walnut	piece 2.4oz/68g	☺	☺+ ×10¼ unit ☺+ ×10½ unit	☹ 1¾	1¾[AG] 3½
Electrolyte replacement drink	glass 8.4oz/240g	☺	☺+ ×9¾ unit ☺+ ×9¾ unit	☺ ☺	☺ ☺
Gatorade®, all flavors	glass 8.4oz/240g	7½ +6¼ unit	☺+ ×1¼ unit ☺+ ×1¼ unit	☺ ☺	41½ 83¼
Gatorade®, from dry mix, all flavors	glass 8.4oz/240g	☺	☺+ ×10½ unit ☺+ ×10½ unit	☺ ☺	☺ ☺
Glaceau® Vitaminwater 10	glass 8.4oz/240g	☺	☹[1] ☹[1]	☹ ☹[2]	☺ ☺
Glaceau® Vitaminwater Energy	glass 8.4oz/240g	☺	☹[2] ☹[2]	☺ ☺	☺ ☺
Glaceau® Vitaminwater Essential	glass 8.4oz/240g	☺	☹[2] ☹[2]	☺ ☺	☺ ☺
Glaceau® Vitaminwater Focus	glass 8.4oz/240g	☺	☹[2] ☹[2]	☺ ☺	☺ ☺
Glaceau® Vitaminwater Power-C	glass 8.4oz/240g	☺	☹[2] ☹[2]	☺ ☺	☺ ☺
Glaceau® Vitaminwater Revive	glass 8.4oz/240g	☺	☹[2] ☹[2]	☺ ☺	☺ ☺
High-protein bar, generic	piece 2.3oz/65g	39¼ +32¾ unit	¾ ¾	☹ 76¾	☺ ☺
Power Bar® 20g Protein Plus, Chocolate Crisp	piece 2.16oz/61g	3 +2½ unit	☹[1] ☹[1]	☹ ☹	17 34¼
Power Bar® 20g Protein Plus, Chocolate Peanut Butter	piece 2.16oz/61g	3 +2½ unit	☹[2] ☹[2]	☹ ☹	17 34¼
Power Bar® 30g Protein Plus, Chocolate Brownie	piece 2.47oz/70g	2 +1½ unit	☺+ ×1½ unit ☺+ ×1½ unit	☹ ☺	11 22¼
Power Bar® Harvest Energy®, Double Chocolate Crisp	piece 2.3oz/65g	2¾ +2¼ unit	☺+ ×5¾ unit ☺+ ×5¾ unit	☹ 10¾	¼[A] ½
Power Bar® Performance Energy®, Banana	piece 2.3oz/65g	☺	¼ ¼	☹ ☺	☺ ☺

Athletes	Unit	Lactose L1 + unit/💊	Fructose* L0 / Fructose L0	Sorbitol L0 / Sorbitol L1	FrucGalactans L0 / FrucGalactans L1 📖
Power Bar® Performance Energy®, Chocolate	piece 2.3oz/65g	☻	¼ ¼	☹ 76¾	☻ ☻
Power Bar® Performance Energy®, Cookie Dough	piece 2.3oz/65g	☻	¼ ¼	☹ ☺	☻ ☻
Power Bar® Performance Energy®, Mixed Berry Blast	piece 2.3oz/65g	☻	¼ ¼	☹ 19	☻ ☻
Power Bar® Performance Energy®, Vanilla Crisp	piece 2.3oz/65g	☻	¼ ¼	☹ ☺	☻ ☻
Powerade®, all flavors	glass 8.4oz/240g	7½ +6¼ unit	☻+ ×1¼ unit ☻+ ×1¼ unit	☻ ☻	41½ 83¼

L0 *Level 0:* lactose measure ×½

L1 *Level 1:* fructose measure ×2

L2 *Level 2:* fructose-/sorbitol measure ×4. the rest ×2

L3 *Level 3:* sorbitol measure ×7. the rest ×3

📖: source of fruc/galactans data

+ Unit/💊: added tolerated amount of unit per strong lactase capsule

Fructose*: fructose, sorbitol adjusted

☻+ ×[Amount] unit: Per unit consumed you can additionally tolerate up to [amount] × fructose(*)-unit of another product.

☹: avoid; ☹[1]: ¼ at TL 1; ☹[2]: ¼ at TL 2; ☹[3]: ¼ at TL 3; ☺: only contains traces; ☻: is free from it

3.3 Beverages

3.3.1 Alcoholic

Alcoholic	Unit	Lactose + unit/	Fructose* Fructose	Sorbitol Sorbitol	FrucGalactans FrucGalactans
Advocaat, regular	glass	¼	☺+ ×4¾ unit	☺	1½
	8.4oz.fl/240ml	+0.24 unit	☺+ ×4¾ unit	☺	3¼
Ale	glass	☺	50	☹	☺
	8.4oz.fl/240ml		☺	10	☺
Amaretto	glass	☺	☺+ ×4½ unit	☹	☺
	8.4oz.fl/240ml		☺+ ×5 unit	¼	☺
Applejack liquor	glass	☺	☺	☺	☺
	8.4oz.fl/240ml		☺	☺	☺
Aquavit	glass	☺	☺	☺	☺
	8.4oz.fl/240ml		☺	☺	☺
Beer	glass	☺	50	☹	☺
	8.4oz.fl/240ml		☺	10	☺
Beer, low alcohol	glass	☺	☺+ ×2¼ unit	☺	☺
	8.4oz.fl/240ml		☺+ ×2¼ unit	☺	☺
Black Russian	glass	☺	☺	☹	☺
	8.4oz.fl/240ml		☺	8¼	☺
Bloody Mary	glass	☺	1¾	☹	☺
	8.4oz.fl/240ml		1¾	½	☺
Bourbon	glass	☺	☺	☺	☺
	8.4oz.fl/240ml		☺	☺	☺
Brandy	glass	☺	☺	☺	☺
	8.4oz.fl/240ml		☺	☺	☺
Brandy, flavored	glass	☺	☺+ ×4½ unit	☹	☺
	8.4oz.fl/240ml		☺+ ×5 unit	¼	☺
Burgundy wine, red	glass	☺	17¾	☹	☺
	8.4oz.fl/240ml		☺	½	☺
Burgundy wine, white	glass	☺	31¼	☹	☺
	8.4oz.fl/240ml		☺	¾	☺
Campari®	glass	☺	☺+ ×4½ unit	☹	☺
	8.4oz.fl/240ml		☺+ ×5 unit	¼	☺
Cape Cod	glass	☺	☺+ ×5 unit	☹	☺
	8.4oz.fl/240ml		☺+ ×5 unit	25	☺
Champagne punch	glass	☺	¾	☹	☺
	8.4oz.fl/240ml		¾	1	☺

Alcoholic	Unit	Lactose [L1] + unit/[capsule]	Fructose* [L0] Fructose [L0]	Sorbitol [L0] Sorbitol [L1]	FrucGalactans [L0] FrucGalactans [L1] 📖
Champagne, white	glass 8.4oz.fl/240ml	😃	31¼ 😃	☹ ¾	😃 😃
Chardonnay	glass 8.4oz.fl/240ml	😃	31¼ 😃	☹ ¾	😃 😃
Club soda	glass 8.4oz.fl/240ml	😃	😃 😃	😃 😃	😃 😃
Cognac	glass 8.4oz.fl/240ml	😃	😃 😃	😃 😃	😃 😃
Cointreau®	glass 8.4oz.fl/240ml	😃	😃+ ×4½ unit 😃+ ×5 unit	☹ ¼	😃 😃
Creme de Cocoa	glass 8.4oz.fl/240ml	😃	☺ ☺	☹ 2½	😃 😃
Creme de menthe	glass 8.4oz.fl/240ml	😃	😃+ ×4½ unit 😃+ ×5 unit	☹ ¼	😃 😃
Curacao	glass 8.4oz.fl/240ml	😃	😃+ ×4½ unit 😃+ ×5 unit	☹ ¼	😃 😃
Daiquiri	glass 8.4oz.fl/240ml	😃	😃 😃	😃 😃	😃 😃
Fruit punch, alcoholic	glass 8.4oz.fl/240ml	😃	¾ ¾	☹ 1	😃 😃
Gibson	glass 8.4oz.fl/240ml	😃	😃 😃	☹ 3¼	😃 😃
Gin	glass 8.4oz.fl/240ml	😃	😃 😃	😃 😃	😃 😃
Grand Marnier®	glass 8.4oz.fl/240ml	😃	😃+ ×4½ unit 😃+ ×5 unit	☹ ¼	😃 😃
Grasshopper	glass 8.4oz.fl/240ml	1¼ +1 unit	😃+ ×1¼ unit 😃+ ×1½ unit	☹ ¾	7 14
Harvey Wallbanger	glass 8.4oz.fl/240ml	😃	16½ ☺	☹ ¼	😃 😃
Kamikaze	glass 8.4oz.fl/240ml	😃	😃+ ×1½ unit 😃+ ×1¾ unit	☹ 1	😃 😃
Kirsch	glass 8.4oz.fl/240ml	😃	😃+ ×4½ unit 😃+ ×5 unit	☹ ¼	😃 😃

[L0] *Level 0:* lactose measure ×½
[L1] *Level 1:* fructose measure ×2
[L2] *Level 2:* fructose-/sorbitol measure ×4. the rest ×2
[L3] *Level 3:* sorbitol measure ×7. the rest ×3
📖: source of fruc/galactans data

+ Unit/[capsule]: added tolerated amount of unit per strong lactase capsule
Fructose*: fructose, sorbitol adjusted

😃+ ×[Amount] unit: Per unit consumed you can additionally tolerate up to [amount] × fructose(*)-unit of another product.

☹: avoid; ☹¹: ¼ at TL 1; ☹²: ¼ at TL 2; ☹³: ¼ at TL 3; ☺: only contains traces; 😃: is free from it

Alcoholic	Unit	Lactose + unit/	Fructose* Fructose	Sorbitol Sorbitol	FrucGalactans FrucGalactans
Liqueur, coffee flavored	glass 8.4oz.fl/240ml	☺	☺ ☺	☹ 2½	☺ ☺
Long Island iced tea	glass 8.4oz.fl/240ml	☺	¾ ¾	☹ 16½	☺ ☺
Mai Tai	glass 8.4oz.fl/240ml	☺	☺+ ×½ unit ☺+ ×½ unit	☹ 1¾	☺ ☺
Malt liquor	glass 8.4oz.fl/240ml	☺	50 ☺	☹ 10	☺ ☺
Manhattan	glass 8.4oz.fl/240ml	☺	½ ½	☹ 2	☺ ☺
Margarita, frozen	glass 8.4oz.fl/240ml	☺	☺+ ×¼ unit ☺+ ×¼ unit	☹ 7	☺ ☺
Martini®	glass 8.4oz.fl/240ml	☺	83¼ ☺	☹ 3¼	☺ ☺
Merlot, red	glass 8.4oz.fl/240ml	☺	17¾ ☺	☹ ½	☺ ☺
Merlot, white	glass 8.4oz.fl/240ml	☺	¾ ¾	☺ ☺	☺ ☺
Mint Julep	glass 8.4oz.fl/240ml	☺	☺ ☺	☺ ☺	☺ ☺
Mojito	glass 8.4oz.fl/240ml	☺	☺ ☺	☺ ☺	☺ ☺
Muscatel	glass 8.4oz.fl/240ml	☺	☹[2] ☹[2]	☹ ½	☺ ☺
Non-alcoholic wine	glass 8.4oz.fl/240ml	☺	2¼ 2¼	☹ 50	☺ ☺
Ouzo	glass 8.4oz.fl/240ml	☺	☺+ ×4½ unit ☺+ ×5 unit	☹ ¼	☺ ☺
Pina colada	glass 8.4oz.fl/240ml	☺	☺+ ×1¼ unit ☺+ ×1¼ unit	☹ 4	☺ ☺
Port wine	glass 8.4oz.fl/240ml	☺	☹[2] ☹[2]	☹ ½	☺ ☺
Riesling	glass 8.4oz.fl/240ml	☺	31¼ ☺	☹ ¾	☺ ☺
Rob Roy	glass 8.4oz.fl/240ml	☺	¼ ¼	☹ 2½	☺ ☺
Rompope (eggnog with alcohol)	glass 8.4oz.fl/240ml	¼ +¼ unit	☺ ☺	☺ ☺	2¾ 5½
Root beer	glass 8.4oz.fl/240ml	☺	½ ½	☺ ☺	☺ ☺

Alcoholic	Unit	Lactose (Level 1) + unit/capsule	Fructose* (Level 0) Fructose (Level 0)	Sorbitol (Level 0) Sorbitol (Level 1)	FrucGalactans (Level 0) FrucGalactans (Level 1) 📖
Rose wine, other types	glass	☺	¾	☺	☺
	8.4oz.fl/240ml		¾	☺	☺
Rum	glass	☺	☺	☺	☺
	8.4oz.fl/240ml		☺	☺	☺
Rum and cola	glass	☺	1	☺	☺
	8.4oz.fl/240ml		1	☺	☺
Rusty nail	glass	☺	☺+ ×1¾ unit	☹	☺
	8.4oz.fl/240ml		☺+ ×2 unit	¾	☺
Sake	glass	☺	☹[2]	☹	☺
	8.4oz.fl/240ml		☹[2]	½	☺
Sambuca	glass	☺	☺+ ×4½ unit	☹	☺
	8.4oz.fl/240ml		☺+ ×5 unit	¼	☺
Sangria	glass	☺	7¾	☹	☺
	8.4oz.fl/240ml		11¼	¾	☺
Schnapps, all flavors	glass	☺	☺+ ×2¼ unit	☹	☺
	8.4oz.fl/240ml		☺+ ×2½ unit	½	☺
Scotch and soda	glass	☺	☺	☺	☺
	8.4oz.fl/240ml		☺	☺	☺
Screwdriver	glass	☺	2	☹	☺
	8.4oz.fl/240ml		2	¼	☺
Seabreeze	glass	☺	☺+ ×5¼ unit	☹	☺
	8.4oz.fl/240ml		☺+ ×5¼ unit	2½	☺
Singapore sling	glass	☺	☺+ ×¼ unit	☹	☺
	8.4oz.fl/240ml		☺+ ×¼ unit	4½	☺
Sloe gin	glass	☺	☺+ ×4½ unit	☹	☺
	8.4oz.fl/240ml		☺+ ×5 unit	¼	☺
Sloe gin fizz	glass	☺	☺+ ×¾ unit	☹	☺
	8.4oz.fl/240ml		☺+ ×¾ unit	1½	☺
Southern Comfort®	glass	☺	☺	☺	☺
	8.4oz.fl/240ml		☺	☺	☺
Sylvaner	glass	☺	31¼	☹	☺
	8.4oz.fl/240ml		☺	¾	☺
Tequila	glass	☺	☺	☺	☺
	8.4oz.fl/240ml		☺	☺	☺

Level 0: lactose measure ×½
Level 1: fructose measure ×2
+ Unit/capsule: added tolerated amount of unit per strong lactase capsule
Fructose*: fructose, sorbitol adjusted

Level 2: fructose-/sorbitol measure ×4. the rest ×2
Level 3: sorbitol measure ×7. the rest ×3
📖: source of fruc/galactans data

☺+ ×[Amount] unit: Per unit consumed you can additionally tolerate up to [amount] × fructose(*)-unit of another product.

☹: avoid; ☹[1]: ¼ at TL 1; ☹[2]: ¼ at TL 2; ☹[3]: ¼ at TL 3; ☺: only contains traces; ☺: is free from it

Alcoholic	Unit	Lactose + unit/	Fructose* Fructose	Sorbitol Sorbitol	FrucGalactans FrucGalactans
Tokaji Wine	glass	☺	☹[2]	☹	☺
	8.4oz.fl/240ml		☹[2]	½	☺
Tom Collins	glass	☺	31¼	☹	☺
	8.4oz.fl/240ml		31¼	16½	☺
Triple Sec	glass	☺	☺+ ×4½ unit	☹	☺
	8.4oz.fl/240ml		☺+ ×5 unit	¼	☺
Vodka	glass	☺	☺	☺	☺
	8.4oz.fl/240ml		☺	☺	☺
Whiskey	glass	☺	☺	☺	☺
	8.4oz.fl/240ml		☺	☺	☺
Whiskey sour	glass	☺	9½	☹	☺
	8.4oz.fl/240ml		9½	6¼	☺
White Russian	glass	1½	☺	☹	9
	8.4oz.fl/240ml	+1¼ unit	☺	8¼	18¼
Wine spritzer	glass	☺	27¾	☹	☺
	8.4oz.fl/240ml		☺	1	☺

3.3.2 Hot beverages

Hot beverages	Unit	Lactose 1 + unit/capsule	Fructose* 0 Fructose 0	Sorbitol 0 Sorbitol 1	FrucGalactans 0 FrucGalactans 1 📖
Americano, decaf, without flavored syrup	cup 5.2oz.fl/150ml	☺	☺ ☺	☺ ☺	☺ ☺
Americano, with flavored syrup	cup 5.2oz.fl/150ml	☺	☺ ☺	☺ ☺	☺ ☺
Americano, without flavored syrup	cup 5.2oz.fl/150ml	☺	☺ ☺	☺ ☺	☺ ☺
Brown sugar	tbsp. 0.5oz/14.21ml	☺	☺ ☺	☺ ☺	☺ ☺
Cafe au lait, without flavored syrup	cup 5.2oz.fl/150ml	1 +¾ unit	☺ ☺	☺ ☺	6½ 13
Cafe latte, with flavored syrup	cup 5.2oz.fl/150ml	½ +¼ unit	☺ ☺	☺ ☺	3 6
Cafe latte, without flavored syrup	cup 5.2oz.fl/150ml	¼ +¼ unit	☺ ☺	☺ ☺	2¾ 5½
Camomile tea	glass 8.5oz.fl/242ml	☺	☺ ☺	☺ ☺	☺ G ☺
Cappuccino, bottled or canned	cup 5.2oz.fl/150ml	½ +½ unit	☺ ☺	☺ ☺	4 8
Cappuccino, decaf, with flavored syrup	cup 5.2oz.fl/150ml	½ +¼ unit	☺ ☺	☺ ☺	3 6¼
Cappuccino, decaf, without flavored syrup	cup 5.2oz.fl/150ml	½ +¼ unit	☺ ☺	☺ ☺	2¾ 5¾
Chicory coffee	cup 5.2oz.fl/150ml	☺	☺ ☺	☹ 11	☹ E ☹
Coffee substitute, prepared	cup 5.2oz.fl/150ml	☺	☺ ☺	☺ ☺	☺ ☺
Coffee, prepared from flavored mix, sugar free	cup 5.2oz.fl/150ml	☺	☺ ☺	☹ 66½	☺ ☺
Demitasse	cup 5.2oz.fl/150ml	☺	☺ ☺	☺ ☺	☺ ☺

0 *Level 0:* lactose measure ×½ — + Unit/capsule: added tolerated amount of unit per strong lactase capsule
1 *Level 1:* fructose measure ×2 — Fructose*: fructose, sorbitol adjusted
2 *Level 2:* fructose-/sorbitol measure ×4. the rest ×2
3 *Level 3:* sorbitol measure ×7. the rest ×3
📖: source of fruc/galactans data
☺+ ×[Amount] unit: Per unit consumed you can additionally tolerate up to [amount] × fructose(*)-unit of another product.
☹: avoid; ☹[1]: ¼ at TL 1; ☹[2]: ¼ at TL 2; ☹[3]: ¼ at TL 3; ☺: only contains traces; ☺: is free from it

Hot beverages	Unit	Lactose + unit/	Fructose* Fructose	Sorbitol Sorbitol	FrucGalactans FrucGalactans
Dove® Promises, Milk Chocolate	cup 5.2oz.fl/150ml	¼ +0.21 unit	☺ ☺	☹ ☺	1¾ 3¾
Earl Grey, strong	glass 8.4oz.fl/240ml	☺	½ ½	☺ ☺	☺G ☺
Espresso, without flavored syrup	cup 5.2oz.fl/150ml	☺	☺ ☺	☺ ☺	☺ ☺
Evaporated milk, diluted, skim (fat free)	cup 5.2oz.fl/150ml	¼ +¼ unit	☺ ☺	☺ ☺	1¾ 3¾
Fennel tea	glass 8.6oz.fl/247ml	☺	☺ ☺	☺ ☺	☺G ☺
Frappuccino®	cup 5.2oz.fl/150ml	½ +½ unit	☺ ☺	☺ ☺	3¾ 7½
Frappuccino®, bottled or canned	cup 5.2oz.fl/150ml	½ +½ unit	☺ ☺	☺ ☺	3½ 7
Frappuccino®, bottled or canned, light	cup 5.2oz.fl/150ml	½ +½ unit	☺ ☺	☺ ☺	4 8
Green tea, strong	glass 8.7oz.fl/248ml	☺	☺ ☺	☺ ☺	☺ ☺
Herbal tea	glass 8.6oz.fl/246ml	☺	☺ ☺	☺ ☺	☺G ☺
Hershey's® Bliss Hot Drink White Chocolate, prepared	cup 5.2oz.fl/150ml	¼ +¼ unit	☺+ ×½ unit ☺+ ×½ unit	☺ ☺	1¾ 3¾
Hot chocolate, homemade	cup 5.2oz.fl/150ml	¼ +¼ unit	27¾ 27¾	☹ 66½	1¾ 3¾
Instant coffee mix, unprepared	cup 5.2oz.fl/150ml	☺	8¼ 8¼	☹ ☹[2]	☺ ☺
Irish coffee with alcohol and whipped cream	cup 5.2oz.fl/150ml	3¾ +3 unit	☺ ☺	☺ ☺	21 42
Jasmine tea	glass 8.4oz.fl/241ml	☺	☺ ☺	☺ ☺	☺G ☺
Light cream	portion 0.53oz.fl/15ml	5¼ +4½ unit	☺ ☺	☺ ☺	30¼ 60½
Milk, lactose reduced (Lactaid®), skim (fat free)	cup 5.2oz.fl/150ml	☺	☺+ ×7½ unit ☺+ ×7½ unit	☺ ☺	☺ ☺
Milk, lactose reduced (Lactaid®), whole	cup 5.2oz.fl/150ml	☺	☺+ ×7½ unit ☺+ ×7½ unit	☺ ☺	☺ ☺
Milk, unprepared dry powder, nonfat, instant	portion 0.78oz.fl/22ml	¼ +0.21 unit	☺ ☺	☺ ☺	1¼ 2¾
Mocha, without flavored syrup	cup 5.2oz.fl/150ml	½ +¼ unit	☺+ ×1¾ unit ☺+ ×1¾ unit	☺ ☺	3 6

Hot beverages	Unit	Lactose 1 + unit/capsule	Fructose* 0 Fructose 0	Sorbitol 0 Sorbitol 1	FrucGalactans 0 FrucGalactans 1 📖
Nestle® Hot Cocoa Dark Chocolate, prepared	cup 5.2oz.fl/150ml	¼ +¼ unit	☻+ ×½ unit ☻+ ×½ unit	☹ ☺	23½ 47¼
Nestle® Hot Cocoa Rich Milk Chocolate, prepared	cup 5.2oz.fl/150ml	¼ +¼ unit	☻ ☻	☻ ☻	22¾ 45¾
Nestle® Nesquik®, chocolate flavors	glass 8.4oz/240g	¼ +¼ unit	1½ 1½	☹ 5½	☻ ☻
Soy milk, chocolate, sweetened with sugar, not fortified, ready-to-drink	cup 5.2oz.fl/150ml	☻	☻ ☻	☹ 4¼	¼[A] ½
Splenda®	portion 0oz.fl/0ml	☻	☻ ☻	☻ ☻	☻ ☻
Starbucks® Hot Cocoa Double Chocolate, prepared	cup 5.2oz.fl/150ml	¼ +¼ unit	37 37	☹ 66½	2¼ 4¾
Starbucks® Hot Cocoa Salted Caramel, prepared	cup 5.2oz.fl/150ml	¼ +¼ unit	33¼ 33¼	☹ 66½	2 4¼
Sugar, white granulated	tbsp. 0.5oz/14.21ml	☻	☻ ☻	☻ ☻	☻ ☻
Sweetened condensed milk	portion 1.35oz.fl/38ml	½ +½ unit	☻ ☻	☻ ☻	3¾ 7½
Sweetened condensed milk, reduced fat	portion 1.38oz.fl/39ml	½ +½ unit	☻ ☻	☻ ☻	3½ 7¼
Whipped cream, aerosol	portion 0.25oz.fl/7ml	☺	☻ ☻	☻ ☻	☺ ☺
Whipped cream, aerosol, fat free	portion 0.18oz.fl/5ml	18¾ +15¾ unit	☻+ ×¼ unit ☻+ ×¼ unit	☻ ☻	☺ ☺
Zsweet®	portion 0.18oz.fl/5ml	☻	☻ ☻	☹ ☹	☻ ☻

0 *Level 0:* lactose measure ×½
1 *Level 1:* fructose measure ×2
2 *Level 2*: fructose-/sorbitol measure ×4. the rest ×2
3 *Level 3:* sorbitol measure ×7. the rest ×3
📖: source of fruc/galactans data

+ Unit/capsule: added tolerated amount of unit per strong lactase capsule
Fructose*: fructose, sorbitol adjusted

☻+ ×[Amount] unit: Per unit consumed you can additionally tolerate up to [amount] × fructose(*)-unit of another product.

☹: avoid; ☹[1]: ¼ at TL 1; ☹[2]: ¼ at TL 2; ☹[3]: ¼ at TL 3; ☺: only contains traces; ☻: is free from it

3.3.3 Juices

Juices	Unit	Lactose + unit/	Fructose* Fructose	Sorbitol Sorbitol	FrucGalactans FrucGalactans
Apple banana strawberry juice	glass 8.4oz.fl/240ml	☺	☹[1] ☹[1]	☹ ☹[2]	¾[FB] 1¾
Apple grape juice	glass 8.4oz.fl/240ml	☺	☹[2] ☹[2]	☹ ☹[2]	1½[CB] 3
Apricot nectar	glass 8.4oz.fl/240ml	☺	☺+ ×4¾ unit ☺+ ×5 unit	☹ ¼	☺ ☺
Arby's® orange juice	glass 8.4oz.fl/240ml	☺	1½ 1½	☹ ¼	☺[B] ☺
Black cherry juice	glass 8.4oz.fl/240ml	☺	¼ ¼	☹ 2½	☺ ☺
Black currant juice	glass 8.4oz.fl/240ml	☺	☺+ ×1½ unit ☺+ ×1½ unit	☹ 1½	☺ ☺
Blackberry juice	glass 8.4oz.fl/240ml	☺	¼ ¼	☺ ☺	☺ ☺
Capri Sun®, all flavors	glass 8.4oz.fl/240ml	☺	☺+ ×1 unit ☺+ ×1 unit	☹ 2	☺ ☺
Carrot juice	glass 8.4oz.fl/240ml	☺	☺+ ×1 unit ☺+ ×1 unit	☹ 4	☺[B] ☺
Cranberry juice cocktail, with apple juice	glass 8.4oz.fl/240ml	☺	☹[1] ☹[1]	☹ ☹[2]	1½[CB] 3
Cranberry juice cocktail, with blueberry juice	glass 8.4oz.fl/240ml	☺	☹[1] ☹[1]	☹ ☹[2]	☺ ☺
Fruit drink or punch, ready to drink	glass 8.4oz.fl/240ml	☺	☺+ ×1 unit ☺+ ×1 unit	☹ 2	1½[C] 3
Grapefruit juice, unsweetened, white	glass 8.4oz.fl/240ml	☺	☺+ ×5 unit ☺+ ×5 unit	☹ ¼	1[CB] 2
Kern's® Mango-Orange Nectar	glass 8.4oz.fl/240ml	☺	☹[1] ☹[1]	☹ 2	3[B] 6¼
Kern's® Strawberry Nectar	glass 8.4oz.fl/240ml	☺	☹[1] ☹[1]	☹ ¾	☺[C] ☺
Lemon juice, fresh	glass 8.4oz.fl/240ml	☺	2¼ 2¼	☹ 1½	2¼[B] 4½
Libby's® Apricot Nectar	glass 8.4oz.fl/240ml	☺	☹[1] ☹[1]	☹ ¼	☺ ☺
Libby's® Banana Nectar	glass 8.4oz.fl/240ml	☺	☹[1] ☹[1]	☹ 25	½[FB] 1

Juices	Unit	Lactose L1 + unit/capsule	Fructose* L0 Fructose L0	Sorbitol L0 Sorbitol L1	FrucGalactans L0 FrucGalactans L1 📖
Libby's® Juicy Juice®, Apple Grape	glass 8.4oz.fl/240ml	☺	☹^{1} ☹^{1}	☹ ¼	1½^{CB} 3
Libby's® Juicy Juice®, Grape	glass 8.4oz.fl/240ml	☺	☹^{1} ☹^{1}	☹ ¼	1½^{CB} 3
Libby's® Pear Nectar	glass 8.4oz.fl/240ml	☺	☹^{2} ☹^{2}	☹ ☹^{2}	☺^{B} ☺
Lime juice, fresh	glass 8.4oz.fl/240ml	☺	☺+ ×¾ unit ☺+ ×¾ unit	☺ ☺	2¼^B 4½
Mango nectar	glass 8.4oz.fl/240ml	☺	1 1	☹ 1¼	☺^{B} ☺
Northland® Cranberry Juice, all flavors	glass 8.4oz.fl/240ml	☺	☺+ ×7¼ unit ☺+ ×7¼ unit	☹ 25	☺ ☺
Orange kiwi passion juice	glass 8.4oz.fl/240ml	☺	☺ ☺	☹ ¾	☺^{B} ☺
Passion fruit juice	glass 8.4oz.fl/240ml	☺	☺+ ×3¾ unit ☺+ ×3¾ unit	☺ ☺	☺ ☺
Peach juice	glass 8.4oz.fl/240ml	☺	¾ ¾	☹ ¾	½^B 1¼
Pear juice	glass 8.4oz.fl/240ml	☺	☹^{2} ☹^{2}	☹ ☹^{3}	1½^C 3
Pineapple juice	glass 8.4oz.fl/240ml	☺	☺+ ×3¼ unit ☺+ ×3¼ unit	☹ 1¾	1½^{CB} 3
Pineapple orange drink	glass 8.4oz.fl/240ml	☺	¾ ¾	☺ ☺	1½^{CB} 3
Pomegranate juice	glass 8.4oz.fl/240ml	☺	¾ 2¾	☹ ☹^{2}	☺ ☺
Raspberry juice	glass 8.4oz.fl/240ml	☺	☹^{2} ☹^{2}	☹ ☹^{2}	¾^B 1½
Tomato juice	glass 8.4oz.fl/240ml	☺	1¼ 1¼	☹ ¼	2¾^B 5½
V-8® 100% A-C-E Vitamin Rich Vegetable Juice	glass 8.4oz.fl/240ml	☺	¼ ¼	☹ 3	2¾^B 5½
Veryfine Cranberry Raspberry	glass 8.4oz.fl/240ml	☺	☹^{1} ☹^{1}	☹ ☹^{2}	¾^B 1½

L0 *Level 0:* lactose measure ×½
L1 *Level 1:* fructose measure ×2
+ Unit/capsule: added tolerated amount of unit per strong lactase capsule
Fructose*: fructose, sorbitol adjusted

L2 *Level 2:* fructose-/sorbitol measure ×4. the rest ×2
L3 *Level 3:* sorbitol measure ×7. the rest ×3
📖: source of fruc/galactans data
☺+ ×[Amount] unit: Per unit consumed you can additionally tolerate up to [amount] × fructose(*)-unit of another product.

☹: avoid; ☹^{1}: ¼ at TL 1; ☹^{2}: ¼ at TL 2; ☹^{3}: ¼ at TL 3; ☺: only contains traces; ☺: is free from it

3.3.4 Other beverages

Other beverages	Unit	Lactose + unit/	Fructose* Fructose	Sorbitol Sorbitol	FrucGalactans FrucGalactans
7 UP®	glass 8.4oz.fl/240ml	☺	☹[2] ☹[2]	☺ ☺	☺ ☺
Cherry Coke®	glass 8.4oz.fl/240ml	☺	½ ½	☺ ☺	☺ ☺
Coke Zero®	glass 8.4oz.fl/240ml	☺	☺ ☺	☺ ☺	☺ ☺
Coke®	glass 8.4oz.fl/240ml	☺	½ ½	☺ ☺	☺ ☺
Coke® with Lime	glass 8.4oz.fl/240ml	☺	½ ½	☺ ☺	☺ ☺
Diet 7 UP®	glass 8.4oz.fl/240ml	☺	☺ ☺	☺ ☺	☺ ☺
Diet Coke®	glass 8.4oz.fl/240ml	☺	☺ ☺	☺ ☺	☺ ☺
Diet Dr. Pepper®	glass 8.4oz.fl/240ml	☺	☺ ☺	☺ ☺	☺ ☺
Diet Pepsi®, fountain	glass 8.4oz.fl/240ml	☺	☺ ☺	☺ ☺	☺ ☺
Fanta Zero®, fruit flavors	glass 8.4oz.fl/240ml	☺	☺ ☺	☺ ☺	☺ ☺
Fanta® Red	glass 8.4oz.fl/240ml	☺	☹[1] ☹[1]	☺ ☺	☺ ☺
Fanta®, fruit flavors	glass 8.4oz.fl/240ml	☺	8¼ 8¼	☺ ☺	☺ ☺
Ginger ale	glass 8.4oz.fl/240ml	☺	☹[2] ☹[2]	☺ ☺	☺ ☺
Lipton® Iced Tea Mix, sweetened with sugar, prepared	glass 8.4oz.fl/240ml	☺	☺ ☺	☺ ☺	☺ ☺
Lipton® Instant 100% Tea, unsweetened, prepared	glass 8.4oz.fl/240ml	☺	☺ ☺	☺ ☺	☺ ☺
Mineral Water	glass 8.4oz.fl/240ml	☺	☺ ☺	☺ ☺	☺ ☺
Monster® Energy®	glass 8.4oz.fl/240ml	☺	☺+ ×17½ unit ☺+ ×17½ unit	☺ ☺	☺ ☺
Monster® Khaos	portion 8.47oz.fl/240ml	☺	☺+ ×9 unit ☺+ ×9½ unit	☹ ¼	☺ ☺

Other beverages	Unit	Lactose + unit/	Fructose* Fructose	Sorbitol Sorbitol	FrucGalactans FrucGalactans
Mountain Dew®	glass 8.4oz.fl/240ml	☺	☹[1] ☹[1]	☺ ☺	☺ ☺
Mountain Dew® Code Red	glass 8.4oz.fl/240ml	☺	☹[1] ☹[1]	☺ ☺	☺ ☺
Nestea® 100% Tea, unsweetened, dry	glass 8.4oz.fl/240ml	☺	☺+ ×22 unit ☺+ ×22 unit	☺ ☺	☺ ☺
Nestea® Iced Tea, Sugar Free, dry	glass 8.4oz.fl/240ml	☺	☺+ ×11½ unit ☺+ ×11½ unit	☺ ☺	☺ ☺
Nestea® Iced Tea, Sugar Free, prepared	glass 8.4oz.fl/240ml	☺	☺ ☺	☺ ☺	☺ ☺
Nestea® Iced Tea, sweetened with sugar, dry	glass 8.4oz.fl/240ml	☺	☺ ☺	☺ ☺	☺ ☺
No Fear®	glass 8.4oz.fl/240ml	☺	☺+ ×6¼ unit ☺+ ×6¼ unit	☹ 50	☺ ☺
No Fear® Sugar Free	glass 8.4oz.fl/240ml	☺	☺ ☺	☺ ☺	☺ ☺
Pepsi®	glass 8.4oz.fl/240ml	☺	½ ½	☺ ☺	☺ ☺
Pepsi® Max	glass 8.4oz.fl/240ml	☺	☺ ☺	☺ ☺	☺ ☺
Pepsi® Twist	glass 8.4oz.fl/240ml	☺	½ ½	☺ ☺	☺ ☺
Red Bull® Energy Drink	glass 8.4oz.fl/240ml	☺	☺+ ×7¾ unit ☺+ ×7¾ unit	☺ ☺	☺ ☺
Red Bull® Energy Drink Sugar Free	glass 8.4oz.fl/240ml	☺	☺ ☺	☺ ☺	☺ ☺
Rockstar Original®	glass 8.4oz.fl/240ml	☺	☺+ ×23¾ unit ☺+ ×23¾ unit	☹ 5	☺ ☺
Rockstar Original® Sugar Free	glass 8.4oz.fl/240ml	☺	☺ ☺	☹ 5	☺ ☺
Schweppes® Bitter Lemon	glass 8.4oz.fl/240ml	☺	☹[2] ☹[2]	☺ ☺	☺ ☺
Spearmint tea	glass 8.4oz.fl/240ml	☺	☺ ☺	☺ ☺	☺ ☺

Level 0: lactose measure ×½
Level 1: fructose measure ×2
+ Unit/ : added tolerated amount of unit per strong lactase capsule
Fructose*: fructose, sorbitol adjusted

Level 2: fructose-/sorbitol measure ×4. the rest ×2
Level 3: sorbitol measure ×7. the rest ×3
: source of fruc/galactans data

☺+ ×[Amount] unit: Per unit consumed you can additionally tolerate up to [amount] × fructose(*)-unit of another product.

☹: avoid; ☹[1]: ¼ at TL 1; ☹[2]: ¼ at TL 2; ☹[3]: ¼ at TL 3; ☺: only contains traces; ☺: is free from it

Other beverages	Unit	Lactose + unit/	Fructose* Fructose	Sorbitol Sorbitol	FrucGalactans FrucGalactans
Sprite®	glass	☺	☹[2]	☺	☺
	8.4oz.fl/240ml		☹[2]	☺	☺
Sprite® Zero	glass	☺	☺	☺	☺
	8.4oz.fl/240ml		☺	☺	☺
Tap water	glass	☺	☺	☺	☺
	8.4oz.fl/240ml		☺	☺	☺
Tonic water	glass	☺	☹[2]	☺	☺
	8.4oz.fl/240ml		☹[2]	☺	☺
Tonic water, diet	glass	☺	☺	☺	☺
	8.4oz.fl/240ml		☺	☺	☺
Vanilla Coke®	glass	☺	½	☺	☺
	8.4oz.fl/240ml		½	☺	☺
Yerba® Mate tea	glass	☺	☺	☺	☺
	8.4oz.fl/240ml		☺	☺	☺

3.4 Cold dishes

3.4.1 Bread

Bread	Unit	Lactose L1 + unit/(capsule)	Fructose* L0 Fructose L0	Sorbitol L0 Sorbitol L1	FrucGalactans L0 FrucGalactans L1 (book)
Baguette	slice 1.49oz/42g	☻	☻ ☻	☻ ☻	1¾ A 3½
Cracked wheat bread, with raisins	slice 1.49oz/42g	☻	1¼ 1½	☹ 4¼	1¾ A 3½
English muffin bread	slice 1.49oz/42g	☻	38¼ 38¼	☻ ☻	1¾ A 3½
Focaccia bread	slice 1.49oz/42g	☻	☻ ☻	☻ ☻	1¼ A 2½
French or Vienna roll	slice 1.49oz/42g	☻	☻ ☻	☻ ☻	1¼ A 2½
GG® Scandinavian Bran Crispbread (Health Valley®)	slice 1.49oz/42g	☻	☺ ☺	☻ ☻	¼ A ½
Gluten free bread	slice 1.49oz/42g	☻	☻ ☻	☻ ☻	3½ A 7
Newman's Own® Organic Pretzels, Spelt	slice 1.49oz/42g	☻	☻+ ×½ unit ☻+ ×½ unit	☻ ☻	¾ A 1½
Potato bread	slice 1.2oz/34g	6¼ +5¼ unit	☻ ☻	☹ ☺	1½ A 3
Pumpernickel roll	slice 1.49oz/42g	☻	☻ ☻	☻ ☻	½ A 1¼
Rice bread	slice 1.49oz/42g	☻	☻ ☻	☻ ☻	☻ A ☻
Rye bread	slice 1.49oz/42g	☻	☻ ☻	☻ ☻	¾ A 1¾
Rye roll	slice 1.49oz/42g	☻	☻ ☻	☻ ☻	¾ A 1¾
Sourdough bread	slice 1.49oz/42g	☻	☻ ☻	☻ ☻	¾ A 1½

L0 *Level 0*: lactose measure ×½
L1 *Level 1*: fructose measure ×2
+ Unit/(capsule): added tolerated amount of unit per strong lactase capsule
Fructose*: fructose, sorbitol adjusted
L2 *Level 2*: fructose-/sorbitol measure ×4. the rest ×2
L3 *Level 3*: sorbitol measure ×7. the rest ×3
(book): source of fruc/galactans data
☻+ ×[Amount] unit: Per unit consumed you can additionally tolerate up to [amount] × fructose(*)-unit of another product.
☹: avoid; ☹¹: ¼ at TL 1; ☹²: ¼ at TL 2; ☹³: ¼ at TL 3; ☺: only contains traces; ☻: is free from it

Bread	Unit	Lactose + unit/	Fructose* Fructose	Sorbitol Sorbitol	FrucGalactans FrucGalactans
Soy bread	slice	3½	11	☹	1 A
	1.49oz/42g	+3 unit	11	2	2
Toast, cinnamon and sugar, whole wheat bread	slice	49½	1½	☺	¾ A
	1.49oz/42g	+41¼ unit	1½	☺	1¾
Toast, wheat bread, with butter	slice	62½	1¾	☺	1¼ A
	1.49oz/42g	+52 unit	1¾	☺	2½
Triticale bread	slice	☺	2½	☺	1 A
	1.49oz/42g		2½	☺	2
White bread, store bought	slice	☺	1¼	☺	1¼ A
	1.49oz/42g		1¼	☺	2½
White whole grain wheat bread	slice	☺	¾	☹	¾ A
	1.49oz/42g		¾	26¼	1¾
Whole wheat bread, store bought	slice	☺	1¼	☺	1 A
	1.49oz/42g		1¼	☺	2¼

3.4.2 Cereals

Cereals	Unit	Lactose (Level 1) + unit/capsule	Fructose* (Level 0) Fructose (Level 0)	Sorbitol (Level 0) Sorbitol (Level 1)	FrucGalactans (Level 0) FrucGalactans (Level 1) 🕮
All-Bran® Original (Kellogg's®)	portion 1.06oz/30g	☺	☺+ ×¼ unit ☺+ ×¼ unit	☺ ☺	¼ [A] ¾
Amaranth Flakes (Arrowhead Mills)	portion 1.06oz/30g	☺	3 3¾	☹ 2½	¾ [G] 1½
Cascadian Farm® Organic Chewy Granola Bar, Trail Mix Dark Chocolate Cranberry	piece 1.24oz/35g	☺	☺+ ×4¼ unit ☺+ ×4¼ unit	☹ 71¼	½ [A] 1
Chocolate Chex® (General Mills®)	tbsp. 0.5ozfl/14.21ml	☺	¼ ¼	☹ ☺	1¼ [A] 2¾
Cinnamon toast crunch® (General Mills®)	portion 1.06oz/30g	☺	¼ ¼	☺ ☺	1½ [A] 3
Cinnamon Toasters® (Malt-O-Meal®)	portion 1.06oz/30g	☺	2 2	☺ ☺	1½ [A] 3
Cocoa Krispies® (Kellogg's®)	portion 1.06oz/30g	☺	☺ ☺	☹ ☺	1½ [A] 3
Cocoa Puffs® (General Mills®)	portion 1.06oz/30g	☺	☺+ ×2 unit ☺+ ×2 unit	☹ ☺	½ [A] 1¼
Corn Chex® (General Mills®)	portion 1.06oz/30g	☺	☺ ☺	☹ ☺	½ [A] 1¼
Corn Flakes (Kellogg's®)	portion 1.06oz/30g	☺	☺+ ×1½ unit ☺+ ×1½ unit	☹ ☺	1½ [A] 3
Crunchy Nut Roasted Nut & Honey (Kellogg's®)	portion 1.06oz/30g	☺	23¾ 24	☹ 15	1½ [A] 3
Essentials Oat Bran cereal (Quaker®)	portion 1.95oz/55g	☺	☺ ☺	☺ ☺	1¼ [A] 2¾
Evaporated milk, diluted, skim (fat free)	glass 8.4oz/240g	¼ +0.21 unit	☺ ☺	☺ ☺	1¼ 2¾
Familia Swiss Muesli®, Original Recipe	portion 1.95oz/55g	☺	1 1	☹ 1	¼ [A] ¾
Fiber One Original® (General Mills®)	portion 1.06oz/30g	☺	41½ 41½	☺ ☺	½ [A] 1¼

Level 0: lactose measure ×½
Level 1: fructose measure ×2
Level 2: fructose-/sorbitol measure ×4. the rest ×2
Level 3: sorbitol measure ×7. the rest ×3
🕮: source of fruc/galactans data

+ Unit/capsule: added tolerated amount of unit per strong lactase capsule
Fructose*: fructose, sorbitol adjusted
☺+ ×[Amount] unit: Per unit consumed you can additionally tolerate up to [amount] × fructose(*)-unit of another product.

☹: avoid; ☹[1]: ¼ at TL 1; ☹[2]: ¼ at TL 2; ☹[3]: ¼ at TL 3; ☺: only contains traces; ☺: is free from it

Cereals	Unit	Lactose + unit/	Fructose* Fructose	Sorbitol Sorbitol	FrucGalactans FrucGalactans
Fiber One® Nutty Clusters & Almonds (General Mills®)	portion 1.95oz/55g	☺	☺ ☺	☺ ☺	¼ A ¾
Froot Loops® (Kellogg's®)	portion 1.06oz/30g	☺	☺ ☺	☺ ☺	½ A 1¼
Frosted Flakes® (Kellogg's®)	portion 1.06oz/30g	☺	☺ ☺	☹ ☺	1½ A 3
Frosted Flakes® Reduced Sugar (Kellogg's®)	portion 1.06oz/30g	☺	☺+ ×¼ unit ☺+ ×¼ unit	☹ ☺	1½ A 3
Frosted Mini-Wheats Big Bite® (Kellogg's®)	portion 1.95oz/55g	☺	☺+ ×¼ unit ☺+ ×¼ unit	☺ ☺	¼ A ¾
GoLEAN® Crisp! Cereal, Cinnamon Crumble (Kashi®)	portion 1.95oz/55g	☺	☺+ ×1¼ unit ☺+ ×1¼ unit	☹ 25¾	¼ A ¾
GoLEAN® Crunch! Cereal, Honey Almond Flax (Kashi®)	portion 1.95oz/55g	☺	☺+ ×1 unit ☺+ ×1 unit	☹ 18	¼ A ¾
Health Valley® Multigrain Chewy Granola Bar, Chocolate Chip	piece 1.03oz/29g	29½ +24¾ unit	☺+ ×1 unit ☺+ ×1 unit	☹ ☺	½ A 1¼
Honey	tbsp. 0.5oz/14.21ml	☺	½ ½	☹ 1¾	☺ ☺
Honey Nut Chex® (General Mills®)	portion 1.06oz/30g	☺	☺ ☺	☹ 37	½ A 1¼
Honey Smacks® (Kellogg's®)	portion 1.06oz/30g	☺	☺+ ×12 unit ☺+ ×12 unit	☹ 83¼	½ A 1¼
Kashi® Chewy Granola Bar, Cherry Dark Chocolate	piece 1.24oz/35g	☺	☺+ ×1 unit ☺+ ×1 unit	☹ 1	½ A 1
Maple syrup, pure	tbsp. 0.5oz/14.21ml	☺	☺+ ×¼ unit ☺+ ×¼ unit	☺ ☺	☺ ☺
Milk, lactose reduced (Lactaid®), skim (fat free)	glass 8.4oz/240g	☺	☺+ ×10 unit ☺+ ×10 unit	☺ ☺	☺ ☺
Milk, lactose reduced, skim (fat free), fortified with calcium (Lactaid®)	glass 8.4oz/240g	☺	☺+ ×10 unit ☺+ ×10 unit	☺ ☺	☺ ☺
Mueslix® (Kellogg's®)	portion 1.95oz/55g	☺	☺+ ×¾ unit ☺+ ×¾ unit	☹ 2¾	¼ A ¾
Rice Krispies® (Kellogg's®)	portion 1.06oz/30g	☺	☺ ☺	☺ ☺	1½ A 3
Sorghum	portion 1.06oz/30g	☺	☺ ☺	☺ ☺	☺ ☺
Special K® Blueberry cereal (Kellogg's®)	portion 1.06oz/30g	☺	☺+ ×½ unit ☺+ ×½ unit	☹ 15	½ A 1¼

Cereals	Unit	Lactose + unit/capsule	Fructose* Fructose	Sorbitol Sorbitol	FrucGalactans FrucGalactans
Special K® Cinnamon Pecan cereal (Kellogg's®)	portion 1.06oz/30g	☺	☺ ☺	☺ ☺	½ A 1¼
Special K® Original cereal (Kellogg's®)	portion 1.06oz/30g	13 +10¾ unit	☺ ☺	☺ ☺	½ A 1¼
Special K® Red Berries cereal (Kellogg's®)	portion 1.06oz/30g	☺	☺ ☺	☹ 41½	½ A 1¼
Sprinkles Cookie Crisp® (General Mills®)	portion 1.06oz/30g	☺	☺+ ×¼ unit ☺+ ×¼ unit	☹ ☺	¾ A 1¾
Sunbelt Bakery® Chewy Granola Bar, Banana Harvest	piece 0.89oz/25g	49 +40¾ unit	☺+ ×½ unit ☺+ ×¾ unit	☹ ¾	¾ A 1½
Sunbelt Bakery® Chewy Granola Bar, Blueberry Harvest	piece 0.89oz/25g	49 +40¾ unit	☺+ ×½ unit ☺+ ×¾ unit	☹ ¾	¾ A 1½
Sunbelt Bakery® Chewy Granola Bar, Golden Almond	piece 0.99oz/28g	4 +3¼ unit	1½ ☺+ ×¾ unit	☹ ☹2	½ A 1¼
Sunbelt Bakery® Chewy Granola Bar, Low Fat Oatmeal Raisin	piece 1.06oz/30g	11¾ +9¾ unit	½ ☺	☹ ☹2	½ A 1¼
Sunbelt Bakery® Chewy Granola Bar, Oats & Honey	piece 0.96oz/27g	17½ +14¾ unit	5¾ ☺+ ×¾ unit	☹ ☹2	½ A 1¼
Sunbelt Bakery® Fudge Dipped Chewy Granola Bar, Coconut	piece 1.03oz/29g	17¼ +14½ unit	¾ ☺+ ×1¾ unit	☹ ☹2	½ A 1¼
Weetabix® Organic Crispy Flakes & Fiber (Barbara's Bakery®)	portion 1.95oz/55g	☺	☺+ ×¾ unit ☺+ ×¾ unit	☺ ☺	¼ A ¾
Wheaties® (General Mills®)	portion 1.06oz/30g	c	83¼ 83¼	☺ ☺	½ A 1¼

Level 0: lactose measure ×½
Level 1: fructose measure ×2
+ Unit/capsule: added tolerated amount of unit per strong lactase capsule
Fructose*: fructose, sorbitol adjusted

Level 2: fructose-/sorbitol measure ×4. the rest ×2
Level 3: sorbitol measure ×7. the rest ×3
📖: source of fruc/galactans data
☺+ ×[Amount] unit: Per unit consumed you can additionally tolerate up to [amount] × fructose(*)-unit of another product.

☹: avoid; ☹1: ¼ at TL 1; ☹2: ¼ at TL 2; ☹3: ¼ at TL 3; ☺: only contains traces; ☺: is free from it

3.4.3 Cold cut

Cold cut	Unit	Lactose + unit/	Fructose* Fructose	Sorbitol Sorbitol	FrucGalactans FrucGalactans
Alpine Lace 25% Reduced Fat, Mozzarella	portion 1.06oz/30g	37¼ +31 unit	☺ ☺	☺ ☺	☺ ☺
American cheese, processed	portion 1.06oz/30g	4½ +3¾ unit	☺ ☺	☺ ☺	25¾ 51½
Blue cheese	portion 1.06oz/30g	20 +16½ unit	☺ ☺	☺ ☺	☺ ☺
Bologna, beef ring	portion 1.95oz/55g	☺	☺+ ×5¾ unit ☺+ ×5¾ unit	☺ ☺	☺ ☺
Bologna, combination of meats, light (reduced fat)	portion 1.95oz/55g	☺	☺+ ×½ unit ☺+ ×½ unit	☺ ☺	☺ ☺
Brie cheese	portion 1.06oz/30g	22 +18½ unit	☺ ☺	☺ ☺	☺ ☺
Butter, light, salted	portion 0.5oz/14g	☺	☺ ☺	☺ ☺	☺ ☺
Butter, unsalted	portion 0.5oz/14g	☺	☺ ☺	☺ ☺	☺ ☺
Camembert cheese	portion 1.06oz/30g	21½ +18 unit	☺ ☺	☺ ☺	☺ ☺
Cheddar cheese, natural	portion 1.06oz/30g	43¼ +36 unit	☺ ☺	☺ ☺	☺ ☺
Cheese sauce, store bought	portion 2.33oz/66g	¼ +¼ unit	☺ ☺	☺ ☺	1¾ 3¾
Colby Jack cheese	portion 1.06oz/30g	27¼ +22¾ unit	☺ ☺	☺ ☺	☺ ☺
Cottage cheese, 1% fat, lactose reduced	portion 3.89oz/110g	3¼ +2¾ unit	☺+ ×1¾ unit ☺+ ×1¾ unit	☺ ☺	18¾ 37¾
Cottage cheese, uncreamed dry curd	portion 1.95oz/55g	3½ +2¾ unit	☺ ☺	☺ ☺	19¾ 39½
Cream cheese spread	portion 1.06oz/30g	2¾ +2¼ unit	☺ ☺	☺ ☺	15¾ 31½
Cream cheese, whipped, flavored	portion 1.06oz/30g	2½ +2 unit	☺ ☺	☺ ☺	14 28
Cream cheese, whipped, plain	portion 1.06oz/30g	3 +2½ unit	☺ ☺	☺ ☺	17¼ 34½
Edam cheese	portion 1.06oz/30g	6¾ +5¾ unit	☺ ☺	☺ ☺	38¾ 77½

Cold cut	Unit	Lactose 1 + unit/capsule	Fructose* 0 Fructose 0	Sorbitol 0 Sorbitol 1	FrucGalactans 0 FrucGalactans 1 📖
Fleischmann's® Move Over Butter Margarine, tub, whipped	portion 0.32oz/9g	21¾ +18 unit	☻ ☻	☻ ☻	☺ ☺
Goats cheese, hard	portion 1.06oz/30g	4½ +3¾ unit	☻ ☻	☻ ☻	25½ 51
Gorgonzola cheese	portion 1.06oz/30g	20 +16½ unit	☻ ☻	☻ ☻	☺ ☺
Gouda cheese	portion 1.06oz/30g	4½ +3¾ unit	☻ ☻	☻ ☻	25 50
Honey	portion 0.75oz/21g	☻	¼ ¼	☹ 1¼	☺ ☺
Hot dog, combination of meats, plain	portion 1.95oz/55g	☻	☻+ ×3 unit ☻+ ×3 unit	☻ ☻	☻ ☻
Jam or preserves	portion 0.71oz/20g	☻	☻+ ×2¾ unit ☻+ ×2¾ unit	☹ 1¾	☻ ☻
Jam or preserves, reduced sugar	portion 0.71oz/20g	☻	7 7	☹ 41½	☻ ☻
Jam or preserves, sugar free with aspartame	portion 0.6oz/17g	☻	15¾ 17½	☹ 5¼	☻ ☻
Jam or preserves, sugar free with saccharin	portion 0.5oz/14g	☻	2¼ 2¼	☹ 19¼	☻ ☻
Jam or preserves, sugar free with sucralose	portion 0.6oz/17g	☻	☻ ☻	☹ 65¼	☻ ☻
Jam or preserves, without sugar or artificial sweetener	tbsp. 0.5ozfl/14.21ml	☻	¼ ¼	☹ ☹[2]	☻ ☻
Kraft® Cheese Spread, Roka Blue	portion 1.06oz/30g	1¾ +1¼ unit	☻ ☻	☻ ☻	9¾ 19½
Limburger cheese	portion 1.06oz/30g	20¼ +17 unit	☻ ☻	☻ ☻	☺ ☺
Maple syrup, pure	tbsp. 0.5oz/14.21ml	☻	☻+ ×¼ unit ☻+ ×¼ unit	☻ ☻	☻ ☻
Margarine, diet, fat free	portion 0.5oz/14g	15½ +13 unit	☻ ☻	☻ ☻	86¾ ☺

0 *Level 0:* lactose measure ×½
1 *Level 1:* fructose measure ×2
2 *Level 2:* fructose-/sorbitol measure ×4. the rest ×2
3 *Level 3:* sorbitol measure ×7. the rest ×3
📖: source of fruc/galactans data

+ Unit/capsule: added tolerated amount of unit per strong lactase capsule
Fructose*: fructose, sorbitol adjusted

☻+ ×[Amount] unit: Per unit consumed you can additionally tolerate up to [amount] × fructose(*)-unit of another product.

☹: avoid; ☹[1]: ¼ at TL 1; ☹[2]: ¼ at TL 2; ☹[3]: ¼ at TL 3; ☺: only contains traces; ☻: is free from it

Cold cut	Unit	Lactose + unit/	Fructose* Fructose	Sorbitol Sorbitol	FrucGalactans FrucGalactans
Margarine, tub, salted, sunflower oil	portion 0.5oz/14g	30 +25 unit	☺ ☺	☺ ☺	☺ ☺
Marmalade, sugar free with aspartame	portion 0.6oz/17g	☺	15¾ 17½	☹ 5¼	☺ ☺
Marmalade, sugar free with saccharin	portion 0.57oz/16g	☺	2 2	☹ 16¾	☺ ☺
Marmalade, sugar free with sucralose	portion 0.6oz/17g	☺	☺ ☺	☹ 65¼	☺ ☺
Mascarpone	portion 1.06oz/30g	2½ +2 unit	☺ ☺	☺ ☺	13¾ 27¾
Mortadella	portion 1.95oz/55g	☺	☺+ ×¼ unit ☺+ ×¼ unit	☺ ☺	☺ ☺
Muenster cheese, natural	portion 1.06oz/30g	8¾ +7¼ unit	☺ ☺	☺ ☺	49½ ☺
Nutella® (filbert spread)	portion 1.31oz/37g	32¼ +27 unit	67½ 67½	☹ 20¾	☺ ☺
Roquefort cheese	portion 1.06oz/30g	5 +4 unit	☺ ☺	☺ ☺	27¾ 55½
Smart Balance® Light with Flax Oil Margarine, tub	portion 0.5oz/14g	32¼ +27 unit	☺ ☺	☺ ☺	☺ ☺
Smart Balance® Margarine	portion 0.5oz/14g	31 +25¾ unit	☺ ☺	☺ ☺	☺ ☺
Soy Kaas Fat Free, all flavors	portion 1.06oz/30g	9 +7½ unit	55½ 55½	☹ 18½	1¼[A] 2¾
Swiss cheese, natural	portion 1.06oz/30g	☺	☺+ ×¼ unit ☺+ ×¼ unit	☺ ☺	☺ ☺
Swiss cheese, natural, low sodium	portion 1.06oz/30g	☺	☺+ ×¼ unit ☺+ ×¼ unit	☺ ☺	☺ ☺
Tilsit cheese	portion 1.06oz/30g	5¼ +4¼ unit	☺ ☺	☺ ☺	29½ 59

3.4.4 Dairy products

Dairy products	Unit	Lactose 1 + unit/capsule	Fructose* 0 Fructose 0	Sorbitol 0 Sorbitol 1	FrucGalactans 0 FrucGalactans 1 📖
Almond milk, vanilla or other flavors, unsweetened	glass 8.4oz/240g	☺	☺ ☺	☺ ☺	☹A ☹2
Breyers® Light! Boosts Immunity Yogurt, all flavors	piece 4oz/114g	½ +¼ unit	28¾ 31	☹ 14¼	3 6
Breyers® No Sugar Added Ice Cream, Vanilla	tbsp. 0.5ozfl/14.21ml	3¼ +2½ unit	¾ ☺	☹ ☹2	18¼ 36½
Breyers® YoCrunch Light Nonfat Yogurt, with granola	piece 6.5oz/185g	¼ +0.24 unit	☺ ☺	☹ 6½	1½ 3
Cabot® Non Fat Yogurt, plain	piece 8.01oz/227g	¼ +0.22 unit	☺ ☺	☺ ☺	1¼ 2¾
Cabot® Non Fat Yogurt, vanilla	piece 8.01oz/227g	¼ +¼ unit	30¼ 33¼	☹ 13¼	2¼ 4½
Chobani® Nonfat Greek Yogurt, Black Cherry	tbsp. 0.5ozfl/14.21ml	5¼ +4½ unit	☺ ☺	☹ 3¾	30¼ 60¾
Chobani® Nonfat Greek Yogurt, Lemon	piece 6.04oz/171g	½ +¼ unit	☺+ ×½ unit ☺+ ×½ unit	☺ ☺	3 6
Chobani® Nonfat Greek Yogurt, Peach	piece 6.04oz/171g	¼ +¼ unit	☺+ ×1 unit ☺+ ×1 unit	☹ 4¼	1¾ 3½
Chobani® Nonfat Greek Yogurt, Raspberry	piece 6.04oz/171g	¼ +¼ unit	☺+ ×¾ unit ☺+ ×¾ unit	☹ 20	1¾ 3½
Chobani® Nonfat Greek Yogurt, Strawberry	piece 6.04oz/171g	¼ +¼ unit	☺+ ×¾ unit ☺+ ×¾ unit	☹ 3½	1¾ 3½
Chocolate pudding, store bought	piece 3.5oz/98g	¾ +½ unit	☺ ☺	☹ 25	4¾ 9¾
Chocolate pudding, store bought, sugar free	tbsp. 0.5ozfl/14.21ml	89¼ +74¼ unit	¾ ☺	☹ ☹2	☺ ☺
Cottage cheese, uncreamed dry curd	portion 1.95oz/55g	3½ +2¾ unit	☺ ☺	☺ ☺	19¾ 39½
Danone® Activia® Light Yogurt, vanilla	piece 4oz/115g	¼ +¼ unit	¼ ¼	☺ ☺	2 4

0 *Level 0:* lactose measure ×½
1 *Level 1:* fructose measure ×2
2 *Level 2:* fructose-/sorbitol measure ×4. the rest ×2
3 *Level 3:* sorbitol measure ×7. the rest ×3
📖: source of fruc/galactans data

+ Unit/capsule: added tolerated amount of unit per strong lactase capsule
Fructose*: fructose, sorbitol adjusted
☺+ ×[Amount] unit: Per unit consumed you can additionally tolerate up to [amount] × fructose(*)-unit of another product.

☹: avoid; ☹1: ¼ at TL 1; ☹2: ¼ at TL 2; ☹3: ¼ at TL 3; ☺: only contains traces; ☺: is free from it

Dairy products	**Unit**	**Lactose** **+ unit/**	**Fructose*** **Fructose**	**Sorbitol** **Sorbitol**	**FrucGalactans** **FrucGalactans**
Danone® Activia® Yogurt, plain	piece 4oz/115g	½ +¼ unit	☺ ☺	☺ ☺	2¾ 5½
Danone® Greek Yogurt, Honey	piece 5.3oz/150g	½ +¼ unit	¼ ¼	☹ 3¼	2¾ 5¾
Danone® Greek Yogurt, Plain	piece 5.3oz/150g	½ +¼ unit	☺ ☺	☺ ☺	1¼ 2½
Danone® la Crème Yogurt, fruit flavors	piece 4oz/115g	¼ +¼ unit	¼ ¼	☹ 10¾	2 4
Evaporated milk, diluted, 2% fat (reduced fat)	glass 8.4oz/240g	¼ +0.22 unit	☺ ☺	☺ ☺	1½ 3
Evaporated milk, diluted, skim (fat free)	glass 8.4oz/240g	¼ +0.21 unit	☺ ☺	☺ ☺	1¼ 2¾
Evaporated milk, diluted, whole	glass 8.4oz/240g	¼ +0.24 unit	☺ ☺	☺ ☺	1½ 3
Feta cheese	portion 1.06oz/30g	2¼ +2 unit	☺ ☺	☺ ☺	13½ 27
Feta cheese, fat free	portion 1.06oz/30g	¾ +¾ unit	☺ ☺	☺ ☺	5 10¼
Fondue sauce	portion 1.87oz/53g	☺	☺+ ×¼ unit ☺+ ×¼ unit	☹ 5	☺ ☺
GO Veggie!™ Rice Slices, all flavors	portion 1.06oz/30g	12 +10 unit	☺ ☺	☺ ☺	67¼[A] ☺
Greek yogurt, plain, nonfat,	piece 5.3oz/150g	¼ +¼ unit	☺ ☺	☺ ☺	2½ 5
Half and half	portion 1.06oz/30g	2¼ +1¾ unit	☺ ☺	☺ ☺	12¾ 25¾
Kefir	portion 8.65oz/245g	¼ +¼ unit	☺ ☺	☺ ☺	1¾ 3¾
Laughing Cow® Mini Babybel®, Cheddar	piece 0.75oz/21g	☺	☺ ☺	☺ ☺	☺ ☺
Laughing Cow® Mini Babybel®, Original	piece 0.75oz/21g	12¾ +10½ unit	☺ ☺	☺ ☺	70¾ ☺
Licuado, mango	glass 8.4oz/240g	¼ +¼ unit	¼ ¼	☹ 1	2½ 5
Light cream	portion 0.53oz/15g	5¼ +4½ unit	☺ ☺	☺ ☺	30¼ 60½
Milk, lactose reduced (Lactaid®), skim (fat free)	glass 8.4oz/240g	☺	☺+ ×10 unit ☺+ ×10 unit	☺ ☺	☺ ☺
Milk, lactose reduced (Lactaid®), whole	glass 8.4oz/240g	☺	☺+ ×10 unit ☺+ ×10 unit	☺ ☺	☺ ☺

Dairy products	Unit	Lactose + unit/	Fructose* Fructose	Sorbitol Sorbitol	FrucGalactans FrucGalactans
Milk, lactose reduced, skim (fat free), fortified with calcium (Lactaid®)	glass 8.4oz/240g	☺	☺+ ×10 unit ☺+ ×10 unit	☺ ☺	☺ ☺
Mozzarella cheese, fat free	portion 1.06oz/30g	½ +½ unit	☺ ☺	☺ ☺	3½ 7¼
Mozzarella cheese, whole milk	portion 1.06oz/30g	9¾ +8¼ unit	☺ ☺	☺ ☺	55 ☺
Oat milk	glass 8.4oz/240g	☺	☺ ☺	☺ ☺	¼ A ¾
Parmesan cheese, dry (grated)	portion 0.18oz/5g	☺	☺ ☺	☺ ☺	☺ ☺
Parmesan cheese, dry (grated), nonfat	portion 0.18oz/5g	☺ +75¾ unit	☺ ☺	☺ ☺	☺ ☺
Pudding mix, other flavors, cooked type	portion 0.88oz/24.75g	☺	☺ ☺	☺ ☺	☺ ☺
Rice milk, plain or original, unsweetened, enriched, ready-to-drink	glass 8.4oz/240g	☺	☺+ ×¼ unit ☺+ ×¼ unit	☺ ☺	☺ A ☺
Rice pudding (arroz con leche), coconut, raisins	piece 7.06oz/200g	½ +¼ unit	27¾ ☺	☹ 1¼	3¼ 6½
Rice pudding (arroz con leche), plain	piece 7.06oz/200g	½ +¼ unit	☺+ ×½ unit ☺+ ×½ unit	☺ ☺	2¾ 5¾
Rice pudding (arroz con leche), raisins	piece 7.06oz/200g	½ +¼ unit	3¾ 8	☹ 1¼	3 6
Ricotta cheese, part skim milk	portion 1.95oz/55g	17½ +14½ unit	☺ ☺	☺ ☺	☺ ☺
Slim-Fast® Easy to Digest, Vanilla, ready-to-drink can	glass 8.4oz/240g	2½ +2 unit	☺ ☺	☺ ☺	14¼ 28¾
Sour cream	portion 1.06oz/30g	3¼ +2¾ unit	☺ ☺	☺ ☺	19¼ 38½
Soy milk, plain or original, sweetened with artificial sweetener, ready-to-drink	glass 8.4oz/240g	☺	4¾ 4¾	☹ 1½	☹ A ¼

Level 0: lactose measure ×½ + Unit/ : added tolerated amount of unit per strong lactase capsule

Level 1: fructose measure ×2 Fructose*: fructose, sorbitol adjusted

Level 2: fructose-/sorbitol measure ×4. the rest ×2

Level 3: sorbitol measure ×7. the rest ×3

: source of fruc/galactans data

☺+ ×[Amount] unit: Per unit consumed you can additionally tolerate up to [amount] × fructose(*)-unit of another product.

☹: avoid; ☹[1]: ¼ at TL 1; ☹[2]: ¼ at TL 2; ☹[3]: ¼ at TL 3; ☺: only contains traces; ☺: is free from it

Dairy products	Unit	Lactose + unit/	Fructose* Fructose	Sorbitol Sorbitol	FrucGalactans FrucGalactans
Soy milk, vanilla or other flavors, sweetened with sugar, fat free, ready-to-drink	glass 8.4oz/240g	☺	☺+ ×¾ unit ☺+ ×¾ unit	☹ 7	☹[A] ¼
Stonyfield® Oikos Greek Yogurt, Blueberry	piece 5.3oz/150g	¼ +¼ unit	☺+ ×1 unit ☺+ ×1 unit	☺ ☺	1¾ 3½
Stonyfield® Oikos Greek Yogurt, Caramel	piece 4.03oz/114g	½ +½ unit	☺+ ×½ unit ☺+ ×½ unit	☺ ☺	4 8
Stonyfield® Oikos Greek Yogurt, Chocolate	piece 4.03oz/114g	½ +¼ unit	66½ 66½	☺ ☺	3 6¼
Stonyfield® Oikos Greek Yogurt, Strawberry	piece 5.3oz/150g	¼ +¼ unit	4 4¼	☹ 2	1¾ 3½
Strawberry milk, plain, prepared	glass 8.4oz/240g	¼ +¼ unit	☺ ☺	☺ ☺	1¾ 3½
Sweetened condensed milk	portion 1.35oz/38g	½ +½ unit	☺ ☺	☺ ☺	3¾ 7½
Sweetened condensed milk, reduced fat	portion 1.38oz/39g	½ +½ unit	☺ ☺	☺ ☺	3½ 7¼
Tofu, raw (not silken), cooked, low fat	portion 3oz/85g	☺	2¼ 2¼	☹ ¾	½[A] 1
Whipped cream, aerosol	portion 0.25oz/7g	☺	☺ ☺	☺ ☺	☺ ☺
Whipped cream, aerosol, chocolate	portion 0.18oz/5g	9¾ +8 unit	☺ ☺	☹ ☺	54½ ☺
Whipped cream, aerosol, fat free	portion 0.18oz/5g	18¾ +15¾ unit	☺+ ×¼ unit ☺+ ×¼ unit	☺ ☺	☺ ☺
Yogurt, chocolate or coffee flavors, nonfat, sweetened with aspartame	tbsp. 0.5ozfl/14.21ml	4 +3¼ unit	☺ ☺	☺ ☺	22½ 45
Yogurt, chocolate or coffee flavors, whole milk, sweetened with sucralose	piece 6.04oz/171g	¼ +¼ unit	40 40	☺ ☺	1½ 3¼
Yogurt, fruited, whole milk	tbsp. 0.5ozfl/14.21ml	2¾ +2¼ unit	¾ ¾	☹ 60½	16 32¼

3.4.5 Nuts and snacks

Nuts and snacks	Unit	Lactose (Level 1) + unit/capsule	Fructose* (Level 0) Fructose (Level 0)	Sorbitol (Level 0) Sorbitol (Level 1)	FrucGalactans (Level 0) FrucGalactans (Level 1) (source)
Almonds, raw	hand 1.06oz/30g	☺	☺ ☺	☺ ☺	½ G 1¼
Baby food, double baked (zwieback)	portion 0.25oz/7g	☺	☺ ☺	☺ ☺	1½ A 3
Brazil nuts, unsalted	hand 1.06oz/30g	☺	☺ ☺	☺ ☺	☺ ☺
Caramel or sugar coated popcorn, store bought	hand 0.75oz/21g	☺	☺+ ×1 unit ☺+ ×1 unit	☺ ☺	☺ C ☺
Cashews, raw	hand 1.06oz/30g	☺	☺ ☺	☺ ☺	¼ G ¾
Cheese cracker	piece 0.11oz/3g	☺	☺ ☺	☺ ☺	3½ A 7
Chestnuts, roasted	portion 1.06oz/30g	☺	☺ ☺	☹ 3	☺ ☺
Chia seeds	hand 1.06oz/30g	☺	☺ ☺	☺ ☺	1¼ G 2¾
Coconut cream (liquid from grated meat)	hand 1.06oz/30g	☺	20¾ 20¾	☺ ☺	☺ ☺
Coconut milk, fresh (liquid from grated meat, water added)	glass 8.4oz/240g	☺	☺+ ×1 unit ☺+ ×1 unit	☺ ☺	1¾ G 3½
Coconut, dried, shredded or flaked, unsweetened	hand 1.06oz/30g	☺	☺+ ×¾ unit ☺+ ×¾ unit	☺ ☺	12¼ 24½
Coconut, fresh	portion 0.53oz/15g	☺	☺+ ×¼ unit ☺+ ×¼ unit	☺ ☺	24½ G 49
Doritos® Tortilla Chips, Nacho Cheese	hand 0.75oz/21g	☺	☺ ☺	☹ ☺	10¾ A 21½
Filberts, raw	hand 1.06oz/30g	☺	☺ ☺	☹ 8¼	2¾ G 5¾
Flax seeds, not fortifed	tbsp. 0.5oz/14.21ml	☺	☺ ☺	☺ ☺	2 G 4¼

Level 0: lactose measure ×½ + Unit/capsule: added tolerated amount of unit per strong lactase capsule
Level 1: fructose measure ×2 Fructose*: fructose, sorbitol adjusted
Level 2: fructose-/sorbitol measure ×4. the rest ×2
Level 3: sorbitol measure ×7. the rest ×3
(book): source of fruc/galactans data
☺+ ×[Amount] unit: Per unit consumed you can additionally tolerate up to [amount] × fructose(*)-unit of another product.

☹: avoid; ☹[1]: ¼ at TL 1; ☹[2]: ¼ at TL 2; ☹[3]: ¼ at TL 3; ☺: only contains traces; ☺: is free from it

Nuts and snacks	Unit	Lactose + unit/	Fructose* Fructose	Sorbitol Sorbitol	FrucGalactans FrucGalactans
Ginko nuts, dried	hand 1.06oz/30g	☺	☺ ☺	☺ ☺	☺ ☺
Hickorynuts	hand 1.06oz/30g	☺	☺ ☺	☺ ☺	2¾ G 5¾
Lay's® Potato Chips, Classic	hand 0.75oz/21g	☺	41¾ 41¾	☹ 79¼	10¾ A 21½
Lay's® Potato Chips, Salt & Vinegar	hand 0.75oz/21g	☺	41¾ 41¾	☹ 79¼	10¾ A 21½
Lay's® Potato Chips, Sour Cream & Onion	hand 0.75oz/21g	☺	41¾ 41¾	☹ 79¼	10¾ A 21½
Lay's® Stax Potato Crisps, Cheddar	hand 0.75oz/21g	☺	41¾ 41¾	☹ 79¼	10¾ A 21½
Lay's® Stax Potato Crisps, Hot 'n Spicy Barbecue	hand 0.75oz/21g	☺	54 54	☹ ☺	10¾ A 21½
Macadamia nuts, raw	hand 1.06oz/30g	☺	☺ ☺	☺ ☺	☺ ☺
Melba Toast®, Classic (Old London®)	portion 0.53oz/15g	☺	☺+ ×¼ unit ☺+ ×¼ unit	☹ ☺	½ A 1¼
Old Dutch® Crunch Curls	hand 0.75oz/21g	4 +3¼ unit	☺ ☺	☹ ☺	7¼ A 14½
Peanut butter, unsalted	portion 1.13oz/32g	☺	☺+ ×¼ unit ☺+ ×¼ unit	☺ ☺	☺ G ☺
Peanuts, dry roasted, salted	hand 1.06oz/30g	☺	☺ ☺	☺ ☺	☺ G ☺
Pine nuts, pignolias	hand 1.06oz/30g	☺	☺ ☺	☺ ☺	☺ ☺
Pistachio nuts, raw	hand 0.75oz/21g	☺	☺ ☺	☺ ☺	☺ ☺
Poore Brothers® Potato Chips, Salt & Cracked Pepper	hand 0.75oz/21g	☺	54 54	☹ ☺	10¾ A 21½
Potato chips, salted	hand 0.75oz/21g	☺	41¾ 41¾	☹ 79¼	10¾ A 21½
Potato sticks	hand 0.75oz/21g	☺	☺ ☺	☹ 79¼	10¾ A 21½
Pretzels, hard, unsalted, sticks	hand 0.75oz/21g	☺	☺ ☺	☺ ☺	1½ A 3¼
Pringles® Light Fat Free Potato Crisps, Barbecue	hand 0.75oz/21g	☺	37 37	☹ 79¼	10¾ A 21½
Pringles® Potato Crisps, Loaded Baked Potato	hand 0.75oz/21g	☺	41¾ 41¾	☹ 79¼	10¾ A 21½

Nuts and snacks	Unit	Lactose + unit/capsule	Fructose* / Fructose	Sorbitol / Sorbitol	FrucGalactans / FrucGalactans
Pringles® Potato Crisps, Original	hand	☻	76¾	☹	10¾^{A}
	0.75oz/21g		76¾	☺	21½
Pringles® Potato Crisps, Salt & Vinegar	hand	☻	41¾	☹	10¾^{A}
	0.75oz/21g		41¾	79¼	21½
Pumpkin or squash seeds, shelled, unsalted	hand	☻	☻	☻	2¾^{G}
	1.06oz/30g		☻	☻	5¾
Rice cake	piece	☻	☻	☻	7½^{A}
	0.32oz/9g		☻	☻	15
Ritz Cracker (Nabisco®)	portion	☻	☻	☻	¼^{A}
	1.06oz/30g		☻	☻	½
Sesame sticks	hand	☻	☻	☹	1½^{A}
	0.75oz/21g		☻	☺	3¼
Soy chips	hand	5¼	15	☹	2^{A}
	0.75oz/21g	+4¼ unit	15	1	4
Sunflower seeds, raw	hand	☻	☻	☻	1^{A}
	1.06oz/30g		☻	☻	2¼
Taco John's® nachos	hand	28	☻	☹	10^{A}
	0.75oz/21g	+23¼ unit	☻	☺	20
Tortilla, white, store bought, fried	piece	☻	☻	☻	¾^{A}
	2.05oz/58g		☻	☻	1¾
Walnuts	hand	☻	☺	☻	☻
	1.06oz/30g		☺	☻	☻
Wise Onion Flavored Rings	Portion	☻	☻	☹	10¼^{AC}
	30 g		☻	☺	20¾

Level 0: lactose measure ×½

Level 1: fructose measure ×2

+ Unit/capsule: added tolerated amount of unit per strong lactase capsule

Fructose*: fructose, sorbitol adjusted

Level 2: fructose-/sorbitol measure ×4. the rest ×2

Level 3: sorbitol measure ×7. the rest ×3

(book icon): source of fruc/galactans data

☻+ ×[Amount] unit: Per unit consumed you can additionally tolerate up to [amount] × fructose(*)-unit of another product.

☹: avoid; ☹1: ¼ at TL 1; ☹2: ¼ at TL 2; ☹3: ¼ at TL 3; ☺: only contains traces; ☻: is free from it

3.4.6 Sweet pastries

Sweet pastries	Unit	Lactose + unit/	Fructose* Fructose	Sorbitol Sorbitol	FrucGalactans FrucGalactans
Almond cookies	piece 0.44oz/12.4g	☺	☺ ☺	☺ ☺	3[A] 6
Apple cake, glazed	piece 1.59oz/45g	☺	¾ 1	☹ ½	1¼[A] 2½
Apple strudel	piece 2.26oz/64g	☺	¼ ¼	☹ ¼	¾[A] 1¾
Archway® Oatmeal Raisin Cookies	piece 0.92oz/26g	23¾ +19¾ unit	☺ ☺	☹ 10¼	2¼[A] 4¾
Archway® Peanut Butter Cookies	piece 1.2oz/34g	23¾ +19¾ unit	2 2	☹ 10¾	1½[A] 3
Biscotti, chocolate, nuts	piece 0.73oz/20.5g	☺	☺ ☺	☹ ☺	2½[A] 5
Brownie, chocolate, fat free	piece 1.56oz/44g	3 +2½ unit	71 71	☹ ☺	1[A] 2¼
Butter cracker	piece 0.15oz/4g	☺	☺ ☺	☺ ☺	10[A] 20
Carrot cake, glazed, homemade	piece 0.98oz/27.72g	☺	☺+ ×¼ unit ☺+ ×¼ unit	☹ 8	2[A] 4
Cheesecake, plain or flavored, graham cracker crust, homemade	piece 7.77oz/220g	½ +½ unit	☺+ ×½ unit ☺+ ×½ unit	☺ ☺	☹[A] ¼
Cherry pie, bottom crust only	piece 4.31oz/122g	☺	1 ☺+ ×1½ unit	☹ ☹[2]	¼[A] ¾
Chips Ahoy!® Chewy Gooey Caramel Cookies (Nabisco®)	piece 0.55oz/15.5g	12¼ +10¼ unit	½ ½	☹ ☺	3[A] 6¼
Chocolate cake, glazed, store bought	piece 1.03oz/29g	☺	☺+ ×½ unit ☺+ ×½ unit	☹ ☺	1¾[A] 3¾
Chocolate chip cookies, store bought	piece 0.36oz/10g	☺	☺ ☺	☹ ☺	2½[A] 5¼
Chocolate cookies, iced, store bought	piece 0.36oz/10g	☺	☺ ☺	☹ ☺	5[A] 10¼
Chocolate sandwich cookies, double filling	piece 0.52oz/14.5g	☺	☺ ☺	☹ ☺	3½[A] 7
Chocolate sandwich cookies, sugar free	piece 0.43oz/12g	☺	13¾ ☺	☹ ☹	4¼[A] 8½
Cinnamon Roll with Icing, all flavours	piece 1.56oz/44g	9 +7½ unit	☺+ ×8¼ unit ☺+ ×8¼ unit	☺ ☺	1[A] 2¼

Sweet pastries	Unit	Lactose (Level 1) + unit/capsule	Fructose* (Level 0) Fructose (Level 0)	Sorbitol (Level 0) Sorbitol (Level 1)	FrucGalactans (Level 0) FrucGalactans (Level 1) 📖
Crepe, plain	piece 1.95oz/55g	1¼ +1 unit	☺ ☺	☺ ☺	¾ A 1¾
Croissant, chocolate	piece 2.44oz/69g	3½ +3 unit	☺+ ×1 unit ☺+ ×1 unit	☹ ☺	¾ A 1½
Croissant, fruit	piece 2.62oz/74g	3½ +3 unit	☺+ ×2½ unit ☺+ ×2½ unit	☹ 2	½ A 1¼
Danish pastry, frosted or glazed, with cheese filling	piece 4.41oz/125g	3 +2½ unit	☺ ☺	☺ ☺	¼ D ½
Dare Breaktime Ginger Cookies	piece 0.27oz/7.5g	☺	☺ ☺	☺ ☺	8½ A 17¼
Dare® Lemon Crème Cookies	piece 0.69oz/19.5g	32½ +27 unit	☺ ☺	☺ ☺	2½ A 5¼
Doughnut, raised, glazed, coconut topping	piece 2.79oz/79g	4¾ +4 unit	☺ ☺	☺ ☺	½ A 1¼
Doughnut, raised, glazed, plain	piece 2.72oz/77g	4¾ +4 unit	☺ ☺	☺ ☺	½ A 1¼
Doughnut, raised, sugared	piece 2.56oz/72.5g	4¾ +4 unit	☺ ☺	☺ ☺	¾ A 1½
EGG® bread roll	piece 1.24oz/35g	5¼ +4¼ unit	☺ ☺	☺ ☺	1½ A 3
Elephant ear (crispy)	piece 2.09oz/59g	4¼ +3½ unit	☺ ☺	☺ ☺	1 A 2
English muffin, whole wheat, with raisins	piece 2.33oz/66g	1¼ +1 unit	2 2½	☹ 2¼	¾ A 1½
French toast, homemade, French bread	piece 4.63oz/131g	1¼ +1 unit	☺+ ×½ unit ☺+ ×½ unit	☺ ☺	¼ A ¾
Frozen custard, chocolate or coffee flavors	portion 3.09oz/87.5g	½ +¼ unit	☺+ ×2¼ unit ☺+ ×2¼ unit	☹ ☺	½ A 1
German chocolate cake, glazed, homemade	piece 1.03oz/29g	☺	☺+ ×½ unit ☺+ ×½ unit	☹ ☺	1¾ A 3¾
Girl Scout® Lemonades	piece 0.55oz/15.5g	☺	☺ ☺	☺ ☺	4 A 8¼
Girl Scout® Peanut Butter Patties	piece 0.45oz/12.5g	☺	☺ ☺	☹ ☺	4 A 8¼

Level 0: lactose measure ×½
Level 1: fructose measure ×2
+ Unit/capsule: added tolerated amount of unit per strong lactase capsule
Fructose*: fructose, sorbitol adjusted
Level 2: fructose-/sorbitol measure ×4. the rest ×2
Level 3: sorbitol measure ×7. the rest ×3
📖: source of fruc/galactans data
☺+ ×[Amount] unit: Per unit consumed you can additionally tolerate up to [amount] × fructose(*)-unit of another product.

☹: avoid; ☹¹: ¼ at TL 1; ☹²: ¼ at TL 2; ☹³: ¼ at TL 3; ☺: only contains traces; ☺: is free from it

Sweet pastries	Unit	Lactose + unit/	Fructose* Fructose	Sorbitol Sorbitol	FrucGalactans FrucGalactans
Girl Scout® Samoas®	piece 0.52oz/14.5g	52¼ +43½ unit	10¼ ☺	☹ ¾	3½[A] 7
Girl Scout® Shortbread®	piece 0.4oz/11.34g	18½ +15½ unit	☺ ☺	☺ ☺	3¼[A] 6¾
Girl Scout® Thin Mints	piece 0.29oz/8g	32½ +27 unit	☺ ☺	☹ ☺	6¼[A] 12½
Halvah	portion 1.42oz/40g	☺	☺+ ×1½ unit ☺+ ×1½ unit	☺ ☺	1¼[A] 2¾
Lebkuchen	piece 1.15oz/32.4g	☺	6¼ 6¼	☹ 6½	2[A] 4
Little Debbie® Coffee Cake, Apple Streusel	piece 1.84oz/52g	☺	☺+ ×5¼ unit ☺+ ×5¼ unit	☺ ☺	1[A] 2
Little Debbie® Fudge Brownies with English Walnuts	piece 1.08oz/30.5g	☺	☺+ ×4¼ unit ☺+ ×4¼ unit	☹ ☺	1¾[A] 3½
Long John or bismarck, glazed, cream or custard filled, with nuts	piece 3.71oz/105g	2¼ +2 unit	☺ ☺	☺ ☺	½[A] 1
Molasses cookies, store bought	piece 0.53oz/15g	☺	☺ ☺	☺ ☺	3¼[A] 6¾
Muffins, banana	piece 3.99oz/113g	2½ +2 unit	☺+ ×¼ unit ☺+ ×¼ unit	☹ 29¼	¼[A] ¾
Muffins, blueberry, store bought	piece 3.99oz/113g	1½ +1¼ unit	☺ ☺	☺ ☺	¼[A] ¾
Muffins, carrot, homemade, with nuts	piece 3.99oz/113g	1½ +1¼ unit	☺ ☺	☹ 3¼	¼[A] ¾
Muffins, oat bran or oatmeal, store bought	piece 3.99oz/113g	1¼ +1 unit	☺+ ×¼ unit ☺+ ×¼ unit	☺ ☺	½[A] 1
Muffins, pumpkin, store bought	piece 3.99oz/113g	1¾ +1¼ unit	☺+ ×¼ unit ☺+ ×¼ unit	☹ 14½	¼[A] ¾
Murray® Sugar Free Oatmeal Cookies	piece 0.39oz/11g	☺	½ ☺	☹ ☹[2]	4½[A] 9
Murray® Sugar Free Shortbread	piece 0.14oz/3.75g	☺	1½ ☺	☹ ☹[2]	10½[A] 21¼
Nabisco® 100 Calorie Packs, Honey Maid Cinnamon Roll Thin Crisps	piece 0.46oz/13g	☺	☺ ☺	☹ 42½	4¾[A] 9¾
Nilla Wafers® (Nabisco®)	piece 0.14oz/3.75g	32½ +27 unit	☺ ☺	☺ ☺	12¼[A] 24¾
Nutter Butter® Cookies (Nabisco®)	portion 0.5oz/14g	☺	☺ ☺	☺ ☺	3½[A] 7¼

Sweet pastries	Unit	Lactose + unit/capsule	Fructose* Fructose	Sorbitol Sorbitol	FrucGalactans FrucGalactans
Oatmeal cookies, store bought	piece 0.46oz/13g	45¾ +38 unit	☺ ☺	☺ ☺	3¾ A 7½
Oreo® Brownie Cookies (Nabisco®)	piece 1.5oz/42.5g	☺	¼ ¼	☹ ☺	1 A 2¼
Oreo® Cookies (Nabisco®)	piece 0.43oz/12g	☺	☺ ☺	☹ ☺	4¼ A 8½
Oreo® Cookies, Sugar Free (Nabisco®)	piece 0.43oz/12g	☺	13¾ ☺	☹ ☹	4¼ A 8½
Pancake, buckwheat, from mix, add water only	piece 1.56oz/44g	☺	☺ ☺	☹ 3¾	1¼ A 2½
Pancake, whole wheat, homemade	piece 1.56oz/44g	2½ +2 unit	☺ ☺	☺ ☺	1 A 2¼
Peach pie, bottom crust only	piece 4.31oz/122g	☺	2¾ 5¾	☹ 1	¼ A ¾
Pepperidge Farm® Sweet & Simple, Soft Baked Sugar Cookies	piece 0.48oz/13.5g	☺	☹1 ☹1	☺ ☺	4¾ A 9½
Pepperidge Farm® Turnover, Apple	piece 3.14oz/89g	9 +7½ unit	½ ½	☹ ¼	½ A 1¼
Pillsbury® Big Deluxe White Chunk Macadamia Nut Cookies	piece 1.35oz/38g	6¾ +5½ unit	☺ ☺	☺ ☺	½ A 1¼
Popcorn, store bought (prepopped), "buttered"	portion 1.06oz/30g	36¾ +30¾ unit	☺ ☺	☺ ☺	☺ CB ☺
Rhubarb pie, bottom crust only	piece 4.31oz/122g	☺	☺ ☺	☺ ☺	¼ A ¾
Sandwich cookies, vanilla	piece 0.53oz/15g	9 +7½ unit	☺ ☺	☺ ☺	3 A 6¼
Sticky bun	piece 2.51oz/71g	8¾ +7¼ unit	☺+ ×¾ unit ☺+ ×¾ unit	☺ ☺	½ D 1
Strawberry pie, bottom crust only	piece 4.31oz/122g	☺	1¾ 2	☹ ¾	¼ A ¾
Sugar cookies, iced, store bought	piece 0.53oz/15g	☺	☺ ☺	☺ ☺	3¼ A 6½

Level 0: lactose measure ×½
Level 1: fructose measure ×2
Level 2: fructose-/sorbitol measure ×4. the rest ×2
Level 3: sorbitol measure ×7. the rest ×3
Book: source of fruc/galactans data

+ Unit/capsule: added tolerated amount of unit per strong lactase capsule
Fructose*: fructose, sorbitol adjusted
☺+ ×[Amount] unit: Per unit consumed you can additionally tolerate up to [amount] × fructose(*)-unit of another product.

☹: avoid; ☹1: ¼ at TL 1; ☹2: ¼ at TL 2; ☹3: ¼ at TL 3; ☺: only contains traces; ☺: is free from it

Sweet pastries	Unit	Lactose + unit/	Fructose* Fructose	Sorbitol Sorbitol	FrucGalactans FrucGalactans
Sweet potato bread	slice 1.49oz/42g	☺	☺ ☺	☺ ☺	1½[A] 3¼
Tiramisu	portion 1.95oz/55g	2½ +2 unit	☺ ☺	☺ ☺	13¾[A] 27¾
Twix®	piece 1.8oz/51g	2 +1¾ unit	☺+ ×1½ unit ☺+ ×1½ unit	☺ ☺	2[A] 4
Waffles, bran	piece 3.36oz/95g	¾ +¾ unit	☺+ ×¼ unit ☺+ ×¼ unit	☺ ☺	¼[A] ¾
Waffles, whole wheat, from mix, add milk, fat and egg	piece 3.36oz/95g	1 +¾ unit	☺+ ×¼ unit ☺+ ×¼ unit	☺ ☺	½[A] 1
Windmill cookies	piece(s) 0.75oz/21g	c	☺ ☺	☺ ☺	6¼[A] 12¾

3.4.7 Sweets

Sweets	Unit	Lactose 1 + unit/💊	Fructose* 0 Fructose 0	Sorbitol 0 Sorbitol 1	FrucGalactans 0 FrucGalactans 1 📖
3 Musketeers®	piece 2.14oz/60.4g	1¾ +1½ unit	☻+ ×3¾ unit ☻+ ×3¾ unit	☻ ☻	6¼ 12½
After Eight® Thin Chocolate Mints	piece 0.29oz/8g	10¼ +8½ unit	☻ ☻	☻ ☻	57¾ ☺
Almond paste (Marzipan)	portion 0.99oz/28g	☻	☺ ☺	☹ 20½	½ G 1¼
Almonds, honey roasted	hand 1.06oz/30g	☻	2 2	☹ 5½	½ G 1¼
Breath mint, regular	portion 0.08oz/2g	☻	☻+ ×¼ unit ☻+ ×¼ unit	☻ ☻	☻ ☻
Breath mint, sugar free	portion 0.08oz/2g	☻	¼ ☻	☹ ☹ 3	☻ ☻
Brown sugar	tbsp. 0.5oz/14.21ml	☻	☻ ☻	☻ ☻	☻ ☻
Buttermels® (Switzer's®)	piece 0.25oz/6.9g	8 +6½ unit	☻+ ×½ unit ☻+ ×½ unit	☻ ☻	44¾ 89¾
Candy necklace	piece 0.75oz/21g	☻	☻+ ×3¼ unit ☻+ ×3¼ unit	☻ ☻	☻ ☻
Chewing gum	piece 0.11oz/3g	☻	☻ ☻	☻ ☻	☻ ☻
Chewing gum, sugar free	piece 0.08oz/2g	☻	¼ ☻	☹ ☹ 2	☻ ☻
Chocolate truffles	piece 0.58oz/16.2g	2½ +2 unit	☻ ☻	☻ ☻	14¼ 28¾
Classic Fruit Chocolates (Liberty Orchards®)	piece 0.53oz/15g	56½ +47 unit	☻+ ×¼ unit ☻+ ×¼ unit	☹ 31½	☺ ☺
Coconut bars, nuts	piece 1.49oz/42g	45¼ +37¾ unit	☻ ☻	☻ ☻	☺ ☺
Dark chocolate bar 45%-59% cacoa	bar 4.77oz/135g	1¼ +1 unit	☻ ☻	☹ 8	¼ ¾

0 *Level 0:* lactose measure ×½
1 *Level 1:* fructose measure ×2
+ Unit/💊: added tolerated amount of unit per strong lactase capsule
Fructose*: fructose, sorbitol adjusted

2 *Level 2:* fructose-/sorbitol measure ×4. the rest ×2
3 *Level 3:* sorbitol measure ×7. the rest ×3
📖: source of fruc/galactans data
☻+ ×[Amount] unit: Per unit consumed you can additionally tolerate up to [amount] × fructose(*)-unit of another product.

☹: avoid; ☹ 1: ¼ at TL 1; ☹ 2: ¼ at TL 2; ☹ 3: ¼ at TL 3; ☺: only contains traces; ☻: is free from it

Sweets	Unit	Lactose + unit/	Fructose* Fructose	Sorbitol Sorbitol	FrucGalactans FrucGalactans
Dark chocolate bar 60%-69% cacao	bar 4.77oz/135g	7½ +6¼ unit	☺ ☺	☹ 6½	¼ ¾
Dark chocolate bar 70%-85% cacao	bar 4.77oz/135g	☺	☺ ☺	☹ 5	¼ ¾
Dark chocolate bar, sugar free	piece 0.43oz.fl/12g	26¾ +22¼ unit	34 34	☹ ☹	4¼ 8¾
Dark Fruit Chocolates (Liberty Orchards®)	piece 0.53oz/15g	56½ +47 unit	☺+ ×¼ unit ☺+ ×¼ unit	☹ 31½	☺ ☺
Dark Fruit Chocolates, Sugar Free (Liberty Orchards®)	piece 0.6oz/17g	37¾ +31¼ unit	☹[2] ☺	☹ ☹	☺ ☺
Fifty 50® Sugar Free Low Glycemic Butterscotch Hard Candy	piece 0.14oz/3.75g	☺	☺ ☺	☹ ☹	☺ ☺
French Burnt Peanuts	hand 1.06oz/30g	☺	☺+ ×1¾ unit ☺+ ×1¾ unit	☺ ☺	☺[G] ☺
Gelatin (jello) powder, flavored, sugar free	piece 0.18oz/5g	☺	☺ ☺	☺ ☺	☺ ☺
Gelatin (jello) powder, plain	piece 0.07oz/1.75g	☺	☺ ☺	☺ ☺	☺ ☺
Gum drops	hand 1.06oz/30g	☺	☺+ ×2¼ unit ☺+ ×2¼ unit	☺ ☺	☺ ☺
Gum drops, sugar free	tsp. 0.16ozfl/4.74ml	☺	☺ ☺	☹ ☹	☺ ☺
Gummi bears	hand 1.06oz/30g	☺	☺+ ×3½ unit ☺+ ×3½ unit	☹ ☺	☺ ☺
Gummi bears, sugar free	tsp. 0.16ozfl/4.74ml	☺	10 ☺	☹ ☹[3]	☺ ☺
Gummi dinosaurs	hand 1.06oz/30g	☺	☺+ ×3½ unit ☺+ ×3½ unit	☹ ☺	☺ ☺
Gummi dinosaurs, sugar free	tsp. 0.16ozfl/4.74ml	☺	10 ☺	☹ ☹[3]	☺ ☺
Gummi worms	hand 1.06oz/30g	☺	☺+ ×3½ unit ☺+ ×3½ unit	☹ ☺	☺ ☺
Gummi worms, sugar free	tsp. 0.16ozfl/4.74ml	☺	10 ☺	☹ ☹[3]	☺ ☺
Hard candy	piece 0.22oz/6g	☺	☺+ ×¾ unit ☺+ ×¾ unit	☺ ☺	☺ ☺
Hard candy, sugar free	piece 0.11oz/3g	☺	☹[1] ☺	☹ ☹	☺ ☺

Sweets	Unit	Lactose + unit/capsule	Fructose* Fructose	Sorbitol Sorbitol	FrucGalactans FrucGalactans
Hershey's® Caramel Filled Chocolates Sugar Free	piece 0.31oz/8.6g	74½ +62 unit	21¾ ☺	☹ ☹	☺ ☺
Hershey's® Milk Chocolate Bar	bar 4.77oz/135g	¼ +¼ unit	☺ ☺	☺ ☺	¼[G] ¾
Jelly beans®	hand 1.06oz/30g	☺	☺+ ×9¾ unit ☺+ ×9¾ unit	☺ ☺	☺ ☺
Jelly beans®, sugar free	tsp. 0.16ozfl/4.74ml	☺	12¼ ☺	☹ ☹	☺ ☺
Jujyfruits®	hand 1.06oz/30g	☺	☺+ ×12¼ unit ☺+ ×12¼ unit	☺ ☺	☺ ☺
Kit Kat®	piece 1.52oz/43g	2 +1¾ unit	☺ ☺	☹ ☺	2[A] 4¼
Kit Kat® White	piece 1.49oz/42g	¾ +½ unit	☺ ☺	☺ ☺	1½[A] 3¼
Licorice	piece 0.39oz/11g	☺	☺+ ×1½ unit ☺+ ×1½ unit	☺ ☺	☺ ☺
Little Debbie® Nutty Bars	piece 1.01oz/28.5g	☺	☺+ ×13¾ unit ☺+ ×13¾ unit	☹ ☺	4¼[A] 8½
M & M's® Peanut	portion 1.42oz/40g	2½ +2 unit	☺ ☺	☺ ☺	8¾ 17¾
Mamba® Fruit Chews	portion 1.42oz/40g	☺	☺ ☺+ ×22¼ unit	☹ ☹	☺ ☺
Mamba® Sour Fruit Chews	portion 1.42oz/40g	☺	☹[2] ☺+ ×17½ unit	☹ ☹	☺ ☺
Marshmallow	portion 1.06oz/30g	☺	☺+ ×4½ unit ☺+ ×4½ unit	☺ ☺	☺ ☺
Mentos®	piece 0.11oz/3g	☺	☺ ☺	☺ ☺	☺ ☺
Milk chocolate bar, cereal	bar 4.77oz/135g	½ +½ unit	☺ ☺	☹ 40	¼[A] ¾
Milk chocolate bar, cereal, sugar free	piece 0.43oz.fl/12g	26½ +22 unit	80 80	☹ ☹	4½[A] 9
Milk chocolate bar, sugar free	piece 0.43oz.fl/12g	32½ +27 unit	80 80	☹ ☹	4½ 9

Level 0: lactose measure ×½
Level 1: fructose measure ×2
Level 2: fructose-/sorbitol measure ×4. the rest ×2
Level 3: sorbitol measure ×7. the rest ×3
(book): source of fruc/galactans data

+ Unit/capsule: added tolerated amount of unit per strong lactase capsule
Fructose*: fructose, sorbitol adjusted
☺+ ×[Amount] unit: Per unit consumed you can additionally tolerate up to [amount] × fructose(*)-unit of another product.

☹: avoid; ☹[1]: ¼ at TL 1; ☹[2]: ¼ at TL 2; ☹[3]: ¼ at TL 3; ☺: only contains traces; ☺: is free from it

Sweets	Unit	Lactose + unit/	Fructose* Fructose	Sorbitol Sorbitol	FrucGalactans FrucGalactans
Milk chocolate bar, sugar free	piece 0.43oz.fl/12g	32½ +27 unit	80 80	☹ ☹	4½ 9
Milk Chocolate covered raisins	hand 1.06oz/30g	2¾ +2¼ unit	☺+ ×¼ unit ☺+ ×¼ unit	☹ 3¼	16 32
Molasses, dark	tbsp. 0.5oz/14.21ml	☺	3¾ 3¾	☺ ☺	☺ ☺
Nougat	bar 4.77oz/135g	☺	☺+ ×18 unit ☺+ ×18 unit	☺ ☺	☺ ☺
Pecan praline	piece 1.95oz/55g	3½ +2¾ unit	☺+ ×1¼ unit ☺+ ×1¼ unit	☺ ☺	19½ 39¼
Riesen®	piece 0.32oz/9g	12¾ +10½ unit	½ ☺+ ×2¾ unit	☹ ☹[3]	71 ☺
Smarties®	hand 1.06oz/30g	☺	☺+ ×55 unit ☺+ ×55 unit	☺ ☺	☺ ☺
Snickers®	piece 2.08oz/58.7g	1½ +1¼ unit	☺+ ×7 unit ☺+ ×7 unit	☺ ☺	8¾ 17½
Snickers®, Almond	piece 1.77oz/49.9g	1¾ +1½ unit	☺+ ×8¾ unit ☺+ ×8¾ unit	☺ ☺	6½[G] 13¼
Splenda®	portion 0oz/0g	☺	☺ ☺	☺ ☺	☺ ☺
Starburst®, Original	piece 0.18oz/5g	☺	☺+ ×½ unit ☺+ ×½ unit	☹ 30¼	☺ ☺
Suckers®, sugar free	piece 0.5oz/14g	☺	☹ ☺	☹ ☹	☺ ☺
Sugar, white granulated	tbsp. 0.5oz/14.21ml	☺	☺ ☺	☺ ☺	☺ ☺
Taffy	piece 0.31oz/8.6g	☺	☺+ ×4¼ unit ☺+ ×4¼ unit	☺ ☺	☺ ☺
Tic Tacs®	2 piece 0.05oz/1.15g	☺	☺ ☺	☺ ☺	☺ ☺
Toblerone® Swiss Dark Chocolate with Honey & Almond Nougat	piece 0.89oz/25g	7¼ +6 unit	☺ ☺	☹ 40	40¼ 80¾
Toblerone® Swiss Milk Chocolate with Honey & Almond Nougat	piece 0.89oz/25g	1½ +1¼ unit	☺ ☺	☺ ☺	8¾ 17½
Toblerone® Swiss White Confection with Honey & Almond Nougat	piece 0.89oz/25g	1 +1 unit	☺ ☺	☺ ☺	6¾ 13½

Sweets	Unit	Lactose L1 / + unit/(capsule)	Fructose* L0 / Fructose L0	Sorbitol L0 / Sorbitol L1	FrucGalactans L0 / FrucGalactans L1 📖
Toffee	piece 0.25oz/7g	40¾ +34 unit	😊 😊	😊 😊	☺ ☺
Toffifay®	piece 0.29oz/8.2g	7½ +6¼ unit	½ 😊+ ×¼ unit	☹ ☹²	42¾ 85½
Tootsie Pops®	piece 0.6oz/17g	😊	😊+ ×2½ unit 😊+ ×2½ unit	😊 😊	😊 😊
Werther's® Original Caramel Coffee Hard Candies	piece 0.15oz/4g	17¾ +14¾ unit	😊+ ×½ unit 😊+ ×½ unit	😊 😊	☺ ☺
White chocolate bar	piece 0.43oz.fl/12g	2½ +2 unit	😊 😊	😊 😊	14 28¼
Wild 'n Fruity Gummi Bears (Brach's®)	hand 1.06oz/30g	😊	😊+ ×3½ unit 😊+ ×3½ unit	☹ ☺	😊 😊
Zsweet®	portion 0.18oz/5g	😊	😊 😊	☹ ☹	😊 😊

L0 *Level 0:* lactose measure ×½
L1 *Level 1:* fructose measure ×2
L2 *Level 2:* fructose-/sorbitol measure ×4. the rest ×2
L3 *Level 3:* sorbitol measure ×7. the rest ×3
📖: source of fruc/galactans data

+ Unit/(capsule): added tolerated amount of unit per strong lactase capsule
Fructose*: fructose, sorbitol adjusted
😊+ ×[Amount] unit: Per unit consumed you can additionally tolerate up to [amount] × fructose(*)-unit of another product.

☹: avoid; ☹¹: ¼ at TL 1; ☹²: ¼ at TL 2; ☹³: ¼ at TL 3; ☺: only contains traces; 😊: is free from it

3.5 Warm dishes

3.5.1 Meals

Meals	Unit	Lactose + unit/	Fructose* Fructose	Sorbitol Sorbitol	FrucGalactans FrucGalactans
Arby's® macaroni and cheese	portion 7.66oz/217g	21½ +18 unit	☺ ☺	☺ ☺	½[A] 1¼
Asian noodle bowl, vegetables only	portion 7.06oz/200g	☺	☺+ ×1 unit ☺+ ×1 unit	☹ 10	1½[A] 3¼
Baby food, Gerber Graduates® Organic Pasta Pick-Ups Three Cheese Ravioli	Portion 170 g	88	☺ ☺	☺ ☺	¾[A] 1½
Beef with noodles soup, condensed	portion 4.45oz/126g	☺	☺ ☺	☹ 4¼	4[A] 8¼
Butternut squash soup	portion 8.65oz/245g	13½ +11¼ unit	☺ ☺	☹ 2½	½[G] 1
Calzone, cheese	piece 5.93oz/168g	12¼ +10¼ unit	☺ ☺	☹ 2¾	¼[A] ½
Casserole, pasta with turkey, gravy base, vegetables other than dark green, with cheese	portion 8.05oz/228g	3¾ +3 unit	☺ ☺	☹ 1¼	½[A] 1
Casserole rice with beef, tomato base, vegetables other than dark green, with cheese	portion 8.61oz/244g	9¾ +8¼ unit	☺+ ×1 unit ☺+ ×1 unit	☹ ¼	¼[A] ¾
Chicken and dumplings soup, condensed	portion 4.45oz/126g	7¼ +6 unit	☺ ☺	☹ 2¼	2¼ 4½
Chicken noodle soup with vegetables, ready-to-serve can	portion 8.65oz/245g	☺	☺ ☺	☹ 1	1¼ 2½
Chicken wonton soup, prepared from condensed can	portion 8.65oz/245g	☺	☺ ☺	☹ 40¾	☺ ☺
Chili with beans, beef, canned	tbsp. 0.5oz.fl/14.8ml	☺	☺ ☺	☹ 55½	3[AC] 6
Chop suey, chicken, no noodles	portion 5.86oz/166g	☺	☺ ☺	☹ ¼	¼[AB] ¾
Chop suey, tofu, no noodles	portion 5.86oz/166g	☺	☺ ☺	☹ ¼	☺ ☺
Cream of asparagus soup, prepared from condensed can	tbsp. 0.5ozfl/14.21ml	6½ +5½ unit	☺ ☺	☹ ☺	1½ 3
Cream of broccoli soup, condensed	portion 4.45oz/126g	5 +4¼ unit	☺ ☺	☹ 19¾	1[C] 2¼

Meals	Unit	Lactose + unit/	Fructose* Fructose	Sorbitol Sorbitol	FrucGalactans FrucGalactans
Cream of celery soup, home-made	portion 8.65oz/245g	½ +½ unit	☺ ☺	☹ ¼	¼ ½
Cream of chicken soup, con-densed	portion 4.45oz/126g	6½ +5½ unit	☺ ☺	☹ 26¼	37¼ CB 74¾
Cream of mushroom soup, prepared from condensed can	portion 8.65oz/245g	8½ +7 unit	☺ ☺	☹ ¼	½ 1
Cream of potato soup mix, dry	portion 0.82oz/23g	3¼ +2¾ unit	☺ ☺	☹ 3	5 10
Cream of spinach soup mix, dry	portion 0.57oz/16g	☺	☺+ ×¼ unit ☺+ ×¼ unit	☹ 18¼	☺ ☺
Dairy Queen® Foot Long Hot Dog	piece 7.02oz/199g	☺	☺+ ×1¾ unit ☺+ ×1¾ unit	☹ 8¼	¼ A ½
Fettuccini Alfredo®, no meat, vegetables other than dark green	tbsp. 0.5oz.l/14.21ml	66¾ +55½ unit	☺ ☺	☹ 2¾	81½ A ☺
Fettuccini Alfredo®, no meat, with carrots or dark green vegetables	portion 7.06oz/200g	5 +4 unit	☺ ☺	☺ ☺	27¾ 55½
Fruit sauce, jelly-based	portion 1.42oz/40g	☺	☺+ ×5¼ unit ☺+ ×5¼ unit	☹ ¾	☺ ☺
German style potato salad, with bacon and vinegar dress-ing	portion 4.94oz/140g	☺	☺+ ×¼ unit ☺+ ×¼ unit	☹ 4¾	1 CB 2
Green pea soup, prepared from condensed can	tbsp. 0.5ozfl/14.21ml	☺	☺ ☺	☹ 20	3¼ AC 6¾
Hardee's® Loaded Omelet Biscuit	piece 5.58oz/158g	12 +10 unit	☺+ ×9¼ unit ☺+ ×9¼ unit	☺ ☺	¼ A ½
Lasagna, homemade, beef	portion 4.94oz/140g	23¼ +19¼ unit	☺+ ×¼ unit ☺+ ×¼ unit	☹ 1	¾ A 1½
Lasagna, homemade, cheese, no vegetables	portion 4.94oz/140g	25¾ +21½ unit	11 12¼	☹ ¾	¾ A 1½
Lasagna, homemade, spinach, no meat	portion 4.94oz/140g	8½ +7 unit	9¾ 11	☹ ½	¾ A 1½

Level 0: lactose measure ×½
Level 1: fructose measure ×2
Level 2: fructose-/sorbitol measure ×4. the rest ×2
Level 3: sorbitol measure ×7. the rest ×3
: source of fruc/galactans data

+ Unit/: added tolerated amount of unit per strong lactase capsule
Fructose*: fructose, sorbitol adjusted
☺+ ×[Amount] unit: Per unit consumed you can additionally tolerate up to [amount] × fructose(*)-unit of another product.

☹: avoid; ☹[1]: ¼ at TL 1; ☹[2]: ¼ at TL 2; ☹[3]: ¼ at TL 3; ☺: only contains traces; ☺: is free from it

Meals	Unit	Lactose + unit/	Fructose* Fructose	Sorbitol Sorbitol	FrucGalactans FrucGalactans
Lentil soup, condensed	portion 4.45oz/126g	☺	☺ ☺	☹ 1	5½[AC] 11¼
Lyonnaise (potatoes and onions)	portion 2.47oz/70g	☺	☺ ☺	☹ 15¾	☺ ☺
Macaroni or pasta salad, with meat, egg, mayo dressing	portion 4.94oz/140g	☺	☺+ ×¼ unit ☺+ ×½ unit	☹ 1¼	☺[A] ☺
Meat ravioli, with tomato sauce	portion 8.82oz/250g	☺	☺+ ×½ unit ☺+ ×½ unit	☹ ½	¼[A] ¾
Minestrone soup, condensed	portion 4.45oz/126g	☺	☺ ☺	☹ ¾	½ 1
Minestrone soup, homemade	portion 8.65oz/245g	☺	☺ ☺	☹ 1	¼ ½
Noodle soup mix, dry	portion 0.57oz/16g	☺	☺+ ×¼ unit ☺+ ×¼ unit	☺ ☺	☺ ☺
Omelet, made with bacon	portion 3.89oz/110g	34¾ +29 unit	☺+ ×1¾ unit ☺+ ×1¾ unit	☺ ☺	☺ ☺
Omelet, made with sausage, potatoes, onions, cheese	portion 3.89oz/110g	52¼ +43½ unit	☺+ ×1 unit ☺+ ×1 unit	☹ 6¾	¼[CB] ½
Pad thai, without meat	portion 4.94oz/140g	☺	☺ ☺	☹ 3¾	☺[A] ☺
Paella	portion 8.47oz/240g	☺	2¼ 2¼	☹ 2¼	1 2
Pasta salad with vegetables, Italian dressing	portion 4.94oz/140g	☺	3¾ 3¾	☹ 1½	1½[A] 3¼
Pho soup (Vietnamese noodle soup)	portion 8.65oz/245g	☺	☺ ☺	☹ 6¾	¾ 1¾
Pizza Hut® cheese bread stick	piece 1.98oz/56g	61½ +51¼ unit	☺+ ×¼ unit ☺+ ×¼ unit	☺ ☺	1¼[A] 2½
Pizza Hut® Pepperoni Lover's pizza, stuffed crust	portion 4.94oz/140g	30 +25 unit	☺ ☺	☹ 1	¾[A] 1½
Pizza Hut® Personal Pan, supreme	piece 9.03oz/256g	16¾ +14 unit	☺ ☺	☹ ¼	4¾[A] 9½
Pizza, homemade or restaurant, cheese, thin crust	piece 7.38oz/209g	12¼ +10¼ unit	☺+ ×¾ unit ☺+ ×¾ unit	☹ ¾	½[A] 1
Potato salad, with egg, mayo dressing	portion 4.94oz/140g	☺	☺+ ×½ unit ☺+ ×½ unit	☹ 2	1[CB] 2
Potato soup with broccoli and cheese	portion 8.65oz/245g	29¾ +24¾ unit	☺ ☺	☹ 13½	½[AC] 1
Ratatouille	portion 3.89oz/110g	☺	☺ ☺	☹ 1¼	4[B] 8

Meals	Unit	Lactose + unit/capsule	Fructose* Fructose	Sorbitol Sorbitol	FrucGalactans FrucGalactans 🕮
Red beans and rice soup mix, dry	portion 1.8oz/51g	☺	¼ ¼	☹ ¼	1¼ AC 2¾
Scrambled egg with bacon	portion 3.89oz/110g	2¼ +1¾ unit	☺+ ×1¾ unit ☺+ ×1¾ unit	☺ ☺	12½ 25¼
Sesame chicken	portion 8.89oz/252g	☺	☺ ☺	☹ 3¾	☺ ☺
Soup base	tbsp. 0.5oz/14.21ml	☺	64 64	☹ 74	☺ ☺
Spaghetti, with carbonara sauce	portion 7.09oz/201g	13½ +11¼ unit	☺+ ×¾ unit ☺+ ×¾ unit	☹ 6	½ A 1
Spinach ravioli, with tomato sauce	portion 8.82oz/250g	5½ +4½ unit	☺+ ×¼ unit ☺+ ×¼ unit	☹ ½	½ A 1
Spring roll	portion 4.94oz/140g	☺	21 21	☹ 2¾	¼ ½
Squash or pumpkin ravioli, with cream sauce	portion 8.82oz/250g	½ +½ unit	☺+ ×¼ unit ☺+ ×¼ unit	☹ 40	½ A 1
Stewed green peas with sofrito	tbsp. 0.5oz.fl/14.8ml	☺ +2¾ unit	☺ ☺	☹ 5½	1¼ AB 2½
Sushi, with fish	portion 4.94oz/140g	☺	10½ 32¼	☹ 2½	☺ ☺
Sushi, with fish and vegetables in seaweed	portion 4.94oz/140g	☺	☺ ☺	☹ 2	☺ ☺
Sushi, with vegetables in seaweed	portion 4.94oz/140g	☺	☺ ☺	☹ 1½	☺ ☺
Swedish Meatballs	portion 4.94oz/140g	1½ +1¼ unit	☺ ☺	☹ 71¼	9 18
Sweet and sour chicken	tbsp. 0.5ozfl/14.21ml	☺	2½ 2½	☹ ☺	☺ ☺
Taco Bell® 7-Layer Burrito	portion 4.94oz/140g	25½ +21¼ unit	☺ ☺	☹ 5¾	¼ A ¾
Taco Bell® Crunchwrap Supreme	piece 8.65oz/245g	4¼ +3½ unit	☺ ☺	☹ 5	☹ A ¼
Taco Bell® Mexican Pizza	piece 7.52oz/213g	13¾ +11½ unit	23¼ 29¼	☹ 1	¼ A ¾

Level 0: lactose measure ×½
Level 1: fructose measure ×2
Level 2: fructose-/sorbitol measure ×4. the rest ×2
Level 3: sorbitol measure ×7. the rest ×3
🕮: source of fruc/galactans data

+ Unit/capsule: added tolerated amount of unit per strong lactase capsule
Fructose*: fructose, sorbitol adjusted
☺+ ×[Amount] unit: Per unit consumed you can additionally tolerate up to [amount] × fructose(*)-unit of another product.

☹: avoid; ☹[1]: ¼ at TL 1; ☹[2]: ¼ at TL 2; ☹[3]: ¼ at TL 3; ☺: only contains traces; ☺: is free from it

Meals	**Unit**	**Lactose** **+ unit/**	**Fructose*** **Fructose**	**Sorbitol** **Sorbitol**	**FrucGalactans** **FrucGalactans**
Taco Bell® Nachos Supreme	portion 4.94 oz/140g	6¼ +5¼ unit	☺ ☺	☹ 7¾	35¾ [B] 71½
Taco, soft corn shell, with beans, cheese	portion 4,94 oz/140g	☺ +77 unit	12¾ 13	☺ 4¼	¼ [A] ½
Tomato relish	portion 0.53 oz/15g	☺	☺ ☺	☹ 5¼	33 66¼
Tomato soup mix, dry	portion 1.2 oz/34g	¼ +0.24 unit	13 13¾	☹ 2	1¼ [B] 2¾
Vegetable soup, condensed	portion 4.45 oz/126g	☺	☺+ ×¼ unit ☺+ ×¼ unit	☹ 1	19¾ 39½
Vichyssoise soup	portion 8.65 oz/245g	¾ +½ unit	☺+ ×¼ unit ☺+ ×¼ unit	☹ 1¼	4¼ [AB] 8½
Wendy's® Strawberry Shake	glass 8.4 oz/240g	¼ +¼ unit	☺+ ×4¼ unit ☺+ ×4¼ unit	☹ 3¼	1¾ 3¾
White bean stew with sofrito	tbsp. 0.5ozfl/14.21ml	☺	☺ ☺	☹ ☺	3 [AC] 6

3.5.2 Meat and fish

Meat and fish	Unit	Lactose 1 + unit/💊	Fructose* 0 Fructose 0	Sorbitol 0 Sorbitol 1	FrucGalactans 0 FrucGalactans 1 📖
Arby's® Chicken Cordon Bleu Sandwich, crispy	portion 4.94oz/140g	32¼ +27 unit	2 2	😀 😀	1[A] 2¼
Beef bacon (kosher)	portion 0.53oz/15g	😀	😀 😀	😀 😀	😀 😀
Beef steak, chuck, visible fat eaten	portion 3oz/85g	😀	😀 😀	😀 😀	😀 😀
Boston Market® 1/4 white rotisserie chicken, with skin	portion 3oz/85g	😀	😀 😀	😀 😀	😀 😀
Boston Market® roasted turkey breast	portion 3oz/85g	😀	😀 😀	😀 😀	😀 😀
Bratwurst	portion 1.95oz/55g	😀	😀+ ×¼ unit 😀+ ×¼ unit	😀 😀	😀 😀
Bratwurst, beef	portion 1.95oz/55g	😀	😀+ ×1 unit 😀+ ×1 unit	😀 😀	😀 😀
Bratwurst, light (reduced fat)	portion 1.95oz/55g	😀	😀+ ×2¾ unit 😀+ ×2¾ unit	😀 😀	😀 😀
Bratwurst, made with beer	portion 1.95oz/55g	😀	😀+ ×¼ unit 😀+ ×¼ unit	☹ ☺	😀 😀
Bratwurst, made with beer, cheese-filled	portion 1.95oz/55g	☺	😀+ ×½ unit 😀+ ×½ unit	☹ ☺	☺ ☺
Bratwurst, turkey	portion 1.95oz/55g	😀	😀+ ×1½ unit 😀+ ×1½ unit	😀 😀	😀 😀
Braunschweiger (liver sausage)	portion 1.95oz/55g	😀	😀 😀	😀 😀	😀 😀
Caviar	tbsp. 0.5oz/14.21ml	😀	😀 😀	😀 😀	😀 😀
Chicken fricassee with gravy, American style	portion 8.61oz/244g	😀	😀 😀	😀 😀	5¾[C] 11½
Clams, stuffed with mushroom, onions, and bread	portion 4.94oz/140g	24½ +20½ unit	😀 😀	☹ ½	3¼[CB] 6¾

0 *Level 0:* lactose measure ×½
1 *Level 1:* fructose measure ×2
2 *Level 2:* fructose-/sorbitol measure ×4. the rest ×2
3 *Level 3:* sorbitol measure ×7. the rest ×3
📖: source of fruc/galactans data

+ Unit/💊: added tolerated amount of unit per strong lactase capsule
Fructose*: fructose, sorbitol adjusted
😀+ ×[Amount] unit: Per unit consumed you can additionally tolerate up to [amount] × fructose(*)-unit of another product.

☹: avoid; ☹[1]: ¼ at TL 1; ☹[2]: ¼ at TL 2; ☹[3]: ¼ at TL 3; ☺: only contains traces; 😀: is free from it

Meat and fish	Unit	Lactose + unit/	Fructose* Fructose	Sorbitol Sorbitol	FrucGalactans FrucGalactans
Fish croquette	portion 3oz/85g	2¼ +1¾ unit	☺ ☺	☹ ☺	1¾ A 3½
Fish sticks, patties, or nuggets, breaded, regular	portion 3oz/85g	☺	☺ ☺	☺ ☺	2 A 4
Fish with breading	portion 3oz/85g	☺	☺ ☺	☺ ☺	☺ ☺
Gorton's® Battered Fish Fillets - Lemon Pepper	portion 3oz/85g	☺	☺ ☺	☺ ☺	☺ ☺
Gorton's® Popcorn Shrimp, Original	portion 3oz/85g	☺	☺ ☺	☺ ☺	2 A 4
Goulash, with beef, noodles or macaroni, tomato base	tbsp. 0.5ozfl/14.21ml	☺	☺ ☺	☹ 4	☺ ☺
Herring, pickled	portion 1.95oz/55g	☺	☺ ☺	☺ ☺	☺ ☺
Herring, pickled	portion 1.95oz/55g	☺	☺ ☺	☺ ☺	6 12
Liver pudding	portion 1.95oz/55g	☺	☺ ☺	☺ ☺	☺ ☺
Mrs. Paul's® Calamari Rings	portion 3oz/85g	☺	☺ ☺	☺ ☺	2¼ A 4½
Pickled beef	portion 1.95oz/55g	☺	☺ ☺	☺ ☺	☺ ☺
Pork cutlet (sirloin cutlet), visible fat eaten	portion 3oz/85g	☺	☺ ☺	☺ ☺	1¼ A 2¾
Ribs, beef, spare, visible fat eaten	portion 3oz/85g	☺	☺ ☺	☺ ☺	☺ ☺
Salami, beer or beerwurst, beef	portion 1.95oz/55g	☺	☺+ ×1 unit ☺+ ×1 unit	☺ ☺	☺ ☺
Salmon, red (sockeye), smoked	portion 1.95oz/55g	☺	☺ ☺	☺ ☺	☺ ☺
Sauerbraten	portion 5.61oz/159g	☺	34¾ 34¾	☺ ☺	☺ ☺
Scallops	portion 3oz/85g	☺	☺ ☺	☺ ☺	☺ ☺
Sea Pak® Seasoned Shrimp, Roasted Garlic	portion 3oz/85g	☺	☺ ☺	☺ ☺	☺ ☺
Sea Pak® Shrimp Scampi in Italian Parmesan Sauce	portion 3oz/85g	☺	☺ ☺	☺ ☺	☺ ☺
Tuna, canned, light, oil pack, not drained	portion 1.95oz/55g	☺	☺ ☺	☺ ☺	☺ ☺

Meat and fish	Unit	Lactose [1] + unit/💊	Fructose* [0] Fructose [0]	Sorbitol [0] Sorbitol [1]	FrucGalactans [0] FrucGalactans [1] 📖
Venison or deer, stewed	portion 3oz/85g	😊	😊 😊	😊 😊	☺ ☺

3.5.3 Lactose hideouts

Sauces and spices	Unit	Lactose [1] + unit/💊	Fructose* [0] Fructose [0]	Sorbitol [0] Sorbitol [1]	FrucGalactans [0] FrucGalactans [1] 📖
Casserole (hot dish), chicken with pasta, cream or white sauce, with cheese	portion 8.4oz/238g	½ +½ unit	☺ ☺	😊 😊	😊 😊
Chicken cake or patty	portion 3oz/85g	1½ +1¼ unit	14 14	☹ 58¾	3¼ [B] 6½
Chicken with cheese sauce, vegetables other than dark green	portion 7.62oz/216g	1 +¾ unit	5 23	☹ ½	😊 😊
Creamed chicken	portion 8.51oz/241g	½ +¼ unit	😊 😊	☹ 13¾	😊 😊
Fish croquette	portion 3oz/85g	2¼ +1¾ unit	😊 😊	☹ ☺	😊 😊
Fish or seafood with cream or white sauce	portion 6.39oz/181g	1½ +1¼ unit	😊 😊	😊 😊	😊 😊
Ham croquette	portion 3oz/85g	2¼ +1¾ unit	😊 😊	☹ ☺	😊 😊
Loaf cold cut, spiced	portion 1.95oz/55g	2¼ +1¾ unit	😊+ ×¼ unit 😊+ ×¼ unit	😊 😊	😊 😊
Meatloaf, pork	portion 3oz/85g	2¼ +2 unit	😊+ ×¼ unit 😊+ ×¼ unit	☹ 3½	😊 😊
Meatloaf, tuna	portion 3oz/85g	5½ +4½ unit	😊 😊	☹ 14½	😊 😊
Souffle, meat	portion 3.89oz/110g	1¼ +1 unit	😊+ ×½ unit 😊+ ×½ unit	☹ ☺	1¾ [B] 3¾
Swedish Meatballs	portion 4.94oz/140g	1½ +1¼ unit	😊 😊	☹ 71¼	9 18

[0] *Level 0:* lactose measure ×½
[1] *Level 1:* fructose measure ×2
[2] *Level 2:* fructose-/sorbitol measure ×4. the rest ×2
[3] *Level 3:* sorbitol measure ×7. the rest ×3
📖: source of fruc/galactans data

+ Unit/💊: added tolerated amount of unit per strong lactase capsule
Fructose*: fructose, sorbitol adjusted
😊+ ×[Amount] unit: Per unit consumed you can additionally tolerate up to [amount] × fructose(*)-unit of another product.

☹: avoid; ☹[1]: ¼ at TL 1; ☹[2]: ¼ at TL 2; ☹[3]: ¼ at TL 3; ☺: only contains traces; 😊: is free from it

3.5.4 Sauces and spices

Sauces and spices	Unit	Lactose + unit/	Fructose* Fructose	Sorbitol Sorbitol	FrucGalactans FrucGalactans
Arby's® ranch sauce	tbsp. 0.5oz/14.21ml	☺	☺ ☺	☹ 18½	☺ ☺
Balsamic vinegar	portion 0.53oz/15g	☺	☺ ☺	☹ 23	☺ ☺
Barbeque sauce (BBQ), store bought	pinch 0.04oz/1g	☺	☺ ☺	☹ 76¾	☺ ☺
Basil, fresh	pinch 0.04oz/1g	☺	☺ ☺	☺ ☺	☺ ☺
Beef gravy, canned	portion 2.05oz/58g	☺	☺ ☺	☹ ☺	☺ ☺
Bertolli® Classico Olive Oil	portion 0.46oz/13g	☺	☺ ☺	☺ ☺	☺ ☺
Black pepper, ground	pinch 0.04oz/1g	☺	☺ ☺	☺ ☺	☺ ☺
Bouillon, unprepared	portion 0.29oz/8g	☺	☺ ☺	☹ ☺	☺ ☺
Capers	pinch 0.04oz/1g	☺	☺ ☺	☹ 70¼	☺ ☺
Caramel sauce, store bought, fat free	portion 1.45oz/41g	6 +5 unit	☺+ ×6 unit ☺+ ×6 unit	☺ ☺	33¾ 67¾
Chili sauce, store bought	portion 2.4oz/68g	☺	2¾ 2¾	☹ ¼	☺ ☺
Chinese oyster sauce	portion 1.13oz/32g	☺	☺ ☺	☺ ☺	☺ ☺
Chives, raw	pinch 0.04oz/1g	☺	☺ ☺	☺ ☺	☺ B ☺
Chocolate sauce, syrup	tbsp. 0.5oz/14.21ml	☺	☺+ ×1½ unit ☺+ ×1½ unit	☹ ☺	☺ ☺
Cider vinegar	portion 0.5oz/14g	☺	6¼ 16½	☹ 1¾	☺ ☺
Cilantro leaf, fresh	pinch 0.04oz/1g	☺	☺ ☺	☺ ☺	☺ ☺
Cocktail sauce	portion 2.4oz/68g	☺	☺+ ×2 unit ☺+ ×2 unit	☹ ¾	☺ ☺
Coconut oil	pinch 0.04oz/1g	☺	☺ ☺	☺ ☺	☺ ☺

Sauces and spices	Unit	Lactose (Level 1) + unit/capsule	Fructose* (Level 0) Fructose (Level 0)	Sorbitol (Level 0) Sorbitol (Level 1)	FrucGalactans (Level 0) FrucGalactans (Level 1) 📖
Crisco® Pure Corn Oil	portion 0.46oz/13g	☻	☻ ☻	☻ ☻	☻ ☻
Curry sauce, from cream	portion 2.09oz/59g	2 +1½ unit	☻ ☻	☹ 4	11¼ 22½
Dijon mustard	tbsp. 0.5oz/14.21ml	☻	☻ ☻	☹ ☺	☻ ☻
Distilled vinegar	portion 0.5oz/14g	☻	☻ ☻	☻ ☻	☻ ☻
Flax seed oil	portion 0.46oz/13g	☻	☻ ☻	☻ ☻	☻ ☻
French onion soup, condensed	portion 4.45oz/126g	☺	☻+ ×1½ unit ☻+ ×1½ unit	☹ 2	¼[CB] ¾
Gardenburger® Sun-Dried Tomato Basil	portion 3oz/85g	☺	1¼ 1¼	☹ 1	7¾[B] 15¾
Garlic sauce	tbsp. 0.5oz/14.21ml	☺	☻ ☻	☻ ☻	☹[FB] ☹
Garlic, powder	pinch 0.04oz/1g	☻	☺ ☺	☻ ☻	3¼[FB] 6½
Ginger sauce, Asian style	portion 1.13oz/32g	☻	☻ ☻	☹ 9¼	☻[B] ☻
Ginger, ground	pinch 0.04oz/1g	☻	89¼ 89¼	☻ ☻	☻[B] ☻
Girard's® Wasabi and Ginger Vinaigrette	pinch 0.04oz/1g	☻	☺ ☺	☹ ☺	☻[B] ☻
Hamburger gravy	portion 7.17oz/203g	☻	☻ ☻	☹ 12¼	☻ ☻
Heinz® 57 sauce®	portion 0.53oz/15g	☻	☻+ ×¼ unit ☻+ ×½ unit	☹ 3¾	☻ ☻
Hollandaise sauce, store bought	tbsp. 0.5oz/14.21ml	5 +4¼ unit	☻ ☻	☻ ☻	28½ 57
Horseradish	pinch 0.04oz/1g	☻	☻ ☻	☻ ☻	☻ ☻
Ketchup	portion 0.53oz/15g	☻	☻+ ×¼ unit ☻+ ×¼ unit	☹ 3¾	☻ ☻

(Level 0) *Level 0:* lactose measure ×½
(Level 1) *Level 1:* fructose measure ×2
(Level 2) *Level 2*: fructose-/sorbitol measure ×4. the rest ×2
(Level 3) *Level 3:* sorbitol measure ×7. the rest ×3
📖: source of fruc/galactans data

+ Unit/capsule: added tolerated amount of unit per strong lactase capsule
Fructose*: fructose, sorbitol adjusted

☻+ ×[Amount] unit: Per unit consumed you can additionally tolerate up to [amount] × fructose(*)-unit of another product.

☹: avoid; ☹[1]: ¼ at TL 1; ☹[2]: ¼ at TL 2; ☹[3]: ¼ at TL 3; ☺: only contains traces; ☻: is free from it

Sauces and spices	Unit	Lactose + unit/	Fructose* Fructose	Sorbitol Sorbitol	FrucGalactans FrucGalactans
Ketchup, low sodium	portion 0.53oz/15g	☺	☺+ ×¼ unit ☺+ ×¼ unit	☹ 4¼	☺ ☺
Kraft® Balsamic Vinaigrette	portion 1.06oz/30g	☺	☺ ☺	☹ 22	☺ ☺
Kraft® Classic Caesar Dressing	portion 1.06oz/30g	☺	☺+ ×½ unit ☺+ ×½ unit	☹ 12¼	☺ ☺
Kraft® Creamy French Dressing	portion 1.06oz/30g	☺	64 64	☹ ☺	☺ ☺
Kraft® Creamy Italian Dressing	portion 1.06oz/30g	☺	☺+ ×¾ unit ☺+ ×¾ unit	☺ ☺	☺ ☺
Kraft® Fat Free Mayonnaise	portion 0.53oz/15g	☺	☺ ☺	☺ ☺	☺ ☺
Kraft® Free Sour Cream & Onion Ranch Dressing , fat free	portion 1.06oz/30g	☺	4½ 4½	☺ ☺	☺ ☺
Kraft® Mayo with Olive Oil, Reduced Fat	portion 0.53oz/15g	☺	☺ ☺	☺ ☺	☺ ☺
Kraft® Miracle Whip® Free Nonfat Dressing	tbsp. 0.5oz/14.21ml	80 +66½ unit	☺ ☺	☺ ☺	☺ ☺
Kraft® Miracle Whip® Light Dressing	tbsp. 0.5oz/14.21ml	☺	☺ ☺	☺ ☺	☺ ☺
Kraft® Miracle Whip® Salad Dressing	tbsp. 0.5oz/14.21ml	☺	☺ ☺	☺ ☺	☺ ☺
Kraft® Sandwich Spread	tbsp. 0.5oz/14.21ml	☺	☺ ☺	☹ ☺	☺ ☺
Kraft® Thousand Island Dressing®	tbsp. 0.5oz/14.21ml	☺	☺+ ×¼ unit ☺+ ×¼ unit	☺ ☺	☺ ☺
Lemon butter sauce	tbsp. 0.5oz/14.21ml	☺	☺ ☺	☹ 60½	☺ ☺
Long John Silver's® tartar sauce	tbsp. 0.5oz/14.21ml	☺	☺ ☺	☹ ☺	☺ ☺
Mushroom gravy, canned	tbsp. 0.5oz/14.21ml	75¼ +62¾ unit	☺ ☺	☹ 2¼	☺ ☺
Oregano, dried	pinch 0.04oz/1g	☺	☺ ☺	☺ ☺	☺ ☺
Palm kernel oil	tbsp. 0.5oz/14.21ml	☺	☺ ☺	☺ ☺	☺ ☺
Parsley, fresh	pinch 0.04oz/1g	☺	☺ ☺	☹ ☺	☺ ☺
Peanut sauce, store bought	portion 1.24oz/35g	☺	☺ ☺	☹ 8¼	☺[G] ☺

Sauces and spices	Unit	Lactose + unit/capsule	Fructose* Fructose	Sorbitol Sorbitol	FrucGalactans FrucGalactans
Peppermint, fresh	pinch 0.04oz/1g	☻	☻ ☻	☻ ☻	☻ ☻
Pesto sauce, store bought	portion 2.19oz/62g	☺	☺ ☺	☻ ☻	1¾[A] 3¾
Pumpkin seed oil	portion 0.46oz/13g	☻	☻ ☻	☻ ☻	☻ ☻
Red pepper (cayenne), ground	pinch 0.04oz/1g	☻	51 51	☻ ☻	☻ ☻
Red wine vinegar	tbsp. 0.5oz/14.21ml	☻	☺ ☻	☹ 20	☻ ☻
Rosemary, dried	pinch 0.04oz/1g	☻	☻ ☻	☻ ☻	☻ ☻
Safflower oil	portion 0.46oz/13g	☻	☻ ☻	☻ ☻	☻ ☻
Salsa, store bought	tbsp. 0.5oz/14.21ml	☻	6¼ 6¼	☹ 6¾	5½ 11¼
Scallions or spring onions, raw or blanched, tops and bulbs, marinated in oil	piece 0.56oz/15.7g	☻	☻+ ×¼ unit ☻+ ×¼ unit	☹ 6	¼[G] ¾
Soy sauce	tbsp. 0.5oz/14.21ml	☻	☻ ☻	☹ 4½	3[A] 6
Soybean oil, unhydrogenated	tbsp. 0.5oz/14.21ml	☻	☻ ☻	☻ ☻	☻ ☻
Subway® honey mustard sauce, fat free	portion 0.99oz/28g	☻	4¾ 4¾	☻ ☻	☻ ☻
Sunflower oil	tbsp. 0.5oz/14.21ml	☻	☻ ☻	☻ ☻	☻ ☻
Sweet and sour sauce, store bought	tbsp. 0.5oz/14.21ml	☻	½ ½	☹ 83¼	☻ ☻
Tabasco® sauce	tbsp. 0.5oz/14.21ml	☻	☻ ☻	☻ ☻	☻ ☻
Taco sauce, red	portion 1.13oz/32g	☻	2¾ 2¾	☹ 3	11 22

Level 0: lactose measure ×½
Level 1: fructose measure ×2
+ Unit/capsule: added tolerated amount of unit per strong lactase capsule
Fructose*: fructose, sorbitol adjusted
Level 2: fructose-/sorbitol measure ×4. the rest ×2
Level 3: sorbitol measure ×7. the rest ×3
📖: source of fruc/galactans data
☻+ ×[Amount] unit: Per unit consumed you can additionally tolerate up to [amount] × fructose(*)-unit of another product.
☹: avoid; ☹[1]: ¼ at TL 1; ☹[2]: ¼ at TL 2; ☹[3]: ¼ at TL 3; ☺: only contains traces; ☻: is free from it

Sauces and spices	Unit	Lactose + unit/	Fructose* Fructose	Sorbitol Sorbitol	FrucGalactans FrucGalactans
Tahini (sesame butter)	portion 1.06oz/30g	☺	☺ ☺	☺ ☺	☺[G] ☺
Thyme, dried	pinch 0.04oz/1g	☺	☺ ☺	☺ ☺	☺ ☺
Tomato sauce	portion 2.12oz/60g	☺	☺+ ×¾ unit ☺+ ×¾ unit	☹ ¾	9¼[B] 18½
Tzatziki sauce (yogurt and cucumber)	portion 1.06oz/30g	4½ +3¾ unit	38¾ 38¾	☹ 9¼	11½[FB] 23¼
Vanilla sauce	tbsp. 0.5oz/14.21ml	☺	☺ ☺	☺ ☺	☺ ☺
Walnut oil	tbsp. 0.5oz/14.21ml	☺	☺ ☺	☺ ☺	☺ ☺
Watercress, raw	pinch 0.04oz/1g	☺	☺ ☺	☺ ☺	☺ ☺
White sauce, store bought	tbsp. 0.5oz/14.21ml	4 +3¼ unit	☺ ☺	☺ ☺	22¼ 44½

3.5.5 Side dishes

Side dishes	Unit	Lactose + unit/capsule	Fructose* Fructose	Sorbitol Sorbitol	FrucGalactans FrucGalactans 📖
Au gratin potato, prepared from fresh	portion 4.94oz/140g	1 +¾ unit	☺ ☺	☹ 7¾	6¼ B 12½
Basmati rice, cooked in unsalted water	portion 4.94oz/140g	☺	☺ ☺	☺ ☺	☺ A ☺
Boston Market® sweet corn	portion 3oz/85g	☺	☺+ ×¼ unit ☺+ ×½ unit	☹ 4	☺ B ☺
Bulgur, home cooked	portion 4.94oz/140g	☺	☺ ☺	☺ ☺	☺ ☺
Cheese gnocchi	portion 2.47oz/70g	28 +23¼ unit	☺ ☺	☺ ☺	1 A 2¼
Couscous, cooked	portion 4.94oz/140g	☺	☺ ☺	☺ ☺	¼ A ¾
Falafel	portion 1.95oz/55g	☺	☺ ☺	☹ 1¾	☺ G ☺
Fettuccini noodles, whole wheat, cooked in unsalted water	portion 4.94oz/140g	☺	☺+ ×¼ unit ☺+ ×¼ unit	☺ ☺	1 A 2
Garbanzo beans (chickpeas), canned, drained	portion 3.18oz/90g	☺	☺ ☺	☹ 1	1½ A 3
Green peas, raw	tbsp. 0.5ozfl/14.21ml	☺	9½ 12¼	☹ 3½	1¼ A 2½
Kidney beans, cooked from dried	portion 3.18oz/90g	☺	☺ ☺	☺ ☺	¼ A ½
Lentils, cooked from dried	portion 3.18oz/90g	☺	☺ ☺	☺ ☺	¾ A 1½
Plain dumplings for stew, biscuit type	portion 1.95oz/55g	1¾ +1½ unit	☺ ☺	☺ ☺	½ A 1
Polenta	portion 8.47oz/240g	½ +½ unit	☺+ ×¼ unit ☺+ ×¼ unit	☹ 20¾	3¼ B 6¾
Potato dumpling (Kartoffelkloesse)	portion 4.94oz/140g	45½ +37¾ unit	☺+ ×¼ unit ☺+ ×¼ unit	☹ 35½	☺ C ☺

Level 0: lactose measure ×½
Level 1: fructose measure ×2
Level 2: fructose-/sorbitol measure ×4. the rest ×2
Level 3: sorbitol measure ×7. the rest ×3
📖: source of fruc/galactans data

+ Unit/capsule: added tolerated amount of unit per strong lactase capsule
Fructose*: fructose, sorbitol adjusted

☺+ ×[Amount] unit: Per unit consumed you can additionally tolerate up to [amount] × fructose(*)-unit of another product.

☹: avoid; ☹[1]: ¼ at TL 1; ☹[2]: ¼ at TL 2; ☹[3]: ¼ at TL 3; ☺: only contains traces; ☺: is free from it

Side dishes	Unit	Lactose + unit/(capsule)	Fructose* Fructose	Sorbitol Sorbitol	FrucGalactans FrucGalactans
Potato gnocchi	portion 6.64oz/188g	2½ +2 unit	☺ ☺	☺ ☺	14[A] 28¼
Potato pancakes	portion 2.47oz/70g	☺	☺+ ×½ unit ☺+ ×½ unit	☹ 12¾	☺[B] ☺
Potato, boiled, with skin	portion 3.89oz/110g	☺	☺ ☺	☹ 45¼	☺[B] ☺
Potato, boiled, without skin	portion 3.89oz/110g	☺	☺ ☺	☹ 45¼	☺[B] ☺
Quinoa, cooked	portion 4.94oz/140g	☺	☺+ ×1¾ unit ☺+ ×1¾ unit	☺ ☺	2½[A] 5
Rice noodles, fried	portion 0.89oz/25g	☺	☺ ☺	☺ ☺	☺[A] ☺
Spaetzle (spatzen)	portion 4.94oz/140g	5¼ +4¼ unit	☺+ ×¼ unit ☺+ ×¼ unit	☺ ☺	1[A] 2

3.6 Fast food chains

3.6.1 Burger King®

Burger King®	Unit	Lactose L1 + unit/capsule	Fructose* L0 Fructose L0	Sorbitol L0 Sorbitol L1	FrucGalactans L0 FrucGalactans L1 📖
Bacon EGG® and Cheese BK Muffin®	piece 4.63oz/131g	11½ +9½ unit	☺+ ×1 unit ☺+ ×1 unit	☺ ☺	¼[A] ¾
Barbecue sauce	portion 1.1oz.fl/31ml	☺	☺+ ×1¼ unit ☺+ ×1¼ unit	☹ 2¼	☺ ☺
BBQ roasted jalapeno sauce	portion 1.1oz.fl/31ml	☺	☺+ ×1 unit ☺+ ×1 unit	☹ 2¾	☺ ☺
BK Big Fish®	piece 8.05oz/228g	☺	☺ ☺	☹ 21¾	☹[A] ¼
BK Fresh Apple Slices	portion 4.94oz/140g	☺	☹[2] ☹[2]	☹ ☹[2]	☺ ☺
BLT Salad® with TenderCrisp chicken (no dressing or croutons)	portion 4.94oz/140g	79¼ +66 unit	5¾ 5¾	☹ 3	☺ ☺
Caesar Salad (no dressing or croutons)	portion 3.53oz/100g	26½ +22 unit	1½ 1½	☹ 4¼	☺ ☺
Cheeseburger	piece 4.27oz/121g	11½ +9½ unit	51½ 59	☹ 3¼	¼[A] ¾
French fries	portion 2.47oz/70g	☺	☺ ☺	☹ 35½	☺ ☺
Hamburger	piece 3.85oz/109g	☺	57¼ 65½	☹ 3¼	½[A] 1
Ken's® Apple Cider Vinaigrette salad dressing	portion 1.06oz.fl/30ml	☺	☺ ☺	☺ ☺	☺ ☺
Onion rings	portion 2.47oz/70g	☺	☺+ ×1½ unit ☺+ ×1½ unit	☹ ¾	¼[AC] ½
Original Chicken Crisp® Sandwich	piece 5.26oz/149g	☺	1½ 1½	☹ 67	5¾[A] 11½
Pancakes and syrup	piece 6.6oz/187g	½ +½ unit	☺+ ×6 unit ☺+ ×6 unit	☺ ☺	¼[A] ½

L0 *Level 0:* lactose measure ×½
L1 *Level 1:* fructose measure ×2
L2 *Level 2:* fructose-/sorbitol measure ×4. the rest ×2
L3 *Level 3:* sorbitol measure ×7. the rest ×3
📖: source of fruc/galactans data

+ Unit/capsule: added tolerated amount of unit per strong lactase capsule
Fructose*: fructose, sorbitol adjusted
☺+ ×[Amount] unit: Per unit consumed you can additionally tolerate up to [amount] × fructose(*)-unit of another product.

☹: avoid; ☹[1]: ¼ at TL 1; ☹[2]: ¼ at TL 2; ☹[3]: ¼ at TL 3; ☺: only contains traces; ☺: is free from it

Burger King®	**Unit**	**Lactose** **+ unit/**	**Fructose*** **Fructose**	**Sorbitol** **Sorbitol**	**FrucGalactans** **FrucGalactans**
Picante taco sauce sauce	portion 1.24oz.fl/35ml	☺	2½ 2½	☹ 2¾	☺ ☺
Ranch Crispy Chicken Wrap	piece 4.84oz/137g	5 +4¼ unit	☺ ☺	☹ 36¼	¼[A] ½
Shake, chocolate	portion 8.15oz.fl/231ml	☹[2] +0.15 unit	☺+ ×7¼ unit ☺+ ×7¼ unit	☺ ☺	½ 1
Shake, strawberry	portion 8.08oz.fl/229ml	☹[2] +0.15 unit	☺+ ×5¼ unit ☺+ ×5¼ unit	☹ 3¼	1 2
Shake, vanilla or other	portion 8.4oz.fl/238ml	☹[2] +0.13 unit	☺+ ×5¾ unit ☺+ ×5¾ unit	☺ ☺	¾ 1¾
Sundaes®, caramel	portion 4.98oz.fl/141ml	¼ +¼ unit	☺+ ×8½ unit ☺+ ×8½ unit	☺ ☺	2 4
Sundaes®, chocolate fudge	portion 4.98oz.fl/141ml	¼ +¼ unit	☺+ ×6¾ unit ☺+ ×6¾ unit	☺ ☺	1¾ 3¾
Sundaes®, mini M & M's®	portion 7.2oz.fl/204ml	¼ +0.23 unit	☺+ ×6¾ unit ☺+ ×6¾ unit	☺ ☺	1½ 3
Sundaes®, Oreo®	portion 7.2oz.fl/204ml	¼ +¼ unit	☺+ ×7¼ unit ☺+ ×7¼ unit	☹ 49	1¾ 3¾
Sundaes®, strawberry	portion 4.98oz.fl/141ml	¼ +¼ unit	☺+ ×2½ unit ☺+ ×2½ unit	☹ 2½	2¼ 4¾
Sweet and sour sauce	portion 1.06oz.fl/30ml	☺	¼ ¼	☹ 41½	☺ ☺
TenderCrisp® Chicken Sandwich	piece 9.32oz/264g	☺	8 8½	☹ 2½	☹[A] ¼
Whopper® with cheese	piece 11.12oz/315g	5¾ +4¾ unit	2¾ 2¾	☹ 1	☹[A] ¼
Zesty onion ring sauce	portion 1.1oz.fl/31ml	☺	☺ ☺	☹ 64½	☺ ☺

3.6.2 KFC®

KFC®	Unit	Lactose (Level 1) / + unit/capsule	Fructose* (Level 0) / Fructose (Level 0)	Sorbitol (Level 0) / Sorbitol (Level 1)	FrucGalactans (Level 0) / FrucGalactans (Level 1) 📖
Caesar salad dressing	portion	4¾	☺	☺	26½
	1.06oz.fl/30ml	+3¾ unit	☺	☺	53
Chicken breast, spicy crispy	piece	☺	☺	☺	¾ A
	6.18oz/175g		☺	☺	1¾
Chicken Littles with sauce	piece	☺	3	☹	½ A
	3.57oz/101g		3	33	1
Cole slaw	portion	☺	☺+ ×¼ unit	☹	1 B
	3.53oz/100g		☺+ ×¼ unit	2¾	2
Creamy buffalo sauce	portion	6	☺+ ×1 unit	☺	34½
	1.04ozfl/29.4ml	+5 unit	☺+ ×1 unit	☺	69
Crispy Chicken Caesar Salad	portion	🙂	2¼	☹	1 A
	4.94oz/140g		2¼	17¾	2¼
Crispy Twister without sauce	piece	☺	19	☹	☹ A
	7.69oz/218g		20¾	2	¼
Crispy Twister® with sauce	piece	☺	17¼	☹	☹ A
	8.47oz/240g		18¾	2	¼
Extra Crispy Tenders	piece	☺	☺	☺	3¼ A
	1.84oz/52g		☺	☺	6½
Honey BBQ sauce	portion	☺	☺+ ×1¼ unit	☹	☺
	1.1oz.fl/31ml		☺+ ×1¼ unit	2¼	☺
Hot wings	portion	☺	☺	☺	☺
	3oz/85g		☺	☺	☺
House side salad	portion	☺	2	☹	☺
	3.53oz/100g		2	4	☺
Mashed potatoes with gravy	portion	½	☺	☹	4
	4.94oz/140g	+½ unit	☺	35½	8¼
Sweet and sour sauce	portion	☺	¼	☹	☺
	1.06oz.fl/30ml		¼	37	☺
Sweet corn	piece	☺	🙂	☹	☺ B
	3.36oz/95g		☺	2½	☺

Level 0: lactose measure ×½ — + Unit/capsule: added tolerated amount of unit per strong lactase capsule

Level 1: fructose measure ×2 — Fructose*: fructose, sorbitol adjusted

Level 2: fructose-/sorbitol measure ×4. the rest ×2

Level 3: sorbitol measure ×7. the rest ×3

📖: source of fruc/galactans data

☺+ ×[Amount] unit: Per unit consumed you can additionally tolerate up to [amount] × fructose(*)-unit of another product.

☹: avoid; ☹[1]: ¼ at TL 1; ☹[2]: ¼ at TL 2; ☹[3]: ¼ at TL 3; 🙂: only contains traces; ☺: is free from it

3.6.3 McDonald's®

McDonald's®	Unit	Lactose / + unit/	Fructose* / Fructose	Sorbitol / Sorbitol	FrucGalactans / FrucGalactans
apple slices	piece	☺	¼	☹	☺
	1.2oz/34g		½	¼	☺
barbecue sauce	portion	☺	☺+ ×1½ unit	☹	☺
	1.1oz.fl/31ml		☺+ ×1½ unit	1¾	☺
Big Mac®	piece	9¾	5	☹	¼[A]
	7.59oz/215g	+8¼ unit	5	6½	½
caramel sundae®	portion	¼	☺+ ×6¾ unit	☺	1¾
	6.42oz.fl/182ml	+¼ unit	☺+ ×6¾ unit	☺	3¾
Cheeseburger	piece	9¾	3¾	☹	¼[A]
	4.03oz/114g	+8¼ unit	3¾	5	¾
Chicken McNuggets®	piece	☺	☺	☺	10¾[A]
	0.58oz/16.25g		☺	☺	21½
chocolate chip cookies	piece	☺	☺+ ×½ unit	☹	¾[A]
	1.17oz/33g		☺+ ×½ unit	☺	1½
chocolate milk	cup	¼	☺+ ×2 unit	☺	1¾
	5.2oz.fl/150ml	+¼ unit	☺+ ×2 unit	☺	3¾
Crispy Chicken Snack Wrap	piece	62	☺	☹	¼[A]
with ranch sauce	4.17oz.fl/118ml	+51½ unit	☺	84½	½
Double Cheeseburger	piece	4¾	4½	☹	¼[A]
	5.83oz/165g	+4 unit	4½	4¼	½
Filet-O-Fish®	piece	19¾	2	☹	¼[A]
	5.01oz/142g	+16½ unit	2	70¼	¾
French fries	portion	☺	☺	☹	☺
	2.47oz/70g		☺	35½	☺
Hamburger	piece	☺	3¾	☹	½[A]
	3.53oz/100g		4	5	1
hot fudge sundae®	portion	¼	☺+ ×7½ unit	☹	1¼[G]
	6.32oz.fl/179ml	+¼ unit	☺+ ×7½ unit	55¾	2½
hot mustard sauce	portion	☺	☺+ ×1¼ unit	☺	☺
	0.71oz.fl/20ml		☺+ ×1¼ unit	☺	☺
M & M's® McFlurry®	portion	☹[2]	☺+ ×3½ unit	☺	1
	8.05oz.fl/228ml	+0.18 unit	☺+ ×3½ unit	☺	2¼
McCafe® shakes, chocolate	cup	¼	☺+ ×4 unit	☹	2¼
flavors	5.2oz.fl/150ml	+¼ unit	☺+ ×4 unit	22	4¾
McCafe® shakes, vanilla or	cup	¼	☺+ ×¼ unit	☹	2¼
other flavors	5.2oz.fl/150ml	+¼ unit	☺+ ×¼ unit	16½	4½

McDonald's®	Unit	Lactose [1] + unit/[capsule]	Fructose* [0] Fructose [0]	Sorbitol [0] Sorbitol [1]	FrucGalactans [0] FrucGalactans [1] [book]
McChicken®	piece 5.05oz/143g	☺	1½ 1½	☹ 69¾	¼ A ¾
McDouble®	piece 5.33oz/151g	9¾ +8¼ unit	4¼ 4¼	☹ 4¼	¼ A ½
McRib®	piece 7.34oz/208g	☺	☺+ ×¾ unit ☺+ ×¾ unit	☹ 1¾	¼ A ½
Newman's Own® Creamy Caesar salad dressing	portion 1.06oz.fl/30ml	18¼ +15¼ unit	26¾ 79¼	☹ 7¼	☺ ☺
Newman's Own® Low Fat Balsamic Vinaigrette salad dressing	portion 1.06oz.fl/30ml	☺	☺ ☺	☺ ☺	☺ ☺
Orange juice	glass 8.4oz.fl/240ml	☺	1½ 1½	☹ ¼	☺ ☺
Quarter Pounder	piece 6.11oz/173g	☺	48 57¾	☹ 2½	¼ A ½
Sausage & EGG® McMuffin®	piece 5.79oz/164g	9¾ +8¼ unit	☺+ ×1 unit ☺+ ×1 unit	☺ ☺	¼ A ½
Side salad	portion 3.53oz/100g	☺	3¾ 3¾	☹ 2½	☺ ☺
Smoothies, all flavors	glass 8.4oz.fl/240ml	2¾ +2¼ unit	3¾ 4¼	☹ 1¼	15½ 31
Southwestern chipotle barbecue sauce	portion 1.1oz.fl/31ml	☺	☺+ ×1¾ unit ☺+ ×1¾ unit	☹ 2¾	☺ ☺
Sweet and sour sauce	portion 1.06oz.fl/30ml	☺	¼ ¼	☹ 41½	☺ ☺

[0] *Level 0:* lactose measure ×½ + Unit/[capsule]: added tolerated amount of unit per strong lactase capsule
[1] *Level 1:* fructose measure ×2 Fructose*: fructose, sorbitol adjusted
[2] *Level 2:* fructose-/sorbitol measure ×4. the rest ×2
[3] *Level 3:* sorbitol measure ×7. the rest ×3
[book]: source of fruc/galactans data
☺+ ×[Amount] unit: Per unit consumed you can additionally tolerate up to [amount] × fructose(*)-unit of another product.

☹: avoid; ☹[1]: ¼ at TL 1; ☹[2]: ¼ at TL 2; ☹[3]: ¼ at TL 3; ☺: only contains traces; ☺: is free from it

3.6.4 Subway®

Subway®	Unit	Lactose + unit/	Fructose* Fructose	Sorbitol Sorbitol	FrucGalactans FrucGalactans
9-grain Wheat bread	piece 2.76oz/78g	☺	1 1	☺ ☺	¼ A ¾
American cheese	portion 1.06oz/30g	4½ +3¾ unit	☺ ☺	☺ ☺	25¾ 51½
Bacon	portion 0.53oz/15g	☺	☺ ☺	☺ ☺	☺ ☺
Cheddar cheese	portion 1.06oz/30g	43¼ +36 unit	☺ ☺	☺ ☺	☺ ☺
Chipotle southwest salad dressing	portion 1.06oz.fl/30ml	7¼ +6 unit	☺ ☺	☺ ☺	40½ 81
Chocolate chip cookie	piece 1.59oz/45g	☺	☺+ ×1 unit ☺+ ×1 unit	☹ ☺	½ A 1
Chocolate chunk cookie	piece 1.59oz/45g	☺	☺+ ×1 unit ☺+ ×1 unit	☹ ☺	½ A 1
Ham Sandwich with Veggies, no mayo	piece 7.73oz/219g	12½ +10½ unit	¾ ¾	☹ 1¼	¼ A ½
Honey mustard salad dressing	portion 1.06oz.fl/30ml	☺	4½ 4½	☺ ☺	☺ ☺
Honey Oat bread	piece 3.14oz/89g	¾ +½ unit	2½ 2½	☹ 6½	¼ A ¾
Italian BMT® Sandwich with Veggies, no mayo	piece 7.98oz/226g	12½ +10½ unit	¾ ¾	☹ 1¼	¼ A ½
M & M's® cookie	piece 1.59oz/45g	9 +7½ unit	☺+ ×½ unit ☺+ ×½ unit	☹ ☺	½ A 1
Mustard	portion 0.18oz/5g	☺	☺ ☺	☺ ☺	☺ ☺
Oven Roasted Chicken Sandwich with Veggies, no mayo	piece 8.22oz/233g	12½ +10½ unit	1¾ 1¾	☹ 1¼	☹ A ¼
Parmesan Oregano bread	piece 2.65oz/75g	☺	☺+ ×½ unit ☺+ ×½ unit	☺ ☺	¾ A 1½
Ranch salad dressing	portion 1.06oz.fl/30ml	☺	☺ ☺	☹ ☺	☺ ☺
Roast Beef Sandwich with Veggies, no mayo	piece 8.22oz/233g	12½ +10½ unit	¾ ¾	☹ 1¼	☹ A ¼
Spicy Italian Sandwich with Veggies, no meat	piece 7.84oz/222g	12½ +10½ unit	¾ ¾	☹ 1¼	¼ A ½

Subway®	Unit	Lactose + unit/capsule	Fructose* Fructose	Sorbitol Sorbitol	FrucGalactans FrucGalactans
Steak & Cheese Sandwich with Veggies, no mayo	piece 8.65oz/245g	☺	1 1	☹ 1¼	☹[A] ¼
Sweet Onion Chicken Teriyaki Sandwich with Veggies, no mayo	piece 9.74oz/276g	12½ +10½ unit	22½ 25¾	☹ 1¼	☹[A] ¼
Sweet onion salad dressing	portion 1.06oz.fl/30ml	☻	☻+ ×1 unit ☻+ ×1 unit	☹ 55½	½ 1¼
Tuna Sandwich with Veggies, no mayo	piece 8.22oz/233g	12½ +10½ unit	¾ ¾	☹ 1¼	☹[A] ¼
Turkey Breast & Ham Sandwich with Veggies, no mayo	piece 7.73oz/219g	12½ +10½ unit	¾ ¾	☹ 1¼	¼[A] ½
Turkey Breast Sandwich with Veggies, no mayo	piece 7.73oz/219g	12½ +10½ unit	¾ ¾	☹ 1¼	¼[A] ½
Veggie Delite Salad, no dressing	portion 3.53oz/100g	34¼ +28½ unit	83¼ ☺	☹ 2¼	☺ ☺
Veggie Delite Sandwich, no mayo	piece 5.72oz/162g	12½ +10½ unit	¾ ¾	☹ 1½	¼[A] ½

Level 0: lactose measure ×½
Level 1: fructose measure ×2
+ Unit/capsule: added tolerated amount of unit per strong lactase capsule
Fructose*: fructose, sorbitol adjusted

Level 2: fructose-/sorbitol measure ×4. the rest ×2
Level 3: sorbitol measure ×7. the rest ×3
📖: source of fruc/galactans data

☻+ ×[Amount] unit: Per unit consumed you can additionally tolerate up to [amount] × fructose(*)-unit of another product.

☹: avoid; ☹[1]: ¼ at TL 1; ☹[2]: ¼ at TL 2; ☹[3]: ¼ at TL 3; ☺: only contains traces; ☻: is free from it

3.7 Fruit and vegetables

3.7.1 Fruit

Fruit	Unit	Lactose + unit/	Fructose* Fructose	Sorbitol Sorbitol	FrucGalactans FrucGalactans
Apple, fresh, with skin	piece 6.42oz/182g	☺	☹² ☹²	☹ ☹²	1¾ CB 3½
Applesauce, canned, sweetened	tbsp. 0.5ozfl/14.21ml	☺	1½ 1¾	☹ ¾	21½ CB 43
Applesauce, canned, unsweetened	tbsp. 0.5ozfl/14.21ml	☺	¾ ¾	☹ 1	21½ CB 43
Apricot, dried, cooked, sweetened	piece 0.71oz/20g	☺	☺+ ×1¼ unit ☺+ ×1½ unit	☹ 1¼	☺ ☺
Apricot, dried, uncooked	piece 0.71oz/20g	☺	☺+ ×7¾ unit ☺+ ×8 unit	☹ ¼	☺ ☺
Apricot, fresh	piece 1.24oz/35g	☺	☺+ ×¾ unit ☺+ ×1 unit	☹ ¾	☺ ☺
Banana, chips	portion 1.42oz/40g	☺	3¾ 3¾	☹ 12½	½ FB 1¼
Banana, fresh	piece 4.17oz/118g	☺	☺+ ×¼ unit ☺+ ×¼ unit	☹ 9¼	¾ FB 1½
Blackberries, fresh	portion 4.94oz/140g	☺	3¾ 3¾	☺ ☺	2¼ B 4½
Blueberries, fresh	portion 4.94oz/140g	☺	3¾ 3¾	☺ ☺	¾ B 1½
Boysenberries, fresh	portion 0.29oz/8g	☺	69¼ 69¼	☺ ☺	☺ ☺
Cantaloupe, fresh	portion 4.94oz/140g	☺	1 1	☹ 14¼	2 B 4¼
Carambola (starfruit), fresh	piece 3.21oz/91g	☺	☺+ ×¼ unit ☺+ ×¼ unit	☹ 1¼	☺ ☺
Clementine, fresh	portion 4.94oz/140g	☺	7 7	☺ ☺	2¼ B 4½
Cranberries, dried (Craisins®)	portion 1.42oz/40g	☺	☺+ ×3¼ unit ☺+ ×3¼ unit	☹ 41½	☺ ☺
Cranberries, fresh	portion 1.95oz/55g	☺	☺+ ×2¾ unit ☺+ ×2¾ unit	☹ 45¼	☺ ☺
Currants, fresh, black	portion 4.94oz/140g	☺	1¼ 1¼	☺ ☺	☺ ☺

Fruit	Unit	Lactose (L1) + unit/[capsule]	Fructose* (L0) Fructose (L0)	Sorbitol (L0) Sorbitol (L1)	FrucGalactans (L0) FrucGalactans (L1) [book]
Currants, fresh, red and white	portion 4.94oz/140g	☺	1 1	☺ ☺	☺ ☺
Dates	portion 1.42oz/40g	☺	☺ ☺	☺ ☺	☺ ☺
Elderberries, fresh	portion 4.94oz/140g	☺	¼ ¼	☺ ☺	☺ ☺
Figs, dried, cooked, sweetened	piece 1.77oz/50g	☺	☺+ ×¾ unit ☺+ ×¾ unit	☺ ☺	☺ ☺
Figs, fresh	piece 1.77oz/50g	☺	☺+ ×2 unit ☺+ ×2 unit	☺ ☺	☺ ☺
Gooseberries, fresh	portion 4.94oz/140g	☺	☺+ ×1 unit ☺+ ×1 unit	☺ ☺	☺ ☺
Grapefruit, fresh, pink or red	portion 4.94oz/140g	☺	2 2	☺ ☺	1½ CB 3
Grapes, fresh	portion 4.94oz/140g	☺	¼ ¼	☹ ½	2¼ B 4½
Guava (guayaba), fresh, common	piece 5.3oz/150g	☺	2¼ 2¼	☹ ½	☺ ☺
Honeydew	portion 4.94oz/140g	☺	¾ ¾	☺ ☺	1½ B 3¼
Jackfruit, fresh	tbsp. 0.5ozfl/14.21ml	☺	☺ ☺	☹ ½	☺ ☺
Kiwi fruit, gold	piece 3.04oz/86g	☺	1 1	☺ ☺	☺ B ☺
Kiwi fruit, green	piece 2.44oz/69g	☺	3 3	☺ ☺	☺ B ☺
Lemon, fresh	piece 2.05oz/58g	☺	☺ ☺	☺ ☺	7¾ B 15½
Lime, fresh	piece 2.37oz/67g	☺	☺ ☺	☺ ☺	6¾ B 13½
Loganberries, fresh	portion 4.94oz/140g	☺	☺+ ×1½ unit ☺+ ×1½ unit	☺ ☺	☺ ☺
Lowbush cranberries (lingonberries)	portion 4.94oz/140g	☺	☺+ ×9¼ unit ☺+ ×9¼ unit	☹ 35½	☺ ☺

(L0) *Level 0:* lactose measure ×½
(L1) *Level 1:* fructose measure ×2
(L2) *Level 2:* fructose-/sorbitol measure ×4. the rest ×2
(L3) *Level 3:* sorbitol measure ×7. the rest ×3
[book]: source of fruc/galactans data

+ Unit/[capsule]: added tolerated amount of unit per strong lactase capsule
Fructose*: fructose, sorbitol adjusted
☺+ ×[Amount] unit: Per unit consumed you can additionally tolerate up to [amount] × fructose(*)-unit of another product.

☹: avoid; ☹¹: ¼ at TL 1; ☹²: ¼ at TL 2; ☹³: ¼ at TL 3; ☺: only contains traces; ☺: is free from it

Fruit	Unit	Lactose + unit/	Fructose* Fructose	Sorbitol Sorbitol	FrucGalactans FrucGalactans
Lychees (litchis), fresh	portion 4.94oz/140g	☺	1 1	☺ ☺	☺ B ☺
lycium (wolf or goji berries)	portion 4.94oz/140g	☺	☺+ ×1 unit ☺+ ×1 unit	☺ ☺	☺ ☺
Mandarin orange, fresh	portion 4.94oz/140g	☺	1¼ 1¼	☺ ☺	2¼ B 4½
Mango, fresh	tbsp. 0.5ozfl/14.21ml	☺	1 1	☹ 4	☺ B ☺
Mangosteen, fresh	portion 4.94oz/140g	☺	35½ 35½	☺ ☺	☺ ☺
Mulberries	portion 4.94oz/140g	☺	½ ½	☺ ☺	☺ ☺
Muskmelon	portion 4.94oz/140g	☺	1¼ 1¼	☺ ☺	1½ B 3¼
Nectarine, fresh	tbsp. 0.5ozfl/14.21ml	☺	8¼ ☺	☹ 1	5½ B 11¼
Orange, fresh	portion 4.94oz/140g	☺	2¼ 2¼	☺ ☺	2¼ B 4½
Papaya, fresh	portion 4.94oz/140g	☺	☺+ ×1 unit ☺+ ×1 unit	☺ ☺	☺ ☺
Passion fruit (maracuya), fresh	portion 4.94oz/140g	☺	☺+ ×2½ unit ☺+ ×2½ unit	☺ ☺	☺ ☺
Peach, fresh	piece 5.3oz/150g	☺	☺+ ×½ unit ☺+ ×1¼ unit	☹ ¼	¾ B 1½
Pear, fresh	tbsp. 0.5ozfl/14.21ml	☺	½ ¾	☹ ¼	☺ B ☺
Persimmon, fresh	piece 4.94oz/140g	☺	2¾ 2¾	☺ ☺	1 C 2
Pineapple, dried	portion 1.42oz/40g	☺	½ ½	☹ ½	2 CB 4
Pineapple, fresh	portion 4.94oz/140g	☺	¾ ¾	☹ ¾	2¼ CB 4½
Plantains, green, boiled	piece 7.87oz/223g	☺	¾ ¾	☺ ☺	¼ FB ¾
Plum, fresh	tbsp. 0.5ozfl/14.21ml	☺	☺+ ×¼ unit ☺+ ×½ unit	☹ ¾	21½ C 43
Pomegranate, fresh (arils-seed/juice sacs)	tbsp. 0.5ozfl/14.21ml	☺	☺+ ×½ unit ☺+ ×½ unit	☹ 2	☺ ☺
Quince, fresh	tbsp. 0.5ozfl/14.21ml	☺	1¼ 1¼	☺ ☺	☺ ☺

Fruit	Unit	Lactose L1 + unit/(capsule)	Fructose* L0 Fructose L0	Sorbitol L0 Sorbitol L1	FrucGalactans L0 FrucGalactans L1 (book)
Raisins, uncooked	portion 1.42oz/40g	☺	½ ½	☹ ½	2[B] 4
Rambutan, canned in syrup	portion 4.94oz/140g	☺	1¼ 1¼	☺ ☺	¾[CB] 1¾
Raspberries, fresh, red	portion 4.94oz/140g	☺	½ ½	☹ 1½	1[B] 2¼
Rhubarb, fresh	portion 4.94oz/140g	☺	☺ ☺	☺ ☺	☺ ☺
Rose hips	portion 4.94oz/140g	☺	☺+ ×½ unit ☺+ ×½ unit	☺ ☺	☺ ☺
Santa Claus melon	portion 4.94oz/140g	☺	1¼ 1¼	☺ ☺	☺ ☺
Sapodilla, fresh	portion 4.94oz/140g	☺	☺+ ×3½ unit ☺+ ×3½ unit	☺ ☺	☺ ☺
Sour cherries, fresh	tbsp. 0.5ozfl/14.21ml	☺	10 ☺	☹ ½	☺ ☺
Soursop (guanabana), fresh	portion 4.94oz/140g	☺	1¼ 1¼	☺ ☺	☺ ☺
Strawberries, fresh	portion 4.94oz/140g	☺	½ ¾	☹ ¼	☺[C] ☺
Sweet cherries, fresh	tbsp. 0.5ozfl/14.21ml	☺	3¾ ☺+ ×¼ unit	☹ ¼	☺ ☺
Watermelon, fresh	tbsp. 0.5ozfl/14.21ml	☺	1¾ 1¾	☹ ☺	10¼[B] 20¾

L0 *Level 0:* lactose measure ×½
L1 *Level 1:* fructose measure ×2
L2 *Level 2:* fructose-/sorbitol measure ×4. the rest ×2
L3 *Level 3:* sorbitol measure ×7. the rest ×3
(book): source of fruc/galactans data

+ Unit/(capsule): added tolerated amount of unit per strong lactase capsule
Fructose*: fructose, sorbitol adjusted

☺+ ×[Amount] unit: Per unit consumed you can additionally tolerate up to [amount] × fructose(*)-unit of another product.

☹: avoid; ☹[1]: ¼ at TL 1; ☹[2]: ¼ at TL 2; ☹[3]: ¼ at TL 3; ☺: only contains traces; ☺: is free from it

3.7.2 Vegetables

Vegetables	Unit	Lactose + unit/	Fructose* Fructose	Sorbitol Sorbitol	FrucGalactans FrucGalactans
Alfalfa sprouts	portion 3oz/85g	☺	14½ 14½	☺ ☺	☺[G] ☺
Artichoke, globe raw	tbsp. 0.5ozfl/14.21ml	☺	☺ ☺	☹ 23¾	1[FB] 2¼
Asparagus, raw	portion 3oz/85g	☺	1½ 1½	☹ 9¾	½[FB] 1¼
Avocado, green skin, Florida type	portion 1.06oz/30g	☺	☺+ ×1 unit ☺+ ×1 unit	☺ ☺	☺[B] ☺
Bamboo shoots, canned and drained	portion 3oz/85g	☺	19½ 19½	☺ ☺	☺ ☺
Beets, raw	portion 3oz/85g	☺	58¾ ☺	☹ 3¼	1[CB] 2
Black olives	portion 0.53oz/15g	☺	☺ ☺	☹ 33¼	☺ ☺
Bok choy, raw	portion 3oz/85g	☺	☺+ ×¼ unit ☺+ ×¼ unit	☹ 23½	☺[B] ☺
Boston Market® sweet corn	portion 3oz/85g	☺	☺+ ×¼ unit ☺+ ×½ unit	☹ 4	☺[B] ☺
Broccoflower (green cauliflower), cooked from fresh	portion 3oz/85g	☺	1 1	☺ ☺	☺[B] ☺
Broccoli, raw	portion 3oz/85g	16¾ +14 unit	3 3	☺ ☺	½[B] 1¼
Brown mushrooms (Italian or Crimini mushrooms), raw	tbsp. 0.5ozfl/14.21ml	☺	☺+ ×¼ unit ☺+ ×¼ unit	☹ ¾	12¼[B] 24½
Brussels sprouts, cooked from fresh	portion 3oz/85g	☺	☺ ☺	☺ ☺	1[B] 2
Butternut squash	portion 4.59oz/130g	☺	☺ ☺	☺ ☺	½[G] 1¼
Cabbage, green, cooked	portion 3oz/85g	☺	☺+ ×¾ unit ☺+ ×¾ unit	☹ 58¾	1¼[B] 2½
Cabbage, red, cooked	portion 3oz/85g	☺	☺+ ×¼ unit ☺+ ×¼ unit	☺ ☺	1¼[B] 2½
Cabbage, savoy, raw	portion 3oz/85g	☺	☺ ☺	☹ 39	1½[B] 3
Carrots, cooked from fresh	portion 3oz/85g	☺	☺ ☺	☹ ½	☺[B] ☺

Vegetables	Unit	Lactose (1) + unit/💊	Fructose* (0) Fructose (0)	Sorbitol (0) Sorbitol (1)	FrucGalactans (0) FrucGalactans (1) 🕮
Carrots, raw	piece 2.16oz/61g	☺	☺ ☺	☹ ¾	☺ B ☺
Cauliflower, cooked from frozen	portion 3oz/85g	☺	☺ ☺	☹ 2½	☺ CB ☺
Celeriac (celery root), cooked from fresh	tbsp. 0.5ozfl/14.21ml	☺	13¼ 13¼	☹ ¾	☺ ☺
Celery, cooked	tbsp. 0.5ozfl/14.21ml	☺	☺ ☺	☹ 1	☺ C ☺
Chard, raw or blanched, marinated in oil	portion 3oz/85g	☺	☺+ ×½ unit ☺+ ×½ unit	☺ ☺	☺ ☺
Chayote squash, cooked	portion 4.59oz/130g	☺	6¼ 6¼	☺ ☺	☺ B ☺
Chestnuts, boiled, steamed	portion 1.06oz/30g	☺	☺ ☺	☹ 6	☺ ☺
Chicory coffee powder, unprepared	portion 0.08oz/2g	☺	☺ ☺	☹ 8¾	½ E 1
Chicory greens, raw	portion 3oz/85g	☺	5¼ 5¼	☹ 39	2¼ B 4½
Coleslaw, with apples and raisins, mayo dressing	portion 3.53oz/100g	☺	½ ½	☹ ½	1 B 2
Coleslaw, with pineapple, mayo dressing	portion 3.53oz/100g	☺	☺+ ×¼ unit ☺+ ×¼ unit	☹ 3¾	☺ B ☺
Collards, raw	portion 3oz/85g	☺	☺ ☺	☺ ☺	1¼ B 2½
Cucumber, raw, with peel	portion 3oz/85g	☺	5¼ 5¼	☹ 1	☺ B ☺
Cucumber, raw, without peel	portion 3oz/85g	☺	4¾ 4¾	☹ 1	☺ B ☺
Eggplant, cooked	portion 3oz/85g	☺	3½ 3½	☹ 2½	☺ B ☺
Endive, curly, raw	portion 3oz/85g	☺	☺ ☺	☹ 3	3¾ C 7½
Enoki mushrooms, raw	tbsp. 0.5ozfl/14.21ml	☺	☺ ☺	☹ ¾	☺ ☺

(0) *Level 0:* lactose measure ×½
(1) *Level 1:* fructose measure ×2
(2) *Level 2*: fructose-/sorbitol measure ×4. the rest ×2
(3) *Level 3:* sorbitol measure ×7. the rest ×3
🕮: source of fruc/galactans data

+ Unit/💊: added tolerated amount of unit per strong lactase capsule
Fructose*: fructose, sorbitol adjusted
☺+ ×[Amount] unit: Per unit consumed you can additionally tolerate up to [amount] × fructose(*)-unit of another product.

☹: avoid; ☹[1]: ¼ at TL 1; ☹[2]: ¼ at TL 2; ☹[3]: ¼ at TL 3; ☺: only contains traces; ☺: is free from it

Vegetables	Unit	Lactose + unit/	Fructose* Fructose	Sorbitol Sorbitol	FrucGalactans FrucGalactans
Fennel bulb, raw	portion 3oz/85g	☺	☺+ ×¾ unit ☺+ ×¾ unit	☹ 2	1¼ B 2¾
Garbanzo beans (chickpeas), canned, drained	portion 3.18oz/90g	☺	☺ ☺	☹ 1	1½ A 3
Garlic, fresh	portion 0.15oz/4g	☺	☺ ☺	☺ ☺	¾ FB 1½
Ginger root, raw	portion 0.15oz/4g	☺	89¼ 89¼	☺ ☺	☺ B ☺
Green beans (string beans), cooked from fresh	portion 3oz/85g	☺	4½ 4½	☺ ☺	¼ A ¾
Green bell peppers	portion 3oz/85g	☺	☺ ☺	☺ ☺	☺ B ☺
Green olives	portion 0.53oz/15g	☺	☺ ☺	☹ 18	☺ ☺
Green tomato, raw	portion 3oz/85g	☺	3 3¼	☹ ¾	6½ B 13
Hot chili peppers, green, cooked from fresh	piece 1.52oz/43g	☺	4½ 4½	☺ ☺	2½ B 5¼
Hot chili peppers, red, cooked from fresh	piece 1.52oz/43g	☺	2¾ 2¾	☺ ☺	2½ B 5¼
Hubbard squash	portion 3oz/85g	☺	☺ ☺	☺ ☺	☺ B ☺
Jerusalem artichoke (sunchoke), raw	pinch 0.04ozfl/1g	☺	☺ ☺	☺ ☺	3¼ FB 6½
Kale, raw	portion 3oz/85g	☺	☺ ☺	☹ ¾	☺ ☺
Kelp, raw	portion 3oz/85g	☺	☺ ☺	☺ ☺	☺ ☺
Kidney beans, cooked from dried	portion 3.18oz/90g	☺	☺ ☺	☺ ☺	¼ A ½
Kohlrabi, cooked	portion 3oz/85g	☺	☺+ ×¼ unit ☺+ ×¼ unit	☹ 13	☺ ☺
Leeks, leafs	portion 3oz/85g	☺	3¼ 3¼	☹ ¼	¾ G 1½
Leeks, root	tbsp. 0.5ozfl/14.21ml	☺	18½ 18½	☹ 2¼	¼ C ¾
Leeks, whole	portion 3oz/85g	☺	3¼ 3¼	☹ ¼	¼ C ½

Vegetables	Unit	Lactose (Level 1) + unit/capsule	Fructose* (Level 0) / Fructose (Level 0)	Sorbitol (Level 0) / Sorbitol (Level 1)	FrucGalactans (Level 0) / FrucGalactans (Level 1) 🕮
Lentils, cooked from dried	portion	☺	☺	☺	¾[A]
	3.18oz/90g		☺	☺	1½
Lettuce, boston, bibb or butterhead	portion	☺	7¼	☹	☺[B]
	3oz/85g		7¼	19½	☺
Lettuce, green leaf	portion	☺	8¼	☹	☺[CB]
	3oz/85g		8¼	16¾	☺
Lettuce, iceberg	portion	☺	6½	☹	☺[CB]
	3oz/85g		6½	19½	☺
Lettuce, red leaf	portion	☺	7¼	☹	☺[B]
	3oz/85g		7¼	19½	☺
Lettuce, romaine or cos	portion	☺	1¼	☹	☺[CB]
	3oz/85g		1¼	16¾	☺
Lima beans, cooked from dried	portion	☺	½	☺	¼[A]
	3.18oz/90g		½	☺	½
Lotus root, cooked	portion	☺	☺	☺	☺
	3oz/85g		☺	☺	☺
Maitake mushrooms, raw	tbsp.	60½	☺+ ×½ unit	☹	☺
	0.5ozfl/14.21ml	+50½ unit	☺+ ×½ unit	¾	☺
Morel mushrooms, raw	tbsp.	☺	☺	☹	☺
	0.5ozfl/14.21ml		☺	¾	☺
Mung beans, cooked from dried	portion	☺	½	☺	¾[A]
	3.18oz/90g		½	☺	1¾
Mushrooms, batter dipped or breaded	portion	☺	☺	☹	2½[B]
	2.47oz/70g		☺	¼	5¼
Okra, raw	portion	☺	2¼	☺	2[CB]
	3oz/85g		2¼	☺	4¼
Onion, white, yellow or red, raw	tbsp.	☺	☺	☹	1[CB]
	0.5ozfl/14.21ml		☺	6	2
Oyster mushrooms, raw	portion	☺	☺+ ×1¾ unit	☹	☺
	3oz/85g		☺+ ×1¾ unit	¼	☺
Parsnip, cooked	portion	☺	☺+ ×¼ unit	☺	☺[C]
	3oz/85g		☺+ ×¼ unit	☺	☺
Pickled beets	portion	☺	☺	☹	3[CB]
	1.06oz/30g		☺	15	6

Level 0: lactose measure ×½ + Unit/capsule: added tolerated amount of unit per strong lactase capsule
Level 1: fructose measure ×2 Fructose*: fructose, sorbitol adjusted
Level 2: fructose-/sorbitol measure ×4. the rest ×2
Level 3: sorbitol measure ×7. the rest ×3
🕮: source of fruc/galactans data
☺+ ×[Amount] unit: Per unit consumed you can additionally tolerate up to [amount] × fructose(*)-unit of another product.
☹: avoid; ☹¹: ¼ at TL 1; ☹²: ¼ at TL 2; ☹³: ¼ at TL 3; ☺: only contains traces; ☺: is free from it

Vegetables	Unit	Lactose + unit/	Fructose* Fructose	Sorbitol Sorbitol	FrucGalactans FrucGalactans
Portabella mushrooms, cooked from fresh	tbsp. 0.5ozfl/14.21ml	☺	☺+ ×½ unit ☺+ ×½ unit	☹ ½	12¼[B] 24½
Purslane, raw	portion 3oz/85g	☺	58¾ 58¾	☺ ☺	☺ ☺
Radicchio, raw	portion 3oz/85g	☺	2¼ 2¼	☺ ☺	¾ 1½
Radish, raw	portion 3oz/85g	☺	☺+ ×½ unit ☺+ ×½ unit	☹ 1	☺[C] ☺
Rocket (arugula), raw	portion 3oz/85g	☺	4¾ 4¾	☺ ☺	☺ ☺
Rutabaga, raw or blanched, marinated in oil mixture	portion 3oz/85g	☺	☺+ ×1 unit ☺+ ×1 unit	☺ ☺	☺[CB] ☺
Sauerkraut	tbsp. 0.5ozfl/14.21ml	☺	☺ ☺	☹ ¾	7[B] 14¼
Scallop squash	portion 3oz/85g	☺	4 4	☺ ☺	☺[CB] ☺
Shallot, raw	tbsp. 0.5ozfl/14.21ml	☺	☺ ☺	☺ ☺	¼[CB] ½
Shiitake mushrooms, cooked	tbsp. 0.5ozfl/14.21ml	☺	☺+ ×1 unit ☺+ ×1 unit	☹ ½	☺ ☺
Snow peas (edible pea pods), cooked from fresh	portion 3oz/85g	☺	☺+ ×3½ unit ☺+ ×3½ unit	☺ ☺	¾[B] 1¾
Sour pickles	portion 1.06oz/30g	☺	☺+ ×¼ unit ☺+ ×¼ unit	☹ 4¼	☺[CB] ☺
Soybean sprouts, raw	portion 3oz/85g	☺	☺ ☺	☹ ½	3¾[CB] 7½
Soybeans, cooked from dried	tbsp. 0.5oz/14.21ml	☺	9 9	☹ 3	3[A] 6
Spaghetti squash	portion 3oz/85g	☺	☺+ ×¼ unit ☺+ ×¼ unit	☺ ☺	☺[CB] ☺
Spinach, cooked from fresh	portion 3oz/85g	☺	☺ ☺	☹ 13	4[CB] 8¼
Split pea sprouts, cooked	tbsp. 0.5ozfl/14.21ml	☺	☺ ☺	☺ ☺	1¼[A] 2½
Straw mushrooms, canned, drained	portion 3oz/85g	☺	☺ ☺	☹ ¼	☺ ☺
Summer squash, cooked from fresh	portion 3oz/85g	☺	2¼ 2¼	☺ ☺	2[CB] 4
Sun-dried tomatoes, oil pack, drained	portion 1.06oz/30g	☺	¼ ¼	☹ ¼	4½[B] 9¼

Vegetables	Unit	Lactose (L1) + unit/capsule	Fructose* (L0) Fructose (L0)	Sorbitol (L0) Sorbitol (L1)	FrucGalactans (L0) FrucGalactans (L1) 🕮
Tempeh	portion 3oz/85g	☺	3¼ 3¼	☹ ½	½ A 1
Tomato, cooked from fresh	portion 3oz/85g	☺	4¼ 4½	☹ ¾	6½ B 13
Turnip, cooked	portion 3oz/85g	☺	☺+ ×½ unit ☺+ ×½ unit	☹ 2½	☺ CB ☺
Wax beans (yellow beans), canned, drained	portion 3oz/85g	☺	☺ ☺	☺ ☺	¼ A ¾
Winter (dark green or orange) squash, cooked	portion 4.59oz/130g	☺	1¾ 1¾	☺ ☺	☺ CB ☺
Winter melon (waxgourd or chinese preserving melon)	portion 3oz/85g	☺	☺ ☺	☺ ☺	☺ CB ☺
Yams, sweet potato type, boiled	portion 3.89oz/110g	☺	☺ ☺	☺ ☺	☺ B ☺
Yellow bell pepper, raw	portion 3oz/85g	☺	½ ½	☺ ☺	☺ CB ☺
Yellow tomato, raw	portion 3oz/85g	☺	4½ 4¾	☹ 1	6½ B 13

(L0) *Level 0:* lactose measure ×½
(L1) *Level 1:* fructose measure ×2
(L2) *Level 2:* fructose-/sorbitol measure ×4. the rest ×2
(L3) *Level 3:* sorbitol measure ×7. the rest ×3
🕮: source of fruc/galactans data

+ Unit/capsule: added tolerated amount of unit per strong lactase capsule
Fructose*: fructose, sorbitol adjusted
☺+ ×[Amount] unit: Per unit consumed you can additionally tolerate up to [amount] × fructose(*)-unit of another product.

☹: avoid; ☹1: ¼ at TL 1; ☹2: ¼ at TL 2; ☹3: ¼ at TL 3; ☺: only contains traces; ☺: is free from it

3.8 Ice cream

Ice cream	Unit	Lactose + unit/	Fructose* Fructose	Sorbitol Sorbitol	FrucGalactans FrucGalactans
Ben & Jerry's® Ice Cream, Brownie Batter	portion 3.89oz/110g	¼ +¼ unit	☺+ ×3 unit ☺+ ×3 unit	☹ ☺	1¼ 2¾
Ben & Jerry's® Ice Cream, Chocolate Chip Cookie Dough	portion 3.67oz/104g	½ +¼ unit	☺+ ×4¾ unit ☺+ ×4¾ unit	☺ ☺	3¼ 6½
Ben & Jerry's® Ice Cream, Chubby Hubby®	portion 3.78oz/107g	½ +½ unit	☺+ ×5 unit ☺+ ×5 unit	☺ ☺	3½ 7
Ben & Jerry's® Ice Cream, Chunky Monkey®	portion 3.78oz/107g	¼ +¼ unit	☺+ ×2¾ unit ☺+ ×2¾ unit	☹ ☺	2½ 5¼
Ben & Jerry's® Ice Cream, Half Baked	portion 3.81oz/108g	¼ +¼ unit	☺+ ×2¼ unit ☺+ ×2¼ unit	☺ ☺	2¼ 4¾
Ben & Jerry's® Ice Cream, Karamel Sutra®	portion 3.74oz/106g	½ +¼ unit	☺+ ×4¾ unit ☺+ ×4¾ unit	☺ ☺	3 6¼
Ben & Jerry's® Ice Cream, New York Super Fudge Chunk®	portion 3.74oz/106g	½ +½ unit	67¼ 67¼	☹ ☺	3½ 7¼
Ben & Jerry's® Ice Cream, One Sweet Whirled	portion 3.74oz/106g	½ +¼ unit	☺+ ×4¾ unit ☺+ ×4¾ unit	☺ ☺	3 6¼
Ben & Jerry's® Ice Cream, Peanut Butter Cup	portion 4.06oz/115g	½ +¼ unit	☺+ ×5¼ unit ☺+ ×5¼ unit	☺ ☺	3¼ 6½
Ben & Jerry's® Ice Cream, Phish Food®	portion 3.67oz/104g	¼ +¼ unit	☺+ ×2¼ unit ☺+ ×2¼ unit	☺ ☺	2¼ 4¾
Ben & Jerry's® Ice Cream, Vanilla For A Change	portion 3.64oz/103g	½ +¼ unit	☺+ ×4½ unit ☺+ ×4½ unit	☺ ☺	3¼ 6½
Breyers® Ice Cream, Natural Vanilla, Lactose Free	portion 2.3oz/65g	4 +3¼ unit	☺+ ×4¾ unit ☺+ ×4¾ unit	☺ ☺	23¼ 46½
Dreyer's® Grand Ice Cream, Chocolate	portion 2.3oz/65g	1 +1 unit	☺+ ×¾ unit ☺+ ×¾ unit	☹ ☺	6¾ 13¾
Dreyer's® No Sugar Added Ice Cream, Triple Chocolate	tsp. 0.16ozfl/4.74ml	11½ +9½ unit	¾ ☺	☹ ☹[2]	64½ ☺
Drumstick® (sundae cone)	piece 3.39oz/96g	1 +¾ unit	☺+ ×2¼ unit ☺+ ×2¼ unit	☹ ☺	6¼ 12¾
Frozen fruit juice bar	piece 2.72oz/77g	☺	☺+ ×1¼ unit ☺+ ×1¼ unit	☹ 4½	☺ ☺
Haagen-Dazs® Desserts Extraordinaire Ice Cream, Creme Brulee	portion 3.78oz/107g	½ +¼ unit	☺+ ×4¾ unit ☺+ ×4¾ unit	☺ ☺	3 6¼

Ice cream	Unit	Lactose + unit/capsule	Fructose* Fructose	Sorbitol Sorbitol	FrucGalactans FrucGalactans
Haagen-Dazs® Frozen Yogurt, chocolate or coffee flavors	portion 3.74oz/106g	½ +½ unit	☺+ ×¾ unit ☺+ ×¾ unit	☹ ☺	1¾ 3½
Haagen-Dazs® Frozen Yogurt, vanilla or other flavors	portion 3.74oz/106g	½ +½ unit	☺+ ×3 unit ☺+ ×3 unit	☺ ☺	3½ 7
Haagen-Dazs® Ice Cream, Bailey's Irish Cream	portion 3.6oz/102g	½ +¼ unit	☺+ ×2¾ unit ☺+ ×2¾ unit	☹ ☺	1½ 3
Haagen-Dazs® Ice Cream, Black Walnut	portion 3.74oz/106g	½ +½ unit	☺+ ×4¾ unit ☺+ ×4¾ unit	☺ ☺	3½ 7
Haagen-Dazs® Ice Cream, Butter Pecan	portion 3.74oz/106g	½ +½ unit	☺+ ×4¾ unit ☺+ ×4¾ unit	☺ ☺	2¼ 4¾
Haagen-Dazs® Ice Cream, Cherry Vanilla	portion 3.57oz/101g	½ +½ unit	☺+ ×4½ unit ☺+ ×4½ unit	☺ ☺	3¼ 6½
Haagen-Dazs® Ice Cream, Chocolate	portion 3.74oz/106g	¼ +¼ unit	☺+ ×2¾ unit ☺+ ×2¾ unit	☹ ☺	1¼ 2¾
Haagen-Dazs® Ice Cream, Coffee	portion 3.74oz/106g	¼ +¼ unit	☺+ ×2¾ unit ☺+ ×2¾ unit	☹ ☺	2½ 5¼
Haagen-Dazs® Ice Cream, Cookies & Cream	portion 3.6oz/102g	½ +¼ unit	☺+ ×4½ unit ☺+ ×4½ unit	☺ ☺	3¼ 6½
Haagen-Dazs® Ice Cream, Mango	portion 3.74oz/106g	¼ +¼ unit	☺+ ×2¼ unit ☺+ ×2¼ unit	☺ ☺	2¼ 4¾
Haagen-Dazs® Ice Cream, Pistachio	portion 3.74oz/106g	½ +½ unit	☺+ ×4¾ unit ☺+ ×4¾ unit	☺ ☺	½ 1¼
Haagen-Dazs® Ice Cream, Rocky Road	portion 3.67oz/104g	¼ +¼ unit	☺+ ×2¾ unit ☺+ ×2¾ unit	☹ ☺	2½ 5¼
Haagen-Dazs® Ice Cream, Strawberry	portion 3.74oz/106g	½ +¼ unit	☺+ ×4¾ unit ☺+ ×4¾ unit	☺ ☺	3 6¼
Haagen-Dazs® Ice Cream, Vanilla Chocolate Chip	portion 3.74oz/106g	½ +½ unit	☺+ ×4¾ unit ☺+ ×4¾ unit	☺ ☺	3½ 7
Ice cream sandwich	piece 2.54oz/72g	1¼ +1 unit	☺+ ×1½ unit ☺+ ×1½ unit	☺ ☺	7½ 15¼
Ice cream, light, no sugar added, with aspartame, vanilla or other flavors (include chocolate chip)	tsp. 0.16ozfl/4.74ml	9¾ +8 unit	2¼ ☺	☹ ¼	54¾ ☺

Level 0: lactose measure ×½
Level 1: fructose measure ×2
Level 2: fructose-/sorbitol measure ×4. the rest ×2
Level 3: sorbitol measure ×7. the rest ×3
📖: source of fruc/galactans data

+ Unit/capsule: added tolerated amount of unit per strong lactase capsule
Fructose*: fructose, sorbitol adjusted

☺+ ×[Amount] unit: Per unit consumed you can additionally tolerate up to [amount] × fructose(*)-unit of another product.

☹: avoid; ☹¹: ¼ at TL 1; ☹²: ¼ at TL 2; ☹³: ¼ at TL 3; ☺: only contains traces; ☺: is free from it

Ice cream	Unit	Lactose + unit/	Fructose* Fructose	Sorbitol Sorbitol	FrucGalactans FrucGalactans
Sorbet, chocolate	portion	☺	☺+ ×3¼ unit	☺	☺
	3.71oz/105g		☺+ ×3¼ unit	☺	☺
Sorbet, coconut	portion	18¾	☺+ ×5 unit	☺	3¼
	3.74oz/106g	+15½ unit	☺+ ×5 unit	☺	6½
Sorbet, fruit	portion	☺	☺+ ×5½ unit	☺	☺
	3.74oz/106g		☺+ ×5½ unit	☺	☺

3.9 Ingredients

Ice cream	Unit	Lactose + unit/	Fructose* Fructose	Sorbitol Sorbitol	FrucGalactans FrucGalactans
Baking powder	sachet 0.22oz/6g	☺	☺ ☺	☺ ☺	☺ ☺
Barley flour	portion 1.06oz/30g	☺	☺ ☺	☺ ☺	6¼[AD] 12¾
Lemon peel	tbsp. 0.5oz/14.21ml	☺	☺ ☺	☺ ☺	☺ ☺
Orange peel	tbsp. 0.5oz/14.21ml	☺	3¼ 3¼	☺ ☺	☺ ☺
Rye flour,in recipes not containing yeast	portion 1.06oz/30g	☺	27¾ 27¾	☺ ☺	¾[AD] 1¾
Semolina flour	portion 1.06oz/30g	☺	☺ ☺	☺ ☺	1¼[AD] 2¾
Spelt flour	portion 1.06oz/30g	☺	☺+ ×¼ unit ☺+ ×¼ unit	☺ ☺	☺[A] ☺
Streusel topping, crumb	portion 0.68oz/19g	68¼ +57 unit	☺ ☺	☺ ☺	2¾[A] 5¾
Wheat bran, unprocessed	tbsp. 0.5oz/14.21ml	☺	☺ ☺	☺ ☺	☺ ☺
White all-purpose flour, unenriched	portion 1.06oz/30g	☺	☺ ☺	☺ ☺	1[AD] 2
White whole wheat flour	portion 1.06oz/30g	☺	33¼ 33¼	☺ ☺	1¼[AD] 2¾

Level 0: lactose measure ×½
Level 1: fructose measure ×2
+ Unit/: added tolerated amount of unit per strong lactase capsule
Fructose*: fructose, sorbitol adjusted
Level 2: fructose-/sorbitol measure ×4. the rest ×2
Level 3: sorbitol measure ×7. the rest ×3
: source of fruc/galactans data
☺+ ×[Amount] unit: Per unit consumed you can additionally tolerate up to [amount] × fructose(*)-unit of another product.
☹: avoid; ☹[1]: ¼ at TL 1; ☹[2]: ¼ at TL 2; ☹[3]: ¼ at TL 3; ☺: only contains traces; ☺: is free from it

SUGGESTIONS

I hope that the diet has been effective for you and increased the well-being of your tummy. This is the first edition and more are planned to follow. Each input can help to make the book even more practical for those that are affected by an intolerance or irritable bowel syndrome. Your suggestions and tips are therefore highly welcomed. Please tell me about your experiences and wishes. Grey areas remain and new foods arrive on the market continuously. In order to keep the brick dragons chained, it is important for us to create a current knowledgebase regarding the handling of the disease. You can also help others like you, by sharing your personal TLs so that we can improve the BTLs in future versions. To do so please visit www.Laxiba.co.uk/tls.

You want to hire a coach for you to learn and keep the diet strategy or want to book a workshop regarding healthy nutrition and stress management for your firm? Come visit us at www.Laxiba.co.uk. We look forward to getting to know you.

As a closing, I wish you cheerfulness and above all healthfulness.

Your author brightly greets you,

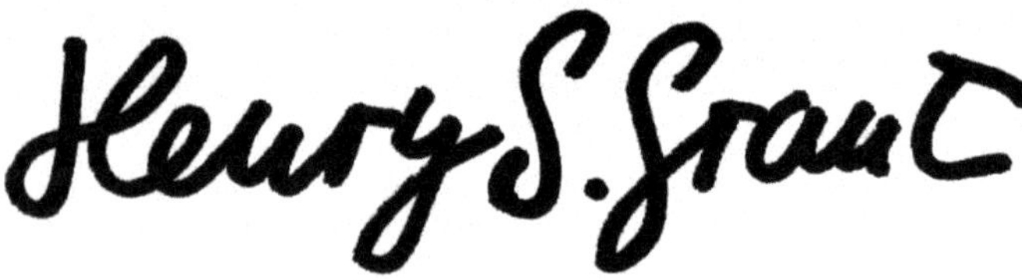

Henry S. Grant
Henry@AmericanDietPublishing.co.uk

This page has been intentionally left blank.

Keyword Index

In the following index, you find the foods once more in alphabetical order. The abbreviations remain the same but the base has changed to TL 1 for all foods.

Keyword Index	Unit	Lactose + unit/	Fructose* Fructose*	Sorbitol Sorbitol	FrucGalactans FrucGalactans
3 Musketeers®	piece 2.14oz/60.4g	1¾ +1½ unit	☺+ ×3¾ unit ☺+ ×1¾ unit	☺ ☺	6¼ 12½
7 UP®	glass 8.4ozfl/240ml	☺	☹[2] ☹[2]	☺ ☺	☺ ☺
Advocaat, regular	glass 8.4ozfl/240ml	¼ +0,24 unit	☺+ ×4¾ unit ☺+ ×2¼ unit	☺ ☺	1½ 3¼
After Eight® Thin Chocolate Mints	piece 0.29oz/8g	10¼ +8½ unit	☺ ☺	☺ ☺	57¾ ☺
Ale	glass 8.4ozfl/240ml	☺	50 ☺	☹ 10	☺ ☺
Alfalfa sprouts	portion 3oz/85g	☺	14½ 29¼	☺ ☺	☺[G] ☺
All-Bran® Original (Kellogg's®)	portion 1.06oz/30g	☺	☺+ ×¼ unit ☺	☺ ☺	¼[A] ¾
Almond cookies	piece 0.44oz/12.4g	☺	☺ ☺	☺ ☺	3[A] 6
Almond milk, vanilla or other flavors, unsweetened	glass 8.4oz/240g	☺	☺ ☺	☺ ☺	☹[A] ☹[2]
Almond paste (Marzipan)	portion 0.99oz/28g	☺	☺ ☺	☹ 20½	½[G] 1¼
Almonds, honey roasted	hand 1.06oz/30g	☺	2 4¼	☹ 5½	½[G] 1¼
Almonds, raw	hand 1.06oz/30g	☺	☺ ☺	☺ ☺	½[G] 1¼
Alpine Lace 25% Reduced Fat, Mozzarella	portion 1.06oz/30g	37¼ +31 unit	☺ ☺	☺ ☺	☺ ☺
Amaranth Flakes (Arrowhead Mills)	portion 1.06oz/30g	☺	3 6¼	☹ 2½	¾[G] 1½
Amaretto	glass 8.4ozfl/240ml	☺	☺+ ×4½ unit ☺+ ×2½ unit	☹ ¼	☺ ☺
American cheese, processed	portion 1.06oz/30g	4½ +3¾ unit	☺ ☺	☺ ☺	25¾ 51½

Keyword Index	Unit	Lactose 1 / + unit/capsule	Fructose* 0 / Fructose* 1	Sorbitol 0 / Sorbitol 1	FrucGalactans 0 / FrucGalactans 1 📖
Americano, decaf, without flavored syrup	cup 5.2ozfl/150ml	🙂	🙂 🙂	🙂 🙂	🙂 🙂
Americano, with flavored syrup	cup 5.2ozfl/150ml	🙂	🙂 🙂	🙂 🙂	🙂 🙂
Americano, without flavored syrup	cup 5.2ozfl/150ml	🙂	🙂 🙂	🙂 🙂	🙂 🙂
Apple banana strawberry juice	glass 8.4ozfl/240ml	🙂	☹[1] ¼	☹ ☹[2]	¾[FB] 1¾
Apple cake, glazed	piece 1.59oz/45g	🙂	¾ 1¾	☹ ½	1¼[A] 2½
Apple grape juice	glass 8.4ozfl/240ml	🙂	☹[2] ☹[2]	☹ ☹[2]	1½[CB] 3
Apple strudel	piece 2.26oz/64g	☺	¼ ½	☹ ¼	¾[A] 1¾
Apple, fresh, with skin	piece 6.42oz/182g	🙂	☹[2] ☹[2]	☹ ☹[2]	1¾[CB] 3½
Applejack liquor	glass 8.4ozfl/240ml	🙂	🙂 🙂	🙂 🙂	🙂 🙂
Applesauce, canned, sweetened	tbsp. 0.5ozfl/14.21ml	🙂	1½ 3	☹ ¾	21½[CB] 43
Applesauce, canned, unsweetened	tbsp. 0.5ozfl/14.21ml	🙂	¾ 1½	☹ 1	21½[CB] 43
Apricot nectar	glass 8.4ozfl/240ml	🙂	🙂+ ×4¾ unit 🙂+ ×2½ unit	☹ ¼	🙂 🙂
Apricot, dried, cooked, sweetened	piece 0.71oz/20g	🙂	🙂+ ×1¼ unit 🙂+ ×¾ unit	☹ 1¼	🙂 🙂
Apricot, dried, uncooked	piece 0.71oz/20g	🙂	🙂+ ×7¾ unit 🙂+ ×4 unit	☹ ¼	🙂 🙂
Apricot, fresh	piece 1.24oz/35g	🙂	🙂+ ×¾ unit 🙂+ ×½ unit	☹ ¾	🙂 🙂
Aquavit	glass 8.4ozfl/240ml	🙂	🙂 🙂	🙂 🙂	🙂 🙂

0 *Level 0:* lactose measure ×½
1 *Level 1:* fructose measure ×2
2 *Level 2*: fructose-/sorbitol measure ×4. the rest ×2
3 *Level 3:* sorbitol measure ×7. the rest ×3
📖: source of fruc/galactans data

+ Unit/capsule: added tolerated amount of unit per strong lactase capsule
Fructose*: fructose, sorbitol adjusted

🙂+ ×[Amount] unit: Per unit consumed you can additionally tolerate up to [amount] × fructose(*)-unit of another product.

☹: avoid; ☹[1]: ¼ at TL 1; ☹[2]: ¼ at TL 2; ☹[3]: ¼ at TL 3; ☺: only contains traces; 🙂: is free from it

KEYWORD INDEX	Unit	Lactose + unit/	Fructose* Fructose*	Sorbitol Sorbitol	FrucGalactans FrucGalactans
Arby's® Chicken Cordon Bleu Sandwich, crispy	portion 4.94oz/140g	32¼ +27 unit	2 4¼	☺ ☺	1[A] 2¼
Arby's® macaroni and cheese	portion 7.66oz/217g	21½ +18 unit	☺ ☺	☺ ☺	½[A] 1¼
Arby's® orange juice	glass 8.4ozfl/240ml	☺	1½ 3¼	☹ ¼	☺[B] ☺
Arby's® ranch sauce	tbsp. 0.5ozfl/14.21ml	☺	☺ ☺	☹ 18½	☺ ☺
Archway® Oatmeal Raisin Cookies	piece 0.92oz/26g	23¾ +19¾ unit	☺ ☺	☹ 10¼	2¼[A] 4¾
Archway® Peanut Butter Cookies	piece 1.2oz/34g	23¾ +19¾ unit	2 4	☹ 10¾	1½[A] 3
Artichoke, globe raw	tbsp. 0.5ozfl/14.21ml	☺	☺ ☺	☹ 23¾	1[FB] 2¼
Asian noodle bowl, vegetables only	portion 7.06oz/200g	☺	☺+ ×1 unit ☺+ ×½ unit	☹ 10	1½[A] 3¼
Asparagus, raw	portion 3oz/85g	☺	1½ 3¼	☹ 9¾	½[FB] 1¼
Au gratin potato, prepared from fresh	portion 4.94oz/140g	1 +¾ unit	☺ ☺	☹ 7¾	6¼[B] 12½
Avocado, green skin, Florida type	portion 1.06oz/30g	☺	☺+ ×1 unit ☺+ ×½ unit	☺ ☺	☺[B] ☺
Baby food, double baked (zwieback)	portion 0.25oz/7g	☺	☺ ☺	☺ ☺	1½[A] 3
Baby food, Gerber Graduates® Organic Pasta Pick-Ups Three Cheese Ravioli	Portion 170 g	88	☺ ☺	☺ ☺	¾[A] 1½
Baguette	slice 1.49oz/42g	☺	☺ ☺	☺ ☺	1¾[A] 3½
Baking powder	sachet 0.22oz/6g	☺	☺ ☺	☺ ☺	☺ ☺
Balsamic vinegar	portion 0.53oz/15g	☺	☺ ☺	☹ 23	☺ ☺
Bamboo shoots, canned and drained	portion 3oz/85g	☺	19½ 39	☺ ☺	☺ ☺
Banana, chips	portion 1.42oz/40g	☺	3¾ 7¾	☹ 12½	½[FB] 1¼
Banana, fresh	piece 4.17oz/118g	☺	☺+ ×¼ unit ☺	☹ 9¼	¾[FB] 1½

Keyword Index	Unit	Lactose (Level 1) + unit/capsule	Fructose* (Level 0) Fructose* (Level 1)	Sorbitol (Level 0) Sorbitol (Level 1)	FrucGalactans (Level 0) FrucGalactans (Level 1) 🕮
Barbeque sauce (BBQ), store bought	pinch 0.04oz/1g	☻	☻ ☻	☹ 76¾	☻ ☻
Barley flour	portion 1.06oz/30g	☻	☻ ☻	☻ ☻	6¼[AD] 12¾
Basil, fresh	pinch 0.04oz/1g	☻	☻ ☻	☻ ☻	☻ ☻
Basmati rice, cooked in unsalted water	portion 4.94oz/140g	☻	☻ ☻	☻ ☻	☻[A] ☻
Beef bacon (kosher)	portion 0.53oz/15g	☻	☻ ☻	☻ ☻	☻ ☻
Beef gravy, canned	portion 2.05oz/58g	☻	☻ ☻	☹ ☺	☻ ☻
Beef steak, chuck, visible fat eaten	portion 3oz/85g	☻	☻ ☻	☻ ☻	☻ ☻
Beef with noodles soup, condensed	portion 4.45oz/126g	☻	☻ ☻	☹ 4¼	4[A] 8¼
Beer	glass 8.4ozfl/240ml	☻	50 ☺	☹ 10	☻ ☻
Beer, low alcohol	glass 8.4ozfl/240ml	☻	☻+ ×2¼ unit ☻+ ×1 unit	☻ ☻	☻ ☻
Beets, raw	portion 3oz/85g	☻	58¾ ☺	☹ 3¼	1¼[B] 2½
Ben & Jerry's® Ice Cream, Brownie Batter	portion 3.89oz/110g	¼ +¼ unit	☻+ ×3 unit ☻+ ×1½ unit	☹ ☺	1¼ 2¾
Ben & Jerry's® Ice Cream, Chocolate Chip Cookie Dough	portion 3.67oz/104g	½ +¼ unit	☻+ ×4¾ unit ☻+ ×2¼ unit	☻ ☻	3¼ 6½
Ben & Jerry's® Ice Cream, Chubby Hubby®	portion 3.78oz/107g	½ +½ unit	☻+ ×5 unit ☻+ ×2½ unit	☻ ☻	3½ 7
Ben & Jerry's® Ice Cream, Chunky Monkey®	portion 3.78oz/107g	¼ +¼ unit	☻+ ×2¾ unit ☻+ ×1¼ unit	☹ ☺	2½ 5¼
Ben & Jerry's® Ice Cream, Half Baked	portion 3.81oz/108g	¼ +¼ unit	☻+ ×2¼ unit ☻+ ×1 unit	☻ ☻	2¼ 4¾

Level 0: lactose measure ×½
Level 1: fructose measure ×2
Level 2: fructose-/sorbitol measure ×4. the rest ×2
Level 3: sorbitol measure ×7. the rest ×3
🕮: source of fruc/galactans data

+ Unit/capsule: added tolerated amount of unit per strong lactase capsule
Fructose*: fructose, sorbitol adjusted

☻+ ×[Amount] unit: Per unit consumed you can additionally tolerate up to [amount] × fructose(*)-unit of another product.

☹: avoid; ☹¹: ¼ at TL 1; ☹²: ¼ at TL 2; ☹³: ¼ at TL 3; ☺: only contains traces; ☻: is free from it

KEYWORD INDEX	Unit	Lactose + unit/	Fructose* Fructose*	Sorbitol Sorbitol	FrucGalactans FrucGalactans
Ben & Jerry's® Ice Cream, Karamel Sutra®	portion 3.74oz/106g	½ +¼ unit	☺+ ×4¾ unit ☺+ ×2¼ unit	☺ ☺	3 6¼
Ben & Jerry's® Ice Cream, New York Super Fudge Chunk®	portion 3.74oz/106g	½ +½ unit	67¼ ☺	☹ ☺	3½ 7¼
Ben & Jerry's® Ice Cream, One Sweet Whirled	portion 3.74oz/106g	½ +¼ unit	☺+ ×4¾ unit ☺+ ×2¼ unit	☺ ☺	3 6¼
Ben & Jerry's® Ice Cream, Peanut Butter Cup	portion 4.06oz/115g	½ +¼ unit	☺+ ×5¼ unit ☺+ ×2½ unit	☺ ☺	3¼ 6½
Ben & Jerry's® Ice Cream, Phish Food®	portion 3.67oz/104g	¼ +¼ unit	☺+ ×2¼ unit ☺+ ×1 unit	☺ ☺	2¼ 4¾
Ben & Jerry's® Ice Cream, Vanilla For A Change	portion 3.64oz/103g	½ +¼ unit	☺+ ×4½ unit ☺+ ×2¼ unit	☺ ☺	3¼ 6½
Bertolli® Classico Olive Oil	portion 0.46oz/13g	☺	☺ ☺	☺ ☺	☺ ☺
Biscotti, chocolate, nuts	piece 0.73oz/20.5g	☺	☺ ☺	☹ ☺	2½[A] 5
Black cherry juice	glass 8.4ozfl/240ml	☺	¼ ¾	☹ 2½	☺ ☺
Black currant juice	glass 8.4ozfl/240ml	☺	☺+ ×1½ unit ☺+ ×¾ unit	☹ 1½	☺ ☺
Black olives	portion 0.53oz/15g	☺	☺ ☺	☹ 33¼	☺ ☺
Black pepper, ground	pinch 0.04oz/1g	☺	☺ ☺	☺ ☺	☺ ☺
Black Russian	glass 8.4ozfl/240ml	☺	☺ ☺	☹ 8¼	☺ ☺
Blackberries, fresh	portion 4.94oz/140g	☺	3¾ 7¾	☺ ☺	2¼[B] 4½
Blackberry juice	glass 8.4ozfl/240ml	☺	¼ ½	☺ ☺	☺ ☺
Bloody Mary	glass 8.4ozfl/240ml	☺	1¾ 3½	☹ ½	☺ ☺
Blue cheese	portion 1.06oz/30g	20 +16½ unit	☺ ☺	☺ ☺	☺ ☺
Blueberries, fresh	portion 4.94oz/140g	☺	3¾ 7¾	☺ ☺	¾[B] 1½
Bok choy, raw	portion 3oz/85g	☺	☺+ ×¼ unit ☺	☹ 23½	☺[B] ☺

KEYWORD INDEX	Unit	Lactose 1 + unit/capsule	Fructose* 0 Fructose* 1	Sorbitol 0 Sorbitol 1	FrucGalactans 0 FrucGalactans 1 📖
Bologna, beef ring	portion 1.95oz/55g	☺	☺+ ×5¾ unit ☺+ ×2¾ unit	☺ ☺	☺ ☺
Bologna, combination of meats, light (reduced fat)	portion 1.95oz/55g	☺	☺+ ×½ unit ☺+ ×¼ unit	☺ ☺	☺ ☺
Boston Market® 1/4 white rotisserie chicken, with skin	portion 3oz/85g	☺	☺ ☺	☺ ☺	☺ ☺
Boston Market® roasted turkey breast	portion 3oz/85g	☺	☺ ☺	☺ ☺	☺ ☺
Boston Market® sweet corn	portion 3oz/85g	☺	☺+ ×¼ unit ☺+ ×¼ unit	☹ 4	☺ B ☺
Bouillon, unprepared	portion 0.29oz/8g	☺	☺ ☺	☹ 🙂	☺ ☺
Bourbon	glass 8.4ozfl/240ml	☺	☺ ☺	☺ ☺	☺ ☺
Boysenberries, fresh	portion 0.29oz/8g	☺	69¼ 🙂	☺ ☺	☺ ☺
Brandy	glass 8.4ozfl/240ml	☺	☺ ☺	☺ ☺	☺ ☺
Brandy, flavored	glass 8.4ozfl/240ml	☺	☺+ ×4½ unit ☺+ ×2½ unit	☹ ¼	☺ ☺
Bratwurst	portion 1.95oz/55g	☺	☺+ ×¼ unit ☺	☺ ☺	☺ ☺
Bratwurst, beef	portion 1.95oz/55g	☺	☺+ ×1 unit ☺+ ×½ unit	☺ ☺	☺ ☺
Bratwurst, light (reduced fat)	portion 1.95oz/55g	☺	☺+ ×2¾ unit ☺+ ×1¼ unit	☺ ☺	☺ ☺
Bratwurst, made with beer	portion 1.95oz/55g	☺	☺+ ×¼ unit ☺	☹ 🙂	☺ ☺
Bratwurst, made with beer, cheese-filled	portion 1.95oz/55g	🙂	☺+ ×½ unit ☺+ ×¼ unit	☹ 🙂	🙂 🙂
Bratwurst, turkey	portion 1.95oz/55g	☺	☺+ ×1½ unit ☺+ ×¾ unit	☺ ☺	☺ ☺

0 *Level 0:* lactose measure ×½ + Unit/capsule: added tolerated amount of unit per strong lactase capsule
1 *Level 1:* fructose measure ×2 Fructose*: fructose, sorbitol adjusted
2 *Level 2:* fructose-/sorbitol measure ×4. the rest ×2
3 *Level 3:* sorbitol measure ×7. the rest ×3
📖: source of fruc/galactans data
☺+ ×[Amount] unit: Per unit consumed you can additionally tolerate up to [amount] × fructose(*)-unit of another product.

☹: avoid; ☹¹: ¼ at TL 1; ☹²: ¼ at TL 2; ☹³: ¼ at TL 3; 🙂: only contains traces; ☺: is free from it

Keyword Index	Unit	Lactose + unit/	Fructose* Fructose*	Sorbitol Sorbitol	FrucGalactans FrucGalactans
Braunschweiger (liver sausage)	portion 1.95oz/55g	☺	☺ ☺	☺ ☺	☺ ☺
Brazil nuts, unsalted	hand 1.06oz/30g	☺	☺ ☺	☺ ☺	☺ ☺
Breath mint, regular	portion 0.08oz/2g	☺	☺+ ×¼ unit ☺	☺ ☺	☺ ☺
Breath mint, sugar free	portion 0.08oz/2g	☺	¼ ½	☹ ☹[3]	☺ ☺
Breyers® Ice Cream, Natural Vanilla, Lactose Free	portion 2.3oz/65g	4 +3¼ unit	☺+ ×4¾ unit ☺+ ×2¼ unit	☺ ☺	23¼ 46½
Breyers® Light! Boosts Immunity Yogurt, all flavors	piece 4oz/114g	½ +¼ unit	28¾ 57¾	☹ 14¼	3 6
Breyers® No Sugar Added Ice Cream, Vanilla	tbsp. 0.5ozfl/14.21ml	3¼ +2½ unit	¾ 1½	☹ ☹[2]	18¼ 36½
Breyers® YoCrunch Light Nonfat Yogurt, with granola	piece 6.5oz/185g	¼ +0,24 unit	☺ ☺	☹ 6½	1½ 3
Brie cheese	portion 1.06oz/30g	22 +18½ unit	☺ ☺	☺ ☺	☺ ☺
Broccoflower (green cauliflower), cooked from fresh	portion 3oz/85g	☺	1 2	☺ ☺	☺[B] ☺
Broccoli, raw	portion 3oz/85g	16¾ +14 unit	3 6	☺ ☺	½[B] 1¼
Brown mushrooms (Italian or Crimini mushrooms), raw	tbsp. 0.5ozfl/14.21ml	☺	☺+ ×¼ unit ☺	☹ ¾	12¼[B] 24½
Brown sugar	tbsp. 0.5ozfl/14.21ml	☺	☺ ☺	☺ ☺	☺ ☺
Brownie, chocolate, fat free	piece 1.56oz/44g	3 +2½ unit	71 ☺	☹ ☺	1[A] 2¼
Brussels sprouts, cooked from fresh	portion 3oz/85g	☺	☺ ☺	☺ ☺	1[B] 2
Bulgur, home cooked	portion 4.94oz/140g	☺	☺ ☺	☺ ☺	☺ ☺
Burger King® Ranch Crispy Chicken Wrap	piece 4.84oz/137g	5 +4¼ unit	☺ ☺	☹ 36¼	¼[A] ½
Burger King® Bacon EGG® and Cheese BK Muffin®	piece 4.63oz/131g	11½ +9½ unit	☺+ ×1 unit ☺+ ×½ unit	☺ ☺	¼[A] ¾
Burger King® barbecue sauce	portion 1.1ozfl/31ml	☺	☺+ ×1¼ unit ☺+ ×½ unit	☹ 2¼	☺ ☺
Burger King® BBQ roasted jalapeno sauce	portion 1.1ozfl/31ml	☺	☺+ ×1 unit ☺+ ×½ unit	☹ 2¾	☺ ☺

Keyword Index	Unit	Lactose (Level 1) + unit/capsule	Fructose* (Level 0) Fructose* (Level 1)	Sorbitol (Level 0) Sorbitol (Level 1)	FrucGalactans (Level 0) FrucGalactans (Level 1) 🕮
Burger King® BK Big Fish®	piece 8.05oz/228g	☺	☺ ☺	☹ 21¾	☹[A] ¼
Burger King® BK Fresh Apple Slices	portion 4.94oz/140g	☺	☹[2] ☹[2]	☹ ☹[2]	☺ ☺
Burger King® BLT Salad® with TenderCrisp chicken (no dressing or croutons)	portion 4.94oz/140g	79¼ +66 unit	5¾ 11½	☹ 3	☺ ☺
Burger King® Caesar Salad (no dressing or croutons)	portion 3.53oz/100g	26½ +22 unit	1½ 3¼	☹ 4¼	☺ ☺
Burger King® Cheeseburger	piece 4.27oz/121g	11½ +9½ unit	51½ ☺	☹ 3¼	¼[A] ¾
Burger King® French fries	portion 2.47oz/70g	☺	☺ ☺	☹ 35½	☺ ☺
Burger King® Hamburger	piece 3.85oz/109g	☺	57¼ ☺	☹ 3¼	½[A] 1
Burger King® Ken's® Apple Cider Vinaigrette salad dressing	portion 1.06ozfl/30ml	☺	☺ ☺	☺ ☺	☺ ☺
Burger King® onion rings	portion 2.47oz/70g	☺	☺+ ×1½ unit ☺+ ×¾ unit	☹ ¾	¼[AC] ½
Burger King® Original Chicken Crisp® Sandwich	piece 5.26oz/149g	☺	1½ 3¼	☹ 67	5¾[A] 11½
Burger King® pancakes and syrup	piece 6.6oz/187g	½ +½ unit	☺+ ×6 unit ☺+ ×3 unit	☺ ☺	¼[A] ½
Burger King® picante taco sauce sauce	portion 1.24ozfl/35ml	☺	2½ 5¼	☹ 2¾	☺ ☺
Burger King® shake, chocolate	portion 8.15ozfl/231ml	☹[2] +0,15 unit	☺+ ×7¼ unit ☺+ ×3½ unit	☺ ☺	½ 1
Burger King® shake, strawberry	portion 8.08ozfl/229ml	☹[2] +0,15 unit	☺+ ×5¼ unit ☺+ ×2½ unit	☹ 3¼	1 2
Burger King® shake, vanilla or other	portion 8.4ozfl/238ml	☹[2] +0,13 unit	☺+ ×5¾ unit ☺+ ×2¾ unit	☺ ☺	¾ 1¾
Burger King® sundaes®, caramel	portion 4.98ozfl/141ml	¼ +¼ unit	☺+ ×8½ unit ☺+ ×4¼ unit	☺ ☺	2 4

Level 0: lactose measure ×½
Level 1: fructose measure ×2
+ Unit/capsule: added tolerated amount of unit per strong lactase capsule
Fructose*: fructose, sorbitol adjusted
Level 2: fructose-/sorbitol measure ×4. the rest ×2
Level 3: sorbitol measure ×7. the rest ×3
🕮: source of fruc/galactans data
☺+ ×[Amount] unit: Per unit consumed you can additionally tolerate up to [amount] × fructose(*)-unit of another product.
☹: avoid; ☹[1]: ¼ at TL 1; ☹[2]: ¼ at TL 2; ☹[3]: ¼ at TL 3; ☺: only contains traces; ☺: is free from it

Keyword Index	Unit	Lactose + unit/	Fructose* Fructose*	Sorbitol Sorbitol	FrucGalactans FrucGalactans
Burger King® sundaes®, chocolate fudge	portion 4.98ozfl/141ml	¼ +¼ unit	☺+ ×6¾ unit ☺+ ×3¼ unit	☺ ☺	1½ 3¼
Burger King® sundaes®, mini M & M's®	portion 7.2ozfl/204ml	¼ +0,23 unit	☺+ ×6¾ unit ☺+ ×3¼ unit	☺ ☺	1¼ 2¾
Burger King® sundaes®, Oreo®	portion 7.2ozfl/204ml	¼ +¼ unit	☺+ ×7¼ unit ☺+ ×3½ unit	☹ 49	1¾ 3½
Burger King® sundaes®, strawberry	portion 4.98ozfl/141ml	¼ +¼ unit	☺+ ×2½ unit ☺+ ×1¼ unit	☹ 2½	2¼ 4¾
Burger King® sweet and sour sauce	portion 1.06ozfl/30ml	☺	¼ ½	☹ 41½	☺ ☺
Burger King® TenderCrisp® Chicken Sandwich	piece 9.32oz/264g	☺	8 16¼	☹ 2½	☹[A] ¼
Burger King® Whopper® with cheese	piece 11.12oz/315g	5¾ +4¾ unit	2¾ 5¾	☹ 1	☹[A] ¼
Burger King® zesty onion ring sauce	portion 1.1ozfl/31ml	☺	☺ ☺	☹ 64½	☺ ☺
Burgundy wine, red	glass 8.4ozfl/240ml	☺	17¾ 35½	☹ ½	☺ ☺
Burgundy wine, white	glass 8.4ozfl/240ml	☺	31¼ 62½	☹ ¾	☺ ☺
Butter cracker	piece 0.15oz/4g	☺	☺ ☺	☺ ☺	10[A] 20
Butter, light, salted	portion 0.5oz/14g	☺	☺ ☺	☺ ☺	☺ ☺
Butter, unsalted	portion 0.5oz/14g	☺	☺ ☺	☺ ☺	☺ ☺
Buttermels® (Switzer's®)	piece 0.25oz/6.9g	8 +6½ unit	☺+ ×½ unit ☺+ ×¼ unit	☺ ☺	44¾ 89¾
Butternut squash	portion 4.59oz/130g	☺	☺ ☺	☺ ☺	½[G] 1¼
Butternut squash soup	portion 8.65oz/245g	13½ +11¼ unit	☺ ☺	☹ 2½	½[G] 1
Cabbage, green, cooked	portion 3oz/85g	☺	☺+ ×¾ unit ☺+ ×¼ unit	☹ 58¾	1¼[B] 2½
Cabbage, red, cooked	portion 3oz/85g	☺	☺+ ×¼ unit ☺	☺ ☺	1¼[B] 2½
Cabbage, savoy, raw	portion 3oz/85g	☺	☺ ☺	☹ 39	1½[B] 3

Keyword Index	Unit	Lactose (Level 1) + unit/capsule	Fructose* (Level 0) Fructose* (Level 1)	Sorbitol (Level 0) Sorbitol (Level 1)	FrucGalactans (Level 0) FrucGalactans (Level 1) (source)
Cabot® Non Fat Yogurt, plain	piece 8.01oz/227g	¼ +0,22 unit	☺ ☺	☺ ☺	1¼ 2¾
Cabot® Non Fat Yogurt, vanilla	piece 8.01oz/227g	¼ +¼ unit	30¼ 60½	☹ 13¼	2¼ 4½
Cafe au lait, without flavored syrup	cup 5.2ozfl/150ml	1 +¾ unit	☺ ☺	☺ ☺	6½ 13
Cafe latte, with flavored syrup	cup 5.2ozfl/150ml	½ +¼ unit	☺ ☺	☺ ☺	3 6
Cafe latte, without flavored syrup	cup 5.2ozfl/150ml	¼ +¼ unit	☺ ☺	☺ ☺	2¾ 5½
Calzone, cheese	piece 5.93oz/168g	12¼ +10¼ unit	☺ ☺	☹ 2¾	¼ A ½
Camembert cheese	portion 1.06oz/30g	21½ +18 unit	☺ ☺	☺ ☺	☺ ☺
Camomile tea	glass 8.5ozfl/242ml	☺	☺ ☺	☺ ☺	½ G 1¼
Campari®	glass 8.4ozfl/240ml	☺	☺+ ×4½ unit ☺+ ×2½ unit	☹ ¼	☺ ☺
Candy necklace	piece 0.75oz/21g	☺	☺+ ×3¼ unit ☺+ ×1½ unit	☺ ☺	☺ ☺
Cantaloupe, fresh	portion 4.94oz/140g	☺	1 2	☹ 14¼	2 B 4¼
Cape Cod	glass 8.4ozfl/240ml	☺	☺+ ×5 unit ☺+ ×2½ unit	☹ 25	☺ ☺
Capers	pinch 0.04oz/1g	☺	☺ ☺	☹ 70¼	☺ ☺
Cappuccino, bottled or canned	cup 5.2ozfl/150ml	½ +½ unit	☺ ☺	☺ ☺	4 8
Cappuccino, decaf, with flavored syrup	cup 5.2ozfl/150ml	½ +¼ unit	☺ ☺	☺ ☺	3 6¼
Cappuccino, decaf, without flavored syrup	cup 5.2ozfl/150ml	½ +¼ unit	☺ ☺	☺ ☺	2¾ 5¾
Capri Sun®, all flavors	glass 8.4ozfl/240ml	☺	☺+ ×1 unit ☺+ ×½ unit	☹ 2	☺ ☺

Level 0: lactose measure ×½
Level 1: fructose measure ×2
+ Unit/capsule: added tolerated amount of unit per strong lactase capsule
Fructose*: fructose, sorbitol adjusted

Level 2: fructose-/sorbitol measure ×4. the rest ×2
Level 3: sorbitol measure ×7. the rest ×3
(book): source of fruc/galactans data

☺+ ×[Amount] unit: Per unit consumed you can additionally tolerate up to [amount] × fructose(*)-unit of another product.

☹: avoid; ☹[1]: ¼ at TL 1; ☹[2]: ¼ at TL 2; ☹[3]: ¼ at TL 3; ☺: only contains traces; ☺: is free from it

Keyword Index	Unit	Lactose + unit/	Fructose* Fructose*	Sorbitol Sorbitol	FrucGalactans FrucGalactans
Carambola (starfruit), fresh	piece 3.21oz/91g	☺	☺+ ×¼ unit ☺	☹ 1¼	☺ ☺
Caramel or sugar coated pop-corn, store bought	hand 0.75oz/21g	☺	☺+ ×1 unit ☺+ ×½ unit	☺ ☺	☺[C] ☺
Caramel sauce, store bought, fat free	portion 1.45oz/41g	6 +5 unit	☺+ ×6 unit ☺+ ×3 unit	☺ ☺	33¾ 67¾
Carrot cake, glazed, homemade	piece 0.98oz/27.72g	☺	☺+ ×¼ unit ☺	☹ 8	2[A] 4
Carrot juice	glass 8.4ozfl/240ml	☺	☺+ ×1 unit ☺+ ×½ unit	☹ 4	☺[B] ☺
Carrots, cooked from fresh	portion 3oz/85g	☺	☺ ☺	☹ ½	☺[B] ☺
Carrots, raw	piece 2.16oz/61g	☺	☺ ☺	☹ ¾	☺[B] ☺
Cascadian Farm® Organic C-hewy Granola Bar, Trail Mix Dark Chocolate Cranberry	piece 1.24oz/35g	☺	☺+ ×4¼ unit ☺+ ×2 unit	☹ 71¼	½[A] 1
Cashews, raw	hand 1.06oz/30g	☺	☺ ☺	☺ ☺	¼[G] ¾
Casserole (hot dish), chicken with pasta, cream or white sauce, with cheese	portion 8.4oz/238g	½ +½ unit	☺ ☺	☺ ☺	☺ ☺
Casserole, pasta with turkey, gravy base, vegetables other than dark green, with cheese	portion 8.05oz/228g	3¾ +3 unit	☺ ☺	☹ 1¼	½[A] 1
Casserole , rice with beef, to-mato base, vegetables other than dark green, with cheese	portion 8.61oz/244g	9¾ +8¼ unit	☺+ ×1 unit ☺+ ×½ unit	☹ ¼	¼[A] ¾
Cauliflower, cooked from frozen	portion 3oz/85g	☺	☺ ☺	☹ 2½	☺[CB] ☺
Caviar	tbsp. 0.5ozfl/14.21ml	☺	☺ ☺	☺ ☺	☺ ☺
Celeriac (celery root), cooked from fresh	tbsp. 0.5ozfl/14.21ml	☺	13¼ 26½	☹ ¾	☺ ☺
Celery, cooked	tbsp. 0.5ozfl/14.21ml	☺	☺ ☺	☹ 1	☺[C] ☺
Champagne punch	glass 8.4ozfl/240ml	☺	¾ 1½	☹ 1	☺ ☺
Champagne, white	glass 8.4ozfl/240ml	☺	31¼ 62½	☹ ¾	☺ ☺

Keyword Index	Unit	Lactose L1 + unit/capsule	Fructose* L0 / Fructose* L1	Sorbitol L0 / Sorbitol L1	FrucGalactans L0 / FrucGalactans L1 (source)
Chard, raw or blanched, marinated in oil	portion 3oz/85g	☺	☺+ ×½ unit ☺+ ×¼ unit	☺ ☺	☺ ☺
Chardonnay	glass 8.4ozfl/240ml	☺	31¼ 62½	☹ ¾	☺ ☺
Chayote squash, cooked	portion 4.59oz/130g	☺	6¼ 12¾	☺ ☺	☺[B] ☺
Cheddar cheese, natural	portion 1.06oz/30g	43¼ +36 unit	☺ ☺	☺ ☺	☺ ☺
Cheese cracker	piece 0.11oz/3g	☺	☺ ☺	☺ ☺	3½[A] 7
Cheese gnocchi	portion 2.47oz/70g	28 +23¼ unit	☺ ☺	☺ ☺	1[A] 2¼
Cheese sauce, store bought	portion 2.33oz/66g	¼ +¼ unit	☺ ☺	☺ ☺	1¾ 3¾
Cheesecake, plain or flavored, graham cracker crust, homemade	piece 7.77oz/220g	½ +½ unit	☺+ ×½ unit ☺+ ×¼ unit	☺ ☺	☹[A] ¼
Cherry Coke®	glass 8.4ozfl/240ml	☺	½ 1¼	☺ ☺	☺ ☺
Cherry pie, bottom crust only	piece 4.31oz/122g	☺	1 2¼	☹ ☹[2]	¼[A] ¾
Chestnuts, boiled, steamed	portion 1.06oz/30g	☺	☺ ☺	☹ 6	☺ ☺
Chestnuts, roasted	portion 1.06oz/30g	☺	☺ ☺	☹ 3	☺ ☺
Chewing gum	piece 0.11oz/3g	☺	☺ ☺	☺ ☺	☺ ☺
Chewing gum, sugar free	piece 0.08oz/2g	☺	¼ ¾	☹ ☹[2]	☺ ☺
Chia seeds	hand 1.06oz/30g	☺	☺ ☺	☺ ☺	1¼[G] 2¾
Chicken and dumplings soup, condensed	portion 4.45oz/126g	7¼ +6 unit	☺ ☺	☹ 2¼	2¼ 4½

L0 *Level 0:* lactose measure ×½
L1 *Level 1:* fructose measure ×2
+ Unit/capsule: added tolerated amount of unit per strong lactase capsule
Fructose*: fructose, sorbitol adjusted
L2 *Level 2:* fructose-/sorbitol measure ×4. the rest ×2
L3 *Level 3:* sorbitol measure ×7. the rest ×3
(book): source of fruc/galactans data
☺+ ×[Amount] unit: Per unit consumed you can additionally tolerate up to [amount] × fructose(*)-unit of another product.

☹: avoid; ☹[1]: ¼ at TL 1; ☹[2]: ¼ at TL 2; ☹[3]: ¼ at TL 3; ☺: only contains traces; ☺: is free from it

Keyword Index	Unit	Lactose + unit/	Fructose* Fructose*	Sorbitol Sorbitol	FrucGalactans FrucGalactans
Chicken cake or patty	portion 3oz/85g	1½ +1¼ unit	14 28	☹ 58¾	3¼[B] 6½
Chicken fricassee with gravy, American style	portion 8.61oz/244g	☺	☺ ☺	☺ ☺	5¾[C] 11½
Chicken noodle soup with vegetables, ready-to-serve can	portion 8.65oz/245g	☺	☺ ☺	☹ 1	1¼ 2½
Chicken with cheese sauce, vegetables other than dark green	portion 7.62oz/216g	1 +¾ unit	5 10	☹ ½	☺ ☺
Chicken wonton soup, prepared from condensed can	portion 8.65oz/245g	☺	☺ ☺	☹ 40¾	☺ ☺
Chicory coffee	cup 5.2ozfl/150ml	☺	☺ ☺	☹ 11	☹[E] ☹
Chicory coffee powder, unprepared	portion 0.08oz/2g	☺	☺ ☺	☹ 8¾	½[E] 1
Chicory greens, raw	portion 3oz/85g	☺	5¼ 10½	☹ 39	2¼[B] 4½
Chili sauce, store bought	portion 2.4oz/68g	☺	2¾ 5½	☹ ¼	☺ ☺
Chili with beans, beef, canned	tbsp. 0.5oz.fl/14.8ml	☺	☺ ☺	☹ 55½	3[AC] 6
Chinese oyster sauce	portion 1.13oz/32g	☺	☺ ☺	☺ ☺	☺ ☺
Chips Ahoy!® Chewy Gooey Caramel Cookies (Nabisco®)	piece 0.55oz/15.5g	12¼ +10¼ unit	½ 1	☹ ☺	3[A] 6¼
Chives, raw	pinch 0.04oz/1g	☺	☺ ☺	☺ ☺	☺[B] ☺
Chobani® Nonfat Greek Yogurt, Black Cherry	tbsp. 0.5ozfl/14.21ml	5¼ +4½ unit	☺ ☺	☹ 3¾	30¼ 60¾
Chobani® Nonfat Greek Yogurt, Lemon	piece 6.04oz/171g	½ +¼ unit	☺+ ×½ unit ☺+ ×¼ unit	☺ ☺	3 6
Chobani® Nonfat Greek Yogurt, Peach	piece 6.04oz/171g	¼ +¼ unit	☺+ ×1 unit ☺+ ×½ unit	☹ 4¼	1¾ 3½
Chobani® Nonfat Greek Yogurt, Raspberry	piece 6.04oz/171g	¼ +¼ unit	☺+ ×¾ unit ☺+ ×¼ unit	☹ 20	1¾ 3½
Chobani® Nonfat Greek Yogurt, Strawberry	piece 6.04oz/171g	¼ +¼ unit	☺+ ×¾ unit ☺+ ×¼ unit	☹ 3½	1¾ 3½
Chocolate cake, glazed, store bought	piece 1.03oz/29g	☺	☺+ ×½ unit ☺+ ×¼ unit	☹ ☺	1¾[A] 3¾

KEYWORD INDEX	Unit	Lactose (1) + unit/[capsule]	Fructose* (0) Fructose* (1)	Sorbitol (0) Sorbitol (1)	FrucGalactans (0) FrucGalactans (1) 📖
Chocolate Chex® (General Mills®)	tbsp. 0.5ozfl/14.21ml	☻	¼ ½	☹ ☺	1¼[A] 2¾
Chocolate chip cookies, store bought	piece 0.36oz/10g	☻	☻ ☻	☹ ☺	2½[A] 5¼
Chocolate cookies, iced, store bought	piece 0.36oz/10g	☻	☻ ☻	☹ ☺	5[A] 10¼
Chocolate pudding, store bought	piece 3.5oz/98g	¾ +½ unit	☻ ☻	☹ 25	1[G] 2¼
Chocolate pudding, store bought, sugar free	tbsp. 0.5ozfl/14.21ml	89¼ +74¼ unit	¾ 1½	☹ ☹[2]	21¼[G] 42½
Chocolate sandwich cookies, double filling	piece 0.52oz/14.5g	☻	☻ ☻	☹ ☺	3½[A] 7
Chocolate sandwich cookies, sugar free	piece 0.43oz/12g	☺	13¾ 27¾	☹ ☹	4¼[A] 8½
Chocolate sauce, syrup	tbsp. 0.5ozfl/14.21ml	☻	☻+ ×1½ unit ☻+ ×¾ unit	☹ ☺	3[G] 6
Chocolate truffles	piece 0.58oz/16.2g	2½ +2 unit	☻ ☻	☻ ☻	2¾ 5½
Chop suey, chicken, no noodles	portion 5.86oz/166g	☻	☻ ☻	☹ ¼	¼[AB] ¾
Chop suey, tofu, no noodles	portion 5.86oz/166g	☻	☻ ☻	☹ ¼	☻ ☻
Cider vinegar	portion 0.5oz/14g	☻	6¼ 12½	☹ 1¾	☻ ☻
Cilantro leaf, fresh	pinch 0.04oz/1g	☻	☻ ☻	☻ ☻	☻ ☻
Cinnamon Roll with Icing, all flavours	piece 1.56oz/44g	9 +7½ unit	☻+ ×8¼ unit ☻+ ×4 unit	☻ ☻	1[A] 2¼
Cinnamon toast crunch® (General Mills®)	portion 1.06oz/30g	☻	¼ ½	☻ ☻	1½[A] 3
Cinnamon Toasters® (Malt-O-Meal®)	portion 1.06oz/30g	☻	2 4¼	☻ ☻	1½[A] 3
Clams, stuffed with mushroom, onions, and bread	portion 4.94oz/140g	24½ +20½ unit	☻ ☻	☹ ½	3¼[CB] 6¾

(0) *Level 0:* lactose measure ×½
(1) *Level 1:* fructose measure ×2
(2) *Level 2:* fructose-/sorbitol measure ×4. the rest ×2
(3) *Level 3:* sorbitol measure ×7. the rest ×3
📖: source of fruc/galactans data

+ Unit/[capsule]: added tolerated amount of unit per strong lactase capsule
Fructose*: fructose, sorbitol adjusted
☻+ ×[Amount] unit: Per unit consumed you can additionally tolerate up to [amount] × fructose(*)-unit of another product.

☹: avoid; ☹[1]: ¼ at TL 1; ☹[2]: ¼ at TL 2; ☹[3]: ¼ at TL 3; ☺: only contains traces; ☻: is free from it

Keyword Index	Unit	Lactose + unit/pill	Fructose* Fructose*	Sorbitol Sorbitol	FrucGalactans FrucGalactans
Classic Fruit Chocolates (Liberty Orchards®)	piece 0.53oz/15g	56½ +47 unit	☺+ ×¼ unit ☺	☹ 31½	5½[G] 11¼
Clementine, fresh	portion 4.94oz/140g	☺	7 14¼	☺ ☺	2¼[B] 4½
Clif Bar®,Chocolate Chip	piece 2.4oz/68g	9 +7½ unit	☺+ ×10 unit ☺+ ×5 unit	☹ 2¼	¾ 1½
Clif Bar®,Crunchy Peanut Butter	piece 2.4oz/68g	☺	☺+ ×10¼ unit ☺+ ×5 unit	☹ 2½	☺ ☺
Clif Bar®,Oatmeal Raisin Walnut	piece 2.4oz/68g	☺	☺+ ×10¼ unit ☺+ ×5¼ unit	☹ 1¾	1¾[AG] 3½
Club soda	glass 8.4ozfl/240ml	☺	☺ ☺	☺ ☺	☺ ☺
Cocktail sauce	portion 2.4oz/68g	☺	☺+ ×2 unit ☺+ ×1 unit	☹ ¾	☺ ☺
Cocoa Krispies® (Kellogg's®)	portion 1.06oz/30g	☺	☺ ☺	☹ ☺	1½[A] 3
Cocoa Puffs® (General Mills®)	portion 1.06oz/30g	☺	☺+ ×2 unit ☺+ ×1 unit	☹ ☺	½[A] 1¼
Coconut bars, nuts	piece 1.49oz/42g	45¼ +37¾ unit	☺ ☺	☺ ☺	☺ ☺
Coconut cream (liquid from grated meat)	hand 1.06oz/30g	☺	20¾ 41½	☺ ☺	☺ ☺
Coconut milk, fresh (liquid from grated meat, water added)	glass 8.4oz/240g	☺	☺+ ×1 unit ☺+ ×½ unit	☺ ☺	1¾[G] 3½
Coconut oil	pinch 0.04oz/1g	☺	☺ ☺	☺ ☺	☺ ☺
Coconut, dried, shredded or flaked, unsweetened	hand 1.06oz/30g	☺	☺+ ×¾ unit ☺+ ×¼ unit	☺ ☺	12¼ 24½
Coconut, fresh	portion 0.53oz/15g	☺	☺+ ×¼ unit ☺	☺ ☺	24½[G] 49
Coffee substitute, prepared	cup 5.2ozfl/150ml	☺	☺ ☺	☺ ☺	☺ ☺
Coffee, prepared from flavored mix, sugar free	cup 5.2ozfl/150ml	☺	☺ ☺	☹ 66½	☺ ☺
Cognac	glass 8.4ozfl/240ml	☺	☺ ☺	☺ ☺	☺ ☺
Cointreau®	glass 8.4ozfl/240ml	☺	☺+ ×4½ unit ☺+ ×2½ unit	☹ ¼	☺ ☺
Coke Zero®	glass 8.4ozfl/240ml	☺	☺ ☺	☺ ☺	☺ ☺

KEYWORD INDEX	Unit	Lactose [1] + unit/(capsule)	Fructose* [0] Fructose* [1]	Sorbitol [0] Sorbitol [1]	FrucGalactans [0] FrucGalactans [1] 📖
Coke®	glass 8.4ozfl/240ml	☺	½ 1¼	☺ ☺	☺ ☺
Coke® with Lime	glass 8.4ozfl/240ml	☺	½ 1¼	☺ ☺	☺ ☺
Colby Jack cheese	portion 1.06oz/30g	27¼ +22¾ unit	☺ ☺	☺ ☺	☺ ☺
Coleslaw, with apples and raisins, mayo dressing	portion 3.53oz/100g	☺	½ 1	☹ ½	1 B 2
Coleslaw, with pineapple, mayo dressing	portion 3.53oz/100g	☺	☺+ ×¼ unit ☺	☹ 3¾	☺ B ☺
Collards, raw	portion 3oz/85g	☺	☺ ☺	☺ ☺	1¼ B 2½
Corn Chex® (General Mills®)	portion 1.06oz/30g	☺	☺ ☺	☹ ☺	½ A 1¼
Corn Flakes (Kellogg's®)	portion 1.06oz/30g	☺	☺+ ×1½ unit ☺+ ×¾ unit	☹ ☺	1½ A 3
Cottage cheese, 1% fat, lactose reduced	portion 3.89oz/110g	3¼ +2¾ unit	☺+ ×1¾ unit ☺+ ×¾ unit	☺ ☺	18¾ 37¾
Cottage cheese, uncreamed dry curd	portion 1.95oz/55g	3½ +2¾ unit	☺ ☺	☺ ☺	19¾ 39½
Couscous, cooked	portion 4.94oz/140g	☺	☺ ☺	☺ ☺	¼ A ¾
Cracked wheat bread, with raisins	slice 1.49oz/42g	☺	1¼ 2¾	☹ 4¼	1¾ A 3½
Cranberries, dried (Craisins®)	portion 1.42oz/40g	☺	☺+ ×3¼ unit ☺+ ×1½ unit	☹ 41½	☺ ☺
Cranberries, fresh	portion 1.95oz/55g	☺	☺+ ×2¾ unit ☺+ ×1¼ unit	☹ 45¼	☺ ☺
Cranberry juice cocktail, with apple juice	glass 8.4ozfl/240ml	☺	☹[1] ¼	☹ ☹[2]	1½ CB 3
Cranberry juice cocktail, with blueberry juice	glass 8.4ozfl/240ml	☺	☹[1] ¼	☹ ☹[2]	☺ ☺
Cream cheese spread	portion 1.06oz/30g	2¾ +2¼ unit	☺ ☺	☺ ☺	15¾ 31½

[0] *Level 0:* lactose measure ×½
[1] *Level 1:* fructose measure ×2
+ Unit/(capsule): added tolerated amount of unit per strong lactase capsule
Fructose*: fructose, sorbitol adjusted

[2] *Level 2:* fructose-/sorbitol measure ×4. the rest ×2
[3] *Level 3:* sorbitol measure ×7. the rest ×3
📖: source of fruc/galactans data
☺+ ×[Amount] unit: Per unit consumed you can additionally tolerate up to [amount] × fructose(*)-unit of another product.

☹: avoid; ☹[1]: ¼ at TL 1; ☹[2]: ¼ at TL 2; ☹[3]: ¼ at TL 3; ☺: only contains traces; ☺: is free from it

Keyword Index	Unit	Lactose + unit/	Fructose* Fructose*	Sorbitol Sorbitol	FrucGalactans FrucGalactans
Cream cheese, whipped, flavored	portion 1.06oz/30g	2½ +2 unit	☺ ☺	☺ ☺	14 28
Cream cheese, whipped, plain	portion 1.06oz/30g	3 +2½ unit	☺ ☺	☺ ☺	17¼ 34½
Cream of asparagus soup, prepared from condensed can	tbsp. 0.5ozfl/14.21ml	6½ +5½ unit	☺ ☺	☹ ☺	1½ 3
Cream of broccoli soup, condensed	portion 4.45oz/126g	5 +4¼ unit	☺ ☺	☹ 19¾	1[C] 2¼
Cream of celery soup, homemade	portion 8.65oz/245g	½ +½ unit	☺ ☺	☹ ¼	¼ ½
Cream of chicken soup, condensed	portion 4.45oz/126g	6½ +5½ unit	☺ ☺	☹ 26¼	37¼[CB] 74¾
Cream of mushroom soup, prepared from condensed can	portion 8.65oz/245g	8½ +7 unit	☺ ☺	☹ ¼	½ 1
Cream of potato soup mix, dry	portion 0.82oz/23g	3¼ +2¾ unit	☺ ☺	☹ 3	5 10
Cream of spinach soup mix, dry	portion 0.57oz/16g	☺	☺+ ×¼ unit ☺	☹ 18¼	3¼ 6¾
Creamed chicken	portion 8.51oz/241g	½ +¼ unit	☺ ☺	☹ 13¾	☺ ☺
Creme de Cocoa	glass 8.4ozfl/240ml	☺	☺ ☺	☹ 2½	☺ ☺
Creme de menthe	glass 8.4ozfl/240ml	☺	☺+ ×4½ unit ☺+ ×2½ unit	☹ ¼	☺ ☺
Crepe, plain	piece 1.95oz/55g	1¼ +1 unit	☺ ☺	☺ ☺	¾[A] 1¾
Crisco® Pure Corn Oil	portion 0.46oz/13g	☺	☺ ☺	☺ ☺	☺ ☺
Croissant, chocolate	piece 2.44oz/69g	3½ +3 unit	☺+ ×1 unit ☺+ ×½ unit	☹ ☺	¾[A] 1½
Croissant, fruit	piece 2.62oz/74g	3½ +3 unit	☺+ ×2½ unit ☺+ ×1¼ unit	☹ 2	½[A] 1¼
Crunchy Nut Roasted Nut & Honey (Kellogg's®)	portion 1.06oz/30g	☺	23¾ 47½	☹ 15	1½[A] 3
Cucumber, raw, with peel	portion 3oz/85g	☺	5¼ 10½	☹ 1	☺[B] ☺
Cucumber, raw, without peel	portion 3oz/85g	☺	4¾ 9¾	☹ 1	☺[B] ☺
Curacao	glass 8.4ozfl/240ml	☺	☺+ ×4½ unit ☺+ ×2½ unit	☹ ¼	☺ ☺

Keyword Index	Unit	Lactose + unit/	Fructose* Fructose*	Sorbitol Sorbitol	FrucGalactans FrucGalactans
Currants, fresh, black	portion 4.94oz/140g	☺	1¼ 2½	☺ ☺	☺ ☺
Currants, fresh, red and white	portion 4.94oz/140g	☺	1 2¼	☺ ☺	☺ ☺
Curry sauce, from cream	portion 2.09oz/59g	2 +1½ unit	☺ ☺	☹ 4	11¼ 22½
Daiquiri	glass 8.4ozfl/240ml	☺	☺ ☺	☺ ☺	☺ ☺
Dairy Queen® Foot Long Hot Dog	piece 7.02oz/199g	☺	☺+ ×1¾ unit ☺+ ×¾ unit	☹ 8¼	¼ A ½
Danish pastry, frosted or glazed, with cheese filling	piece 4.41oz/125g	3 +2½ unit	☺ ☺	☺ ☺	¼ D ½
Danone® Activia® Light Yogurt, vanilla	piece 4oz/115g	¼ +¼ unit	¼ ¾	☺ ☺	2 4
Danone® Activia® Yogurt, plain	piece 4oz/115g	½ +¼ unit	☺ ☺	☺ ☺	2¾ 5½
Danone® Greek Yogurt, Honey	piece 5.3oz/150g	½ +¼ unit	¼ ½	☹ 3¼	2¾ 5¾
Danone® Greek Yogurt, Plain	piece 5.3oz/150g	½ +¼ unit	☺ ☺	☺ ☺	1¼ 2½
Danone® la Crème Yogurt, fruit flavors	piece 4oz/115g	¼ +¼ unit	¼ ½	☹ 10¾	2 4
Dare Breaktime Ginger Cookies	piece 0.27oz/7.5g	☺	☺ ☺	☺ ☺	8½ A 17¼
Dare® Lemon Crème Cookies	piece 0.69oz/19.5g	32½ +27 unit	☺ ☺	☺ ☺	2½ A 5¼
Dark chocolate bar 45%-59% cacoa	bar 4.77oz/135g	1¼ +1 unit	☺ ☺	☹ 8	¼ ¾
Dark chocolate bar 60%-69% cacao	bar 4.77oz/135g	7½ +6¼ unit	☺ ☺	☹ 6½	¼ ¾
Dark chocolate bar 70%-85% cacao	bar 4.77oz/135g	☺	☺ ☺	☹ 5	¼ ¾
Dark chocolate bar, sugar free	piece 0.43ozfl/12g	26¾ +22¼ unit	34 68¼	☹ ☹	4¼ 8¾

0 *Level 0:* lactose measure ×½ + Unit/: added tolerated amount of unit per strong lactase capsule
1 *Level 1:* fructose measure ×2 Fructose*: fructose, sorbitol adjusted
2 *Level 2:* fructose-/sorbitol measure ×4. the rest ×2 ☺+ ×[Amount] unit: Per unit consumed you can additionally tolerate up to [amount] × fructose(*)-unit of another product.
3 *Level 3:* sorbitol measure ×7. the rest ×3
: source of fruc/galactans data
☹: avoid; ☹1: ¼ at TL 1; ☹2: ¼ at TL 2; ☹3: ¼ at TL 3; ☺: only contains traces; ☺: is free from it

Keyword Index	Unit	Lactose + unit/	Fructose* Fructose*	Sorbitol Sorbitol	FrucGalactans FrucGalactans
Dark Fruit Chocolates (Liberty Orchards®)	piece 0.53oz/15g	56½ +47 unit	☺+ ×¼ unit ☺	☹ 31½	5½[G] 11¼
Dark Fruit Chocolates, Sugar Free (Liberty Orchards®)	piece 0.6oz/17g	37¾ +31¼ unit	☹[2] ☹[2]	☹ ☹	4¾[G] 9¾
Dates	portion 1.42oz/40g	☺	☺ ☺	☺ ☺	☺ ☺
Demitasse	cup 5.2ozfl/150ml	☺	☺ ☺	☺ ☺	☺ ☺
Diet 7 UP®	glass 8.4ozfl/240ml	☺	☺ ☺	☺ ☺	☺ ☺
Diet Coke®	glass 8.4ozfl/240ml	☺	☺ ☺	☺ ☺	☺ ☺
Diet Dr. Pepper®	glass 8.4ozfl/240ml	☺	☺ ☺	☺ ☺	☺ ☺
Diet Pepsi®, fountain	glass 8.4ozfl/240ml	☺	☺ ☺	☺ ☺	☺ ☺
Dijon mustard	tbsp. 0.5ozfl/14.21ml	☺	☺ ☺	☹ ☺	☺ ☺
Distilled vinegar	portion 0.5oz/14g	☺	☺ ☺	☺ ☺	☺ ☺
Doritos® Tortilla Chips, Nacho Cheese	hand 0.75oz/21g	☺	☺ ☺	☹ ☺	10¾[A] 21½
Doughnut, raised, glazed, coconut topping	piece 2.79oz/79g	4¾ +4 unit	☺ ☺	☺ ☺	½[A] 1¼
Doughnut, raised, glazed, plain	piece 2.72oz/77g	4¾ +4 unit	☺ ☺	☺ ☺	½[A] 1¼
Doughnut, raised, sugared	piece 2.56oz/72.5g	4¾ +4 unit	☺ ☺	☺ ☺	¾[A] 1½
Dove® Promises, Milk Chocolate	cup 5.2ozfl/150ml	¼ +0.21 unit	☺ ☺	☹ ☺	1¾ 3¾
Dreyer's® Grand Ice Cream, Chocolate	portion 2.3oz/65g	1 +1 unit	☺+ ×¾ unit ☺+ ×¼ unit	☹ ☺	2¾[G] 5¾
Dreyer's® No Sugar Added Ice Cream, Triple Chocolate	tsp. 0.16ozfl/4.74ml	11½ +9½ unit	¾ 1¾	☹ ☹[2]	32¾[G] 65½
Drumstick® (sundae cone)	piece 3.39oz/96g	1 +¾ unit	☺+ ×2¼ unit ☺+ ×1 unit	☹ ☺	6¼ 12¾
Earl Grey, strong	glass 8.4ozfl/240ml	☺	½ 1¼	☺ ☺	1½[G] 3
Edam cheese	portion 1.06oz/30g	6¾ +5¾ unit	☺ ☺	☺ ☺	38¾ 77½

KEYWORD INDEX	Unit	Lactose (L1) + unit/capsule	Fructose* (L0) Fructose* (L1)	Sorbitol (L0) Sorbitol (L1)	FrucGalactans (L0) FrucGalactans (L1) 📖
EGG® bread roll	piece 1.24oz/35g	5¼ +4¼ unit	☺ ☺	☺ ☺	1½ [A] 3
Eggplant, cooked	portion 3oz/85g	☺	3½ 7¼	☹ 2½	☺ [B] ☺
Elderberries, fresh	portion 4.94oz/140g	☺	¼ ½	☺ ☺	☺ ☺
Electrolyte replacement drink	glass 8.4oz/240g	☺	☺+ ×9¾ unit ☺+ ×4¾ unit	☺ ☺	☺ ☺
Elephant ear (crispy)	piece 2.09oz/59g	4¼ +3½ unit	☺ ☺	☺ ☺	1 [A] 2
Endive, curly, raw	portion 3oz/85g	☺	☺ ☺	☹ 3	3¾ [C] 7½
English muffin bread	slice 1.49oz/42g	☺	38¼ 76¾	☺ ☺	1¾ [A] 3½
English muffin, whole wheat, with raisins	piece 2.33oz/66g	1¼ +1 unit	2 4	☹ 2¼	¾ [A] 1½
Enoki mushrooms, raw	tbsp. 0.5ozfl/14.21ml	☺	☺ ☺	☹ ¾	☺ ☺
Espresso, without flavored syrup	cup 5.2ozfl/150ml	☺	☺ ☺	☺ ☺	☺ ☺
Essentials Oat Bran cereal (Quaker®)	portion 1.95oz/55g	☺	☺ ☺	☺ ☺	1¼ [A] 2¾
Evaporated milk, diluted, 2% fat (reduced fat)	glass 8.4oz/240g	¼ +0,22 unit	☺ ☺	☺ ☺	1½ 3
Evaporated milk, diluted, skim (fat free)	glass 8.4oz/240g	¼ +0,21 unit	☺ ☺	☺ ☺	1¼ 2¾
Evaporated milk, diluted, whole	glass 8.4oz/240g	¼ +0,24 unit	☺ ☺	☺ ☺	1½ 3
Falafel	portion 1.95oz/55g	☺	☺ ☺	☹ 1¾	¾ [G] 1½
Familia Swiss Muesli®, Original Recipe	portion 1.95oz/55g	☺	1 2	☹ 1	¼ [A] ¾
Fanta Zero®, fruit flavors	glass 8.4ozfl/240ml	☺	☺ ☺	☺ ☺	☺ ☺

Level 0: lactose measure ×½
Level 1: fructose measure ×2
+ Unit/capsule: added tolerated amount of unit per strong lactase capsule
Fructose*: fructose, sorbitol adjusted
Level 2: fructose-/sorbitol measure ×4. the rest ×2
Level 3: sorbitol measure ×7. the rest ×3
📖: source of fruc/galactans data
☺+ ×[Amount] unit: Per unit consumed you can additionally tolerate up to [amount] × fructose(*)-unit of another product.
☹: avoid; ☹[1]: ¼ at TL 1; ☹[2]: ¼ at TL 2; ☹[3]: ¼ at TL 3; ☺: only contains traces; ☺: is free from it

Keyword Index	Unit	Lactose + unit/	Fructose* Fructose*	Sorbitol Sorbitol	FrucGalactans FrucGalactans
Fanta® Red	glass 8.4ozfl/240ml	☺	☹[1] ¼	☺ ☺	☺ ☺
Fanta®, fruit flavors	glass 8.4ozfl/240ml	☺	8¼ 16½	☺ ☺	☺ ☺
Fennel bulb, raw	portion 3oz/85g	☺	☺+ ×¾ unit ☺+ ×¼ unit	☹ 2	1¼[B] 2¾
Fennel tea	glass 8.6ozfl/247ml	☺	☺ ☺	☺ ☺	½[G] 1¼
Feta cheese	portion 1.06oz/30g	2¼ +2 unit	☺ ☺	☺ ☺	13½ 27
Feta cheese, fat free	portion 1.06oz/30g	¾ +¾ unit	☺ ☺	☺ ☺	5 10¼
Fettuccini Alfredo®, no meat, vegetables other than dark green	tbsp. 0.5ozfl/14.21ml	66¾ +55½ unit	☺ ☺	☹ 2¾	81½[A] ☺
Fettuccini Alfredo®, no meat, with carrots or dark green vegetables	portion 7.06oz/200g	5 +4 unit	☺ ☺	☺ ☺	27¾ 55½
Fettuccini noodles, whole wheat, cooked in unsalted water	portion 4.94oz/140g	☺	☺+ ×¼ unit ☺	☺ ☺	1[A] 2
Fiber One Original® (General Mills®)	portion 1.06oz/30g	☺	41½ 83¼	☺ ☺	½[A] 1¼
Fiber One® Nutty Clusters & Almonds (General Mills®)	portion 1.95oz/55g	☺	☺ ☺	☺ ☺	¼[A] ¾
Fifty 50® Sugar Free Low Glycemic Butterscotch Hard Candy	piece 0.14oz/3.75g	☺	☺ ☺	☹ ☹	☺ ☺
Figs, dried, cooked, sweetened	piece 1.77oz/50g	☺	☺+ ×¾ unit ☺+ ×¼ unit	☺ ☺	☺ ☺
Figs, fresh	piece 1.77oz/50g	☺	☺+ ×2 unit ☺+ ×1 unit	☺ ☺	☺ ☺
Filberts, raw	hand 1.06oz/30g	☺	☺ ☺	☹ 8¼	2¾[G] 5¾
Fish croquette	portion 3oz/85g	2¼ +1¾ unit	☺ ☺	☹ ☺	1¾[A] 3½
Fish or seafood with cream or white sauce	portion 6.39oz/181g	1½ +1¼ unit	☺ ☺	☺ ☺	☺ ☺
Fish sticks, patties, or nuggets, breaded, regular	portion 3oz/85g	☺	☺ ☺	☺ ☺	2[A] 4
Fish with breading	portion 3oz/85g	☺	☺ ☺	☺ ☺	☺ ☺

Keyword Index	Unit	Lactose 1 + unit/💊	Fructose* 0 Fructose* 1	Sorbitol 0 Sorbitol 1	FrucGalactans 0 FrucGalactans 1 📖
Flax seed oil	portion 0.46oz/13g	😀	😀 😀	😀 😀	😀 😀
Flax seeds, not fortifed	tbsp. 0.5ozfl/14.21ml	😀	😀 😀	😀 😀	2 4¼ G
Fleischmann's® Move Over Butter Margarine, tub, whipped	portion 0.32oz/9g	21¾ +18 unit	😀 😀	😀 😀	☺ ☺
Focaccia bread	slice 1.49oz/42g	😀	😀 😀	😀 😀	1¼ A 2½
Fondue sauce	portion 1.87oz/53g	☺	😀+ ×¼ unit 😀	☹ 5	☺ ☺
Frappuccino®	cup 5.2ozfl/150ml	½ +½ unit	😀 😀	😀 😀	3¾ 7½
Frappuccino®, bottled or canned	cup 5.2ozfl/150ml	½ +½ unit	😀 😀	😀 😀	3½ 7
Frappuccino®, bottled or canned, light	cup 5.2ozfl/150ml	½ +½ unit	😀 😀	😀 😀	4 8
French Burnt Peanuts	hand 1.06oz/30g	😀	😀+ ×1¾ unit 😀+ ×¾ unit	😀 😀	😀 G 😀
French onion soup, condensed	portion 4.45oz/126g	☺	😀+ ×1½ unit 😀+ ×¾ unit	☹ 2	¼ CB ¾
French or Vienna roll	slice 1.49oz/42g	😀	😀 😀	😀 😀	1¼ A 2½
French toast, homemade, French bread	piece 4.63oz/131g	1¼ +1 unit	😀+ ×½ unit 😀+ ×¼ unit	😀 😀	¼ A ¾
Froot Loops® (Kellogg's®)	portion 1.06oz/30g	😀	😀 😀	😀 😀	½ A 1¼
Frosted Flakes® (Kellogg's®)	portion 1.06oz/30g	😀	😀 😀	☹ ☺	1½ A 3
Frosted Flakes® Reduced Sugar (Kellogg's®)	portion 1.06oz/30g	😀	😀+ ×¼ unit 😀	☹ ☺	1½ A 3
Frosted Mini-Wheats Big Bite® (Kellogg's®)	portion 1.95oz/55g	😀	😀+ ×¼ unit 😀	😀 😀	¼ A ¾

0 *Level 0:* lactose measure ×½
1 *Level 1:* fructose measure ×2
2 *Level 2*: fructose-/sorbitol measure ×4. the rest ×2
3 *Level 3:* sorbitol measure ×7. the rest ×3
📖: source of fruc/galactans data

+ Unit/💊: added tolerated amount of unit per strong lactase capsule
Fructose*: fructose, sorbitol adjusted

😀+ ×[Amount] unit: Per unit consumed you can additionally tolerate up to [amount] × fructose(*)-unit of another product.

☹: avoid; ☹[1]: ¼ at TL 1; ☹[2]: ¼ at TL 2; ☹[3]: ¼ at TL 3; ☺: only contains traces; 😀: is free from it

Keyword Index	Unit	Lactose + unit/	Fructose* Fructose*	Sorbitol Sorbitol	FrucGalactans FrucGalactans
Frozen custard, chocolate or coffee flavors	portion 3.09oz/87.5g	½ +¼ unit	☺+ ×2¼ unit ☺+ ×1 unit	☹ ☺	½[A] 1
Frozen fruit juice bar	piece 2.72oz/77g	☺	☺+ ×1¼ unit ☺+ ×½ unit	☹ 4½	☺ ☺
Fruit drink or punch, ready to drink	glass 8.4ozfl/240ml	☺	☺+ ×1 unit ☺+ ×½ unit	☹ 2	1½[C] 3
Fruit punch, alcoholic	glass 8.4ozfl/240ml	☺	¾ 1½	☹ 1	☺ ☺
Fruit sauce, jelly-based	portion 1.42oz/40g	☺	☺+ ×5¼ unit ☺+ ×2½ unit	☹ ¾	☺ ☺
Garbanzo beans (chickpeas), canned, drained	portion 3.18oz/90g	☺	☺ ☺	☹ 1	1½[A] 3
Gardenburger® Sun-Dried Tomato Basil	portion 3oz/85g	☺	1¼ 2½	☹ 1	7¾[B] 15¾
Garlic sauce	tbsp. 0.5ozfl/14.21ml	☺	☺ ☺	☺ ☺	☹[FB] ☹
Garlic, fresh	portion 0.15oz/4g	☺	☺ ☺	☺ ☺	¾[FB] 1½
Garlic, powder	pinch 0.04oz/1g	☺	☺ ☺	☺ ☺	3¼[FB] 6½
Gatorade®, all flavors	glass 8.4oz/240g	7½ +6¼ unit	☺+ ×1¼ unit ☺+ ×½ unit	☺ ☺	41½ 83¼
Gatorade®, from dry mix, all flavors	glass 8.4oz/240g	☺	☺+ ×10½ unit ☺+ ×5¼ unit	☺ ☺	☺ ☺
Gelatin (jello) powder, flavored, sugar free	piece 0.18oz/5g	☺	☺ ☺	☺ ☺	☺ ☺
Gelatin (jello) powder, plain	piece 0.07oz/1.75g	☺	☺ ☺	☺ ☺	☺ ☺
German chocolate cake, glazed, homemade	piece 1.03oz/29g	☺	☺+ ×½ unit ☺+ ×¼ unit	☹ ☺	1¾[A] 3¾
German style potato salad, with bacon and vinegar dressing	portion 4.94oz/140g	☺	☺+ ×¼ unit ☺	☹ 4¾	1[CB] 2
GG® Scandinavian Bran Crispbread (Health Valley®)	slice 1.49oz/42g	☺	☺ ☺	☺ ☺	¼[A] ½
Gibson	glass 8.4ozfl/240ml	☺	☺ ☺	☹ 3¼	☺ ☺
Gin	glass 8.4ozfl/240ml	☺	☺ ☺	☺ ☺	☺ ☺
Ginger ale	glass 8.4ozfl/240ml	☺	☹[2] ☹[2]	☺ ☺	☺ ☺

KEYWORD INDEX	Unit	Lactose 1🗲 + unit/capsule	Fructose* 0🗲 Fructose* 1🗲	Sorbitol 0🗲 Sorbitol 1🗲	FrucGalactans 0🗲 FrucGalactans 1🗲 📖
Ginger root, raw	portion 0.15oz/4g	☻	89¼ ☺	☻ ☻	☻^{B} ☻
Ginger sauce, Asian style	portion 1.13oz/32g	☻	☻ ☻	☹ 9¼	☻^{B} ☻
Ginger, ground	pinch 0.04oz/1g	☻	89¼ ☺	☻ ☻	☻^{B} ☻
Ginko nuts, dried	hand 1.06oz/30g	☻	☺ ☺	☻ ☻	☻ ☻
Girard's® Wasabi and Ginger Vinaigrette	pinch 0.04oz/1g	☻	☺ ☺	☹ ☺	☻^{B} ☻
Girl Scout® Lemonades	piece 0.55oz/15.5g	☻	☻ ☻	☻ ☻	4^{A} 8¼
Girl Scout® Peanut Butter Patties	piece 0.45oz/12.5g	☻	☻ ☻	☹ ☺	4^{A} 8¼
Girl Scout® Samoas®	piece 0.52oz/14.5g	52¼ +43½ unit	10¼ 20½	☹ ¾	3½^{A} 7
Girl Scout® Shortbread®	piece 0.4oz/11.34g	18½ +15½ unit	☻ ☻	☻ ☻	3¼^{A} 6¾
Girl Scout® Thin Mints	piece 0.29oz/8g	32½ +27 unit	☺ ☺	☹ ☺	6¼^{A} 12½
Glaceau® Vitaminwater 10	glass 8.4oz/240g	☻	☹^{1} ¼	☹ ☹^{2}	☻ ☻
Glaceau® Vitaminwater Energy	glass 8.4oz/240g	☻	☹^{2} ☹^{2}	☻ ☻	☻ ☻
Glaceau® Vitaminwater Essential	glass 8.4oz/240g	☻	☹^{2} ☹^{2}	☻ ☻	☻ ☻
Glaceau® Vitaminwater Focus	glass 8.4oz/240g	☻	☹^{2} ☹^{2}	☻ ☻	☻ ☻
Glaceau® Vitaminwater Power-C	glass 8.4oz/240g	☻	☹^{2} ☹^{2}	☻ ☻	☻ ☻
Glaceau® Vitaminwater Revive	glass 8.4oz/240g	☻	☹^{2} ☹^{2}	☻ ☻	☻ ☻
Gluten free bread	slice 1.49oz/42g	☻	☻ ☻	☻ ☻	3½^{A} 7

0🗲 *Level 0:* lactose measure ×½
1🗲 *Level 1:* fructose measure ×2
+ Unit/capsule: added tolerated amount of unit per strong lactase capsule
Fructose*: fructose, sorbitol adjusted

2🗲 *Level 2:* fructose-/sorbitol measure ×4. the rest ×2
3🗲 *Level 3:* sorbitol measure ×7. the rest ×3
📖: source of fruc/galactans data

☻+ ×[Amount] unit: Per unit consumed you can additionally tolerate up to [amount] × fructose(*)-unit of another product.

☹: avoid; ☹^{1}: ¼ at TL 1; ☹^{2}: ¼ at TL 2; ☹^{3}: ¼ at TL 3; ☺: only contains traces; ☻: is free from it

KEYWORD INDEX	Unit	Lactose + unit/	Fructose* Fructose*	Sorbitol Sorbitol	FrucGalactans FrucGalactans
GO Veggie!™ Rice Slices, all flavors	portion 1.06oz/30g	12 +10 unit	☺ ☺	☺ ☺	67¼[A] ☺
Goats cheese, hard	portion 1.06oz/30g	4½ +3¾ unit	☺ ☺	☺ ☺	25½ 51
GoLEAN® Crisp! Cereal, Cinnamon Crumble (Kashi®)	portion 1.95oz/55g	☺	☺+ ×1¼ unit ☺+ ×½ unit	☹ 25¾	¼[A] ¾
GoLEAN® Crunch! Cereal, Honey Almond Flax (Kashi®)	portion 1.95oz/55g	☺	☺+ ×1 unit ☺+ ×½ unit	☹ 18	¼[A] ¾
Gooseberries, fresh	portion 4.94oz/140g	☺	☺+ ×1 unit ☺+ ×½ unit	☺ ☺	☺ ☺
Gorgonzola cheese	portion 1.06oz/30g	20 +16½ unit	☺ ☺	☺ ☺	☺ ☺
Gorton's® Battered Fish Fillets - Lemon Pepper	portion 3oz/85g	☺	☺ ☺	☺ ☺	☺ ☺
Gorton's® Popcorn Shrimp, Original	portion 3oz/85g	☺	☺ ☺	☺ ☺	2[A] 4
Gouda cheese	portion 1.06oz/30g	4½ +3¾ unit	☺ ☺	☺ ☺	25 50
Goulash, with beef, noodles or macaroni, tomato base	tbsp. 0.5ozfl/14.21ml	☺	☺ ☺	☹ 4	☺ ☺
Grand Marnier®	glass 8.4ozfl/240ml	☺	☺+ ×4½ unit ☺+ ×2½ unit	☹ ¼	☺ ☺
Grapefruit juice, unsweetened, white	glass 8.4ozfl/240ml	☺	☺+ ×5 unit ☺+ ×2½ unit	☹ ¼	1[CB] 2
Grapefruit, fresh, pink or red	portion 4.94oz/140g	☺	2 4¼	☺ ☺	1½[CB] 3
Grapes, fresh	portion 4.94oz/140g	☺	¼ ½	☹ ½	2¼[B] 4½
Grasshopper	glass 8.4ozfl/240ml	1¼ +1 unit	☺+ ×1¼ unit ☺+ ×¾ unit	☹ ¾	7 14
Greek yogurt, plain, nonfat,	piece 5.3oz/150g	¼ +¼ unit	☺ ☺	☺ ☺	2½ 5
Green beans (string beans), cooked from fresh	portion 3oz/85g	☺	4½ 9	☺ ☺	¼[A] ¾
Green bell peppers	portion 3oz/85g	☺	☺ ☺	☺ ☺	☺[B] ☺
Green olives	portion 0.53oz/15g	☺	☺ ☺	☹ 18	☺ ☺
Green pea soup, prepared from condensed can	tbsp. 0.5ozfl/14.21ml	☺	☺ ☺	☹ 20	3¼[AC] 6¾

KEYWORD INDEX	Unit	Lactose (Level 1) + unit/capsule	Fructose* (Level 0) Fructose* (Level 1)	Sorbitol (Level 0) Sorbitol (Level 1)	FrucGalactans (Level 0) FrucGalactans (Level 1) 📖
Green tea, strong	glass 8.7ozfl/248ml	☺	☺ ☺	☺ ☺	☺ G ☺
Green tomato, raw	portion 3oz/85g	☺	3 6¼	☹ ¾	6½ B 13
Guava (guayaba), fresh, common	piece 5.3oz/150g	☺	2¼ 5	☹ ½	☺ ☺
Gum drops	hand 1.06oz/30g	☺	☺+ ×2¼ unit ☺+ ×1 unit	☺ ☺	☺ ☺
Gum drops, sugar free	tsp. 0.16ozfl/4.74ml	☺	☺ ☺	☹ ☹	☺ ☺
Gummi bears	hand 1.06oz/30g	☺	☺+ ×3½ unit ☺+ ×1¾ unit	☹ ☺	☺ ☺
Gummi bears, sugar free	tsp. 0.16ozfl/4.74ml	☺	10 20¼	☹ ☹3	☺ ☺
Gummi dinosaurs	hand 1.06oz/30g	☺	☺+ ×3½ unit ☺+ ×1¾ unit	☹ ☺	☺ ☺
Gummi dinosaurs, sugar free	tsp. 0.16ozfl/4.74ml	☺	10 20¼	☹ ☹3	☺ ☺
Gummi worms	hand 1.06oz/30g	☺	☺+ ×3½ unit ☺+ ×1¾ unit	☹ ☺	☺ ☺
Gummi worms, sugar free	tsp. 0.16ozfl/4.74ml	☺	10 20¼	☹ ☹3	☺ ☺
Haagen-Dazs® Desserts Extraordinaire Ice Cream, Creme Brulee	portion 3.78oz/107g	½ +¼ unit	☺+ ×4¾ unit ☺+ ×2¼ unit	☺ ☺	3 6¼
Haagen-Dazs® Frozen Yogurt, chocolate or coffee flavors	portion 3.74oz/106g	½ +½ unit	☺+ ×¾ unit ☺+ ×¼ unit	☹ ☺	1¾ 3½
Haagen-Dazs® Frozen Yogurt, vanilla or other flavors	portion 3.74oz/106g	½ +½ unit	☺+ ×3 unit ☺+ ×1½ unit	☺ ☺	3½ 7
Haagen-Dazs® Ice Cream, Bailey's Irish Cream	portion 3.6oz/102g	½ +¼ unit	☺+ ×2¾ unit ☺+ ×1¼ unit	☹ ☺	1½ 3
Haagen-Dazs® Ice Cream, Black Walnut	portion 3.74oz/106g	½ +½ unit	☺+ ×4¾ unit ☺+ ×2¼ unit	☺ ☺	1½ 3

Level 0: lactose measure ×½ + Unit/capsule: added tolerated amount of unit per strong lactase capsule
Level 1: fructose measure ×2 Fructose*: fructose, sorbitol adjusted

Level 2: fructose-/sorbitol measure ×4. the rest ×2
Level 3: sorbitol measure ×7. the rest ×3
📖: source of fruc/galactans data

☺+ ×[Amount] unit: Per unit consumed you can additionally tolerate up to [amount] × fructose(*)-unit of another product.

☹: avoid; ☹1: ¼ at TL 1; ☹2: ¼ at TL 2; ☹3: ¼ at TL 3; ☺: only contains traces; ☺: is free from it

KEYWORD INDEX	Unit	Lactose + unit/	Fructose* Fructose*	Sorbitol Sorbitol	FrucGalactans FrucGalactans
Haagen-Dazs® Ice Cream, Butter Pecan	portion 3.74oz/106g	½ +½ unit	☺+ ×4¾ unit ☺+ ×2¼ unit	☺ ☺	2¼ 4¾
Haagen-Dazs® Ice Cream, Cherry Vanilla	portion 3.57oz/101g	½ +½ unit	☺+ ×4½ unit ☺+ ×2¼ unit	☺ ☺	3¼ 6½
Haagen-Dazs® Ice Cream, Chocolate	portion 3.74oz/106g	¼ +¼ unit	☺+ ×2¾ unit ☺+ ×1¼ unit	☹ ☺	1¼ 2¾
Haagen-Dazs® Ice Cream, Coffee	portion 3.74oz/106g	¼ +¼ unit	☺+ ×2¾ unit ☺+ ×1¼ unit	☹ ☺	2½ 5¼
Haagen-Dazs® Ice Cream, Cookies & Cream	portion 3.6oz/102g	½ +¼ unit	☺+ ×4½ unit ☺+ ×2¼ unit	☺ ☺	3¼ 6½
Haagen-Dazs® Ice Cream, Mango	portion 3.74oz/106g	¼ +¼ unit	☺+ ×2¼ unit ☺+ ×1 unit	☺ ☺	2¼ 4¾
Haagen-Dazs® Ice Cream, Pistachio	portion 3.74oz/106g	½ +½ unit	☺+ ×4¾ unit ☺+ ×2¼ unit	☺ ☺	½ 1¼
Haagen-Dazs® Ice Cream, Rocky Road	portion 3.67oz/104g	¼ +¼ unit	☺+ ×2¾ unit ☺+ ×1¼ unit	☹ ☺	2½ 5¼
Haagen-Dazs® Ice Cream, Strawberry	portion 3.74oz/106g	½ +¼ unit	☺+ ×4¾ unit ☺+ ×2¼ unit	☺ ☺	3 6¼
Haagen-Dazs® Ice Cream, Vanilla Chocolate Chip	portion 3.74oz/106g	½ +½ unit	☺+ ×4¾ unit ☺+ ×2¼ unit	☺ ☺	3½ 7
Half and half	portion 1.06oz/30g	2¼ +1¾ unit	☺ ☺	☺ ☺	12¾ 25¾
Halvah	portion 1.42oz/40g	☺	☺+ ×1½ unit ☺+ ×¾ unit	☺ ☺	1¼ [A] 2¾
Ham croquette	portion 3oz/85g	2¼ +1¾ unit	☺ ☺	☹ ☺	☺ ☺
Hamburger gravy	portion 7.17oz/203g	☺	☺ ☺	☹ 12¼	☺ ☺
Hard candy	piece 0.22oz/6g	☺	☺+ ×¾ unit ☺+ ×¼ unit	☺ ☺	☺ ☺
Hard candy, sugar free	piece 0.11oz/3g	☺	☹ [1] ¼	☹ ☹	☺ ☺
Hardee's® Loaded Omelet Biscuit	piece 5.58oz/158g	12 +10 unit	☺+ ×9¼ unit ☺+ ×4½ unit	☺ ☺	¼ [A] ½
Harvey Wallbanger	glass 8.4ozfl/240ml	☺	16½ 33¼	☹ ¼	☺ ☺
Health Valley® Multigrain Chewy Granola Bar, Chocolate Chip	piece 1.03oz/29g	29½ +24¾ unit	☺+ ×1 unit ☺+ ×½ unit	☹ ☺	½ [A] 1¼

Keyword Index	Unit	Lactose 1 + unit/capsule	Fructose* 0 Fructose* 1	Sorbitol 0 Sorbitol 1	FrucGalactans 0 FrucGalactans 1 📖
Hershey's® Caramel Filled Chocolates Sugar Free	piece 0.31oz/8.6g	74½ +62 unit	21¾ 43½	☹ ☹	☺ ☺
Hershey's® Milk Chocolate Bar	bar 4.77oz/135g	¼ +¼ unit	☺ ☺	☺ ☺	¼[G] ¾
Hickorynuts	hand 1.06oz/30g	☺	☺ ☺	☺ ☺	2¾[G] 5¾
High-protein bar, generic	piece 2.3oz/65g	39¼ +32¾ unit	¾ 1¾	☹ 76¾	☺ ☺
Hollandaise sauce, store bought	tbsp. 0.5ozfl/14.21ml	5 +4¼ unit	☺ ☺	☺ ☺	28½ 57
Honey	tbsp. 0.5ozfl/14.21ml	☺	½ 1¼	☹ 1¾	☺ ☺
Honey Nut Chex® (General Mills®)	portion 1.06oz/30g	☺	☺ ☺	☹ 37	½[A] 1¼
Honey Smacks® (Kellogg's®)	portion 1.06oz/30g	☺	☺+ ×12 unit ☺+ ×6 unit	☹ 83¼	½[A] 1¼
Honeydew	portion 4.94oz/140g	☺	¾ 1½	☺ ☺	1½[B] 3¼
Horseradish	pinch 0.04oz/1g	☺	☺ ☺	☺ ☺	☺ ☺
Hot chili peppers, green, cooked from fresh	piece 1.52oz/43g	☺	4½ 9¼	☺ ☺	2½[B] 5¼
Hot chili peppers, red, cooked from fresh	piece 1.52oz/43g	☺	2¾ 5½	☺ ☺	2½[B] 5¼
Hot chocolate, homemade	cup 5.2ozfl/150ml	¼ +¼ unit	27¾ 27¾	☹ 66½	1¾ 3¾
Hot dog, combination of meats, plain	portion 1.95oz/55g	☺	☺+ ×3 unit ☺+ ×1½ unit	☺ ☺	☺ ☺
Hubbard squash	portion 3oz/85g	☺	☺ ☺	☺ ☺	☺[B] ☺
Ice cream sandwich	piece 2.54oz/72g	1¼ +1 unit	☺+ ×1½ unit ☺+ ×¾ unit	☺ ☺	6¼ 12½

0 *Level 0:* lactose measure ×½
1 *Level 1:* fructose measure ×2
2 *Level 2:* fructose-/sorbitol measure ×4. the rest ×2
3 *Level 3:* sorbitol measure ×7. the rest ×3
📖: source of fruc/galactans data

+ Unit/capsule: added tolerated amount of unit per strong lactase capsule
Fructose*: fructose, sorbitol adjusted

☺+ ×[Amount] unit: Per unit consumed you can additionally tolerate up to [amount] × fructose(*)-unit of another product.

☹: avoid; ☹[1]: ¼ at TL 1; ☹[2]: ¼ at TL 2; ☹[3]: ¼ at TL 3; ☺: only contains traces; ☺: is free from it

KEYWORD INDEX	Unit	Lactose + unit/	Fructose* Fructose*	Sorbitol Sorbitol	FrucGalactans FrucGalactans
Ice cream, light, no sugar added, with aspartame, vanilla or other flavors (include chocolate chip)	tsp. 0.16ozfl/4.74ml	9¾ +8 unit	2¼ 4¾	☹ ¼	54¾ ☺
Instant coffee mix, unprepared	cup 5.2ozfl/150ml	☺	8¼ 16½	☹ ☹2	☺ ☺
Irish coffee with alcohol and whipped cream	cup 5.2ozfl/150ml	3¾ +3 unit	☺ ☺	☺ ☺	21 42
Jackfruit, fresh	tbsp. 0.5ozfl/14.21ml	☺	☺ ☺	☹ ½	☺ ☺
Jam or preserves	portion 0.71oz/20g	☺	☺+ ×2¾ unit ☺+ ×1¼ unit	☹ 1¾	☺ ☺
Jam or preserves, reduced sugar	portion 0.71oz/20g	☺	7 14	☹ 41½	☺ ☺
Jam or preserves, sugar free with aspartame	portion 0.6oz/17g	☺	15¾ 31¾	☹ 5¼	☺ ☺
Jam or preserves, sugar free with saccharin	portion 0.5oz/14g	☺	2¼ 4¾	☹ 19¼	☺ ☺
Jam or preserves, sugar free with sucralose	portion 0.6oz/17g	☺	☺ ☺	☹ 65¼	☺ ☺
Jam or preserves, without sugar or artificial sweetener	tbsp. 0.5ozfl/14.21ml	☺	¼ ½	☹ ☹2	☺ ☺
Jasmine tea	glass 8.4ozfl/240ml	☺	☺ ☺	☺ ☺	☺ ☺
Jelly beans®	hand 1.06oz/30g	☺	☺+ ×9¾ unit ☺+ ×4¾ unit	☺ ☺	☺ ☺
Jelly beans®, sugar free	tsp. 0.16ozfl/4.74ml	☺	12¼ 24½	☹ ☹	☺ ☺
Jerusalem artichoke (sunchoke), raw	pinch 0.04ozfl/1g	☺	☺ ☺	☺ ☺	3¼ FB 6½
Jujyfruits®	hand 1.06oz/30g	☺	☺+ ×12¼ unit ☺+ ×6 unit	☺ ☺	☺ ☺
Kale, raw	portion 3oz/85g	☺	☺ ☺	☹ ¾	☺ ☺
Kamikaze	glass 8.4ozfl/240ml	☺	☺+ ×1½ unit ☺+ ×¾ unit	☹ 1	☺ ☺
Kashi® Chewy Granola Bar, Cherry Dark Chocolate	piece 1.24oz/35g	☺	☺+ ×1 unit ☺+ ×½ unit	☹ 1	½ A 1
Kefir	portion 8.65oz/245g	¼ +¼ unit	☺ ☺	☺ ☺	1¾ 3¾

Keyword Index	Unit	Lactose (Level 1) + unit/capsule	Fructose* (Level 0) Fructose* (Level 1)	Sorbitol (Level 0) Sorbitol (Level 1)	FrucGalactans (Level 0) FrucGalactans (Level 1) 📖
Kelp, raw	portion 3oz/85g	☺	☺ ☺	☺ ☺	☺ ☺
Kern's® Mango-Orange Nectar	glass 8.4ozfl/240ml	☺	☹[1] ¼	☹ 2	3[B] 6¼
Kern's® Strawberry Nectar	glass 8.4ozfl/240ml	☺	☹[1] ¼	☹ ¾	☺[C] ☺
Ketchup	portion 0.53oz/15g	☺	☺+ ×¼ unit ☺	☹ 3¾	☺ ☺
Ketchup, low sodium	portion 0.53oz/15g	☺	☺+ ×¼ unit ☺	☹ 4¼	☺ ☺
KFC® honey BBQ sauce	portion 1.1ozfl/31ml	☺	☺+ ×1¼ unit ☺+ ×½ unit	☹ 2¼	☺ ☺
KFC® Caesar salad dressing	portion 1.06ozfl/30ml	4¾ +3¾ unit	☺ ☺	☺ ☺	26½ 53
KFC® chicken breast, spicy crispy	piece 6.18oz/175g	☺	☺ ☺	☺ ☺	¾[A] 1¾
KFC® Chicken Littles with sauce	piece 3.57oz/101g	☺	3 6¼	☹ 33	½[A] 1
KFC® cole slaw	portion 3.53oz/100g	☺	☺+ ×¼ unit ☺	☹ 2¾	1[B] 2
KFC® creamy buffalo sauce	portion 1.04ozfl/29.4ml	6 +5 unit	☺+ ×1 unit ☺+ ×½ unit	☺ ☺	34½ 69
KFC® Crispy Chicken Caesar Salad	portion 4.94oz/140g	☺	2¼ 4½	☹ 17¾	1[A] 2¼
KFC® Crispy Twister without sauce	piece 7.69oz/218g	☺	19 38	☹ 2	☹[A] ¼
KFC® Crispy Twister® with sauce	piece 8.47oz/240g	☺	17¼ 34½	☹ 2	☹[A] ¼
KFC® hot wings	portion 3oz/85g	☺	☺ ☺	☺ ☺	☺ ☺
KFC® house side salad	portion 3.53oz/100g	☺	2 4¼	☹ 4	☺ ☺

Level 0: lactose measure ×½
Level 1: fructose measure ×2
Level 2: fructose-/sorbitol measure ×4. the rest ×2
Level 3: sorbitol measure ×7. the rest ×3
📖: source of fruc/galactans data

+ Unit/capsule: added tolerated amount of unit per strong lactase capsule
Fructose*: fructose, sorbitol adjusted
☺+ ×[Amount] unit: Per unit consumed you can additionally tolerate up to [amount] × fructose(*)-unit of another product.

☹: avoid; ☹[1]: ¼ at TL 1; ☹[2]: ¼ at TL 2; ☹[3]: ¼ at TL 3; ☺: only contains traces; ☺: is free from it

Keyword Index	Unit	Lactose + unit/	Fructose* Fructose*	Sorbitol Sorbitol	FrucGalactans FrucGalactans
KFC® mashed potatoes with gravy	portion 4.94oz/140g	½ +½ unit	☺ ☺	☹ 35½	4 8¼
KFC® sweet and sour sauce	portion 1.06ozfl/30ml	☺	¼ ½	☹ 37	☺ ☺
KFC® sweet corn	piece 3.36oz/95g	☺	☺ ☺	☹ 2½	1¼[G] 2½
KFC®, Extra Crispy Tenders	piece 1.84oz/52g	☺	☺ ☺	☺ ☺	3¼[A] 6½
Kidney beans, cooked from dried	portion 3.18oz/90g	☺	☺ ☺	☺ ☺	¼[A] ½
Kirsch	glass 8.4ozfl/240ml	☺	☺+ ×4½ unit ☺+ ×2½ unit	☹ ¼	☺ ☺
Kit Kat®	piece 1.52oz/43g	2 +1¾ unit	☺ ☺	☹ ☺	2[A] 4¼
Kit Kat® White	piece 1.49oz/42g	¾ +½ unit	☺ ☺	☺ ☺	1½[A] 3¼
Kiwi fruit, gold	piece 3.04oz/86g	☺	1 2¼	☺ ☺	☺[B] ☺
Kiwi fruit, green	piece 2.44oz/69g	☺	3 6	☺ ☺	☺[B] ☺
Kohlrabi, cooked	portion 3oz/85g	☺	☺+ ×¼ unit ☺	☹ 13	☺ ☺
Kraft® Balsamic Vinaigrette	portion 1.06oz/30g	☺	☺ ☺	☹ 22	☺ ☺
Kraft® Cheese Spread, Roka Blue	portion 1.06oz/30g	1¾ +1¼ unit	☺ ☺	☺ ☺	9¾ 19½
Kraft® Classic Caesar Dressing	portion 1.06oz/30g	☺	☺+ ×½ unit ☺+ ×¼ unit	☹ 12¼	☺ ☺
Kraft® Creamy French Dressing	portion 1.06oz/30g	☺	64 ☺	☹ ☺	☺ ☺
Kraft® Creamy Italian Dressing	portion 1.06oz/30g	☺	☺+ ×¾ unit ☺+ ×¼ unit	☺ ☺	☺ ☺
Kraft® Fat Free Mayonnaise	portion 0.53oz/15g	☺	☺ ☺	☺ ☺	☺ ☺
Kraft® Free Sour Cream & Onion Ranch Dressing , fat free	portion 1.06oz/30g	☺	4½ 9	☺ ☺	☺ ☺
Kraft® Mayo with Olive Oil, Reduced Fat	portion 0.53oz/15g	☺	☺ ☺	☺ ☺	☺ ☺
Kraft® Miracle Whip® Free Nonfat Dressing	tbsp. 0.5ozfl/14.21ml	80 +66½ unit	☺ ☺	☺ ☺	☺ ☺

Keyword Index	Unit	Lactose (Level 1) / + unit/capsule	Fructose* (Level 0) / Fructose* (Level 1)	Sorbitol (Level 0) / Sorbitol (Level 1)	FrucGalactans (Level 0) / FrucGalactans (Level 1) 🕮
Kraft® Miracle Whip® Light Dressing	tbsp. 0.5ozfl/14.21ml	☺	☻ ☻	☻ ☻	☺ ☺
Kraft® Miracle Whip® Salad Dressing	tbsp. 0.5ozfl/14.21ml	☺	☻ ☻	☻ ☻	☺ ☺
Kraft® Sandwich Spread	tbsp. 0.5ozfl/14.21ml	☺	☻ ☻	☹ ☺	☺ ☺
Kraft® Thousand Island Dressing®	tbsp. 0.5ozfl/14.21ml	☻	☻+ ×¼ unit ☻	☻ ☻	☻ ☻
Lasagna, homemade, beef	portion 4.94oz/140g	23¼ +19¼ unit	☻+ ×¼ unit ☻	☹ 1	¾ [A] 1½
Lasagna, homemade, cheese, no vegetables	portion 4.94oz/140g	25¾ +21½ unit	11 22¼	☹ ¾	¾ [A] 1½
Lasagna, homemade, spinach, no meat	portion 4.94oz/140g	8½ +7 unit	9¾ 19¾	☹ ½	¾ [A] 1½
Laughing Cow® Mini Babybel®, Cheddar	piece 0.75oz/21g	☺	☻ ☻	☻ ☻	☺ ☺
Laughing Cow® Mini Babybel®, Original	piece 0.75oz/21g	12¾ +10½ unit	☻ ☻	☻ ☻	70¾ ☺
Lay's® Potato Chips, Classic	hand 0.75oz/21g	☻	41¾ 83½	☹ 79¼	10¾ [A] 21½
Lay's® Potato Chips, Salt & Vinegar	hand 0.75oz/21g	☻	41¾ 83½	☹ 79¼	10¾ [A] 21½
Lay's® Potato Chips, Sour Cream & Onion	hand 0.75oz/21g	☻	41¾ 83½	☹ 79¼	10¾ [A] 21½
Lay's® Stax Potato Crisps, Cheddar	hand 0.75oz/21g	☻	41¾ 83½	☹ 79¼	10¾ [A] 21½
Lay's® Stax Potato Crisps, Hot 'n Spicy Barbecue	hand 0.75oz/21g	☻	54 ☺	☹ ☺	10¾ [A] 21½
Lebkuchen	piece 1.15oz/32.4g	☺	6¼ 12¾	☹ 6½	2 [A] 4
Leeks, leafs	piece 3.14oz/89g	☻	3 6	☹ ¼	¾ [G] 1½
Leeks, root	tbsp. 0.5ozfl/14.21ml	☻	18½ 37	☹ 2¼	¼ [C] ¾

Level 0: lactose measure ×½
Level 1: fructose measure ×2
+ Unit/capsule: added tolerated amount of unit per strong lactase capsule
Fructose*: fructose, sorbitol adjusted
Level 2: fructose-/sorbitol measure ×4. the rest ×2
Level 3: sorbitol measure ×7. the rest ×3
🕮: source of fruc/galactans data
☻+ ×[Amount] unit: Per unit consumed you can additionally tolerate up to [amount] × fructose(*)-unit of another product.

☹: avoid; ☹[1]: ¼ at TL 1; ☹[2]: ¼ at TL 2; ☹[3]: ¼ at TL 3; ☺: only contains traces; ☻: is free from it

Keyword Index	Unit	Lactose + unit/	Fructose* Fructose*	Sorbitol Sorbitol	FrucGalactans FrucGalactans
Leeks, whole	piece	☺	3	☹	¼[C]
	3.14oz/89g		6	¼	½
Lemon butter sauce	tbsp.	☺	☺	☹	☺
	0.5ozfl/14.21ml		☺	60½	☺
Lemon juice, fresh	glass	☺	2¼	☹	2¼[B]
	8.4ozfl/240ml		5	1½	4½
Lemon peel	tbsp.	☺	☺	☺	☺
	0.5ozfl/14.21ml		☺	☺	☺
Lemon, fresh	piece	☺	☺	☺	7¾[B]
	2.05oz/58g		☺	☺	15½
Lentil soup, condensed	portion	☺	☺	☹	5½[AC]
	4.45oz/126g		☺	1	11¼
Lentils, cooked from dried	portion	☺	☺	☺	¾[A]
	3.18oz/90g		☺	☺	1½
Lettuce, boston, bibb or	portion	☺	7¼	☹	☺[B]
butterhead	3oz/85g		14½	19½	☺
Lettuce, green leaf	portion	☺	8¼	☹	☺[CB]
	3oz/85g		16¾	16¾	☺
Lettuce, iceberg	portion	☺	6½	☹	☺[CB]
	3oz/85g		13	19½	☺
Lettuce, red leaf	portion	☺	7¼	☹	☺[B]
	3oz/85g		14½	19½	☺
Lettuce, romaine or cos	portion	☺	1¼	☹	☺[CB]
	3oz/85g		2¾	16¾	☺
Libby's® Apricot Nectar	glass	☺	☹[1]	☹	☺
	8.4ozfl/240ml		¼	¼	☺
Libby's® Banana Nectar	glass	☺	☹[1]	☹	½[FB]
	8.4ozfl/240ml		¼	25	1
Libby's® Juicy Juice®, Apple	glass	☺	☹[1]	☹	1½[CB]
Grape	8.4ozfl/240ml		¼	¼	3
Libby's® Juicy Juice®, Grape	glass	☺	☹[1]	☹	1½[CB]
	8.4ozfl/240ml		¼	¼	3
Libby's® Pear Nectar	glass	☺	☹[2]	☹	☺[B]
	8.4ozfl/240ml		☹[2]	☹[2]	☺
Licorice	piece	☺	☺+ ×1½ unit	☺	☺
	0.39oz/11g		☺+ ×¾ unit	☺	☺
Licuado, mango	glass	¼	¼	☹	2½
	8.4oz/240g	+¼ unit	½	1	5
Light cream	portion	5¼	☺	☺	30¼
	0.53ozfl/15ml	+4½ unit	☺	☺	60½

KEYWORD INDEX	Unit	Lactose L1 + unit/capsule	Fructose* L0 Fructose* L1	Sorbitol L0 Sorbitol L1	FrucGalactans L0 FrucGalactans L1 📖
Lima beans, cooked from dried	portion 3.18oz/90g	☻	½ 1¼	☻ ☻	¼[A] ½
Limburger cheese	portion 1.06oz/30g	20¼ +17 unit	☻ ☻	☻ ☻	☺ ☺
Lime juice, fresh	glass 8.4ozfl/240ml	☻	☻+ ×¾ unit ☻+ ×¼ unit	☻ ☻	2¼[B] 4½
Lime, fresh	piece 2.37oz/67g	☻	☻ ☻	☻ ☻	6¾[B] 13½
Lipton® Iced Tea Mix, sweetened with sugar, prepared	glass 8.4ozfl/240ml	☻	☻ ☻	☻ ☻	☻ ☻
Lipton® Instant 100% Tea, unsweetened, prepared	glass 8.4ozfl/240ml	☻	☻ ☻	☻ ☻	☻ ☻
Liqueur, coffee flavored	glass 8.4ozfl/240ml	☻	☺ ☺	☹ 2½	☻ ☻
Little Debbie® Coffee Cake, Apple Streusel	piece 1.84oz/52g	☻	☻+ ×5¼ unit ☻+ ×2½ unit	☻ ☻	1[A] 2
Little Debbie® Fudge Brownies with English Walnuts	piece 1.08oz/30.5g	☻	☻+ ×4¼ unit ☻+ ×2 unit	☹ ☺	1¾[A] 3½
Little Debbie® Nutty Bars	piece 1.01oz/28.5g	☻	☻+ ×13¾ unit ☻+ ×6¾ unit	☹ ☺	4¼[A] 8½
Liver pudding	portion 1.95oz/55g	☻	☻ ☻	☻ ☻	☻ ☻
Loaf cold cut, spiced	portion 1.95oz/55g	2¼ +1¾ unit	☻+ ×¼ unit ☻	☻ ☻	☻ ☻
Loganberries, fresh	portion 4.94oz/140g	☻	☻+ ×1½ unit ☻+ ×¾ unit	☻ ☻	☻ ☻
Long Island iced tea	glass 8.4ozfl/240ml	☻	¾ 1¾	☹ 16½	☻ ☻
Long John or bismarck, glazed, cream or custard filled, with nuts	piece 3.71oz/105g	2¼ +2 unit	☻ ☻	☻ ☻	½[A] 1
Long John Silver's® tartar sauce	tbsp. 0.5ozfl/14.21ml	☺	☻ ☻	☹ ☺	☺ ☺

L0 *Level 0:* lactose measure ×½
L1 *Level 1:* fructose measure ×2
L2 *Level 2:* fructose-/sorbitol measure ×4. the rest ×2
L3 *Level 3:* sorbitol measure ×7. the rest ×3
📖: source of fruc/galactans data

+ Unit/capsule: added tolerated amount of unit per strong lactase capsule
Fructose*: fructose, sorbitol adjusted

☻+ ×[Amount] unit: Per unit consumed you can additionally tolerate up to [amount] × fructose(*)-unit of another product.

☹: avoid; ☹[1]: ¼ at TL 1; ☹[2]: ¼ at TL 2; ☹[3]: ¼ at TL 3; ☺: only contains traces; ☻: is free from it

Keyword Index	Unit	Lactose + unit/	Fructose* Fructose*	Sorbitol Sorbitol	FrucGalactans FrucGalactans
Long John Silver's® tartar sauce	tbsp. 0.5ozfl/14.21ml	☺	☺ ☺	☹ ☺	☺ ☺
Lotus root, cooked	portion 3oz/85g	☺	☺ ☺	☺ ☺	☺ ☺
Lowbush cranberries (lingonberries)	portion 4.94oz/140g	☺	☺+ ×9¼ unit ☺+ ×4½ unit	☹ 35½	☺ ☺
Lychees (litchis), fresh	portion 4.94oz/140g	☺	1 2¼	☺ ☺	☺[B] ☺
lycium (wolf or goji berries)	portion 4.94oz/140g	☺	☺+ ×1 unit ☺+ ×½ unit	☺ ☺	☺ ☺
Lyonnaise (potatoes and onions)	portion 2.47oz/70g	☺	☺ ☺	☹ 15¾	☺ ☺
M & M's® Peanut	portion 1.42oz/40g	2½ +2 unit	☺ ☺	☺ ☺	8¾ 17¾
Macadamia nuts, raw	hand 1.06oz/30g	☺	☺ ☺	☺ ☺	☺ ☺
Macaroni or pasta salad, with meat, egg, mayo dressing	portion 4.94oz/140g	☺	☺+ ×¼ unit ☺+ ×¼ unit	☹ 1¼	1½[A] 3
Mai Tai	glass 8.4ozfl/240ml	☺	☺+ ×½ unit ☺+ ×¼ unit	☹ 1¾	☺ ☺
Maitake mushrooms, raw	tbsp. 0.5ozfl/14.21ml	60½ +50½ unit	☺+ ×½ unit ☺+ ×¼ unit	☹ ¾	☺ ☺
Malt liquor	glass 8.4ozfl/240ml	☺	50 ☺	☹ 10	☺ ☺
Mamba® Fruit Chews	portion 1.42oz/40g	☺	☺ ☺+ ×11 unit	☹ ☹	☺ ☺
Mamba® Sour Fruit Chews	portion 1.42oz/40g	☺	☹[2] ☹[2]	☹ ☹	☺ ☺
Mandarin orange, fresh	portion 4.94oz/140g	☺	1¼ 2½	☺ ☺	2¼[B] 4½
Mango nectar	glass 8.4ozfl/240ml	☺	1 2	☹ 1¼	☺[B] ☺
Mango, fresh	tbsp. 0.5ozfl/14.21ml	☺	1 2¼	☹ 4	☺[B] ☺
Mangosteen, fresh	portion 4.94oz/140g	☺	35½ 71¼	☺ ☺	☺ ☺
Manhattan	glass 8.4ozfl/240ml	☺	½ 1	☹ 2	☺ ☺
Maple syrup, pure	tbsp. 0.5ozfl/14.21ml	☺	☺+ ×¼ unit ☺	☺ ☺	☺ ☺

Keyword Index	Unit	Lactose ¹ / + unit/💊	Fructose* ⁰ Fructose* ¹	Sorbitol ⁰ Sorbitol ¹	FrucGalactans ⁰ FrucGalactans ¹ 🕮
Margarine, diet, fat free	portion 0.5oz/14g	15½ +13 unit	☻ ☻	☻ ☻	86¾ ☺
Margarine, tub, salted, sun-flower oil	portion 0.5oz/14g	30 +25 unit	☻ ☻	☻ ☻	☺ ☺
Margarita, frozen	glass 8.4ozfl/240ml	☻	☻+ ×¼ unit ☻	☹ 7	☻ ☻
Marmalade, sugar free with aspartame	portion 0.6oz/17g	☻	15¾ 31¾	☹ 5¼	☻ ☻
Marmalade, sugar free with saccharin	portion 0.57oz/16g	☻	2 4¼	☹ 16¾	☻ ☻
Marmalade, sugar free with sucralose	portion 0.6oz/17g	☻	☻ ☻	☹ 65¼	☻ ☻
Marshmallow	portion 1.06oz/30g	☻	☻+ ×4½ unit ☻+ ×2¼ unit	☻ ☻	☻ ☻
Martini®	glass 8.4ozfl/240ml	☻	83¼ ☺	☹ 3¼	☻ ☻
Mascarpone	portion 1.06oz/30g	2½ +2 unit	☻ ☻	☻ ☻	13¾ 27¾
McDonald's® apple slices	piece 1.2oz/34g	☻	¼ ¾	☹ ¼	☻ ☻
McDonald's® barbecue sauce	portion 1.1ozfl/31ml	☻	☻+ ×1½ unit ☻+ ×¾ unit	☹ 1¾	☻ ☻
McDonald's® Big Mac®	piece 7.59oz/215g	9¾ +8¼ unit	5 10¼	☹ 6½	¼ A ½
McDonald's® caramel sundae®	portion 6.42ozfl/182ml	¼ +¼ unit	☻+ ×6¾ unit ☻+ ×3¼ unit	☻ ☻	1¾ 3¾
McDonald's® Cheeseburger	piece 4.03oz/114g	9¾ +8¼ unit	3¾ 7¾	☹ 5	¼ A ¾
McDonald's® Chicken McNuggets®	piece 0.58oz/16.25g	☻	☻ ☻	☻ ☻	10¾ A 21½
McDonald's® chocolate chip cookies	piece 1.17oz/33g	☻	☻+ ×½ unit ☻+ ×¼ unit	☹ ☺	¾ A 1½

⁰ *Level 0:* lactose measure ×½
¹ *Level 1:* fructose measure ×2
² *Level 2*: fructose-/sorbitol measure ×4. the rest ×2
³ *Level 3:* sorbitol measure ×7. the rest ×3
🕮: source of fruc/galactans data

+ Unit/💊: added tolerated amount of unit per strong lactase capsule
Fructose*: fructose, sorbitol adjusted

☻+ ×[Amount] unit: Per unit consumed you can additionally tolerate up to [amount] × fructose(*)-unit of another product.

☹: avoid; ☹¹: ¼ at TL 1; ☹²: ¼ at TL 2; ☹³: ¼ at TL 3; ☺: only contains traces; ☻: is free from it

Keyword Index	Unit	Lactose + unit/	Fructose* Fructose*	Sorbitol Sorbitol	FrucGalactans FrucGalactans
McDonald's® chocolate milk	cup 5.2ozfl/150ml	¼ +¼ unit	☺+ ×2 unit ☺+ ×1 unit	☺ ☺	1¾ 3¾
McDonald's® Crispy Chicken Snack Wrap with ranch sauce	piece 4.17ozfl/118ml	62 +51½ unit	☺ ☺	☹ 84½	¼ A ½
McDonald's® Double Cheeseburger	piece 5.83oz/165g	4¾ +4 unit	4½ 9	☹ 4¼	¼ A ½
McDonald's® Filet-O-Fish®	piece 5.01oz/142g	19¾ +16½ unit	2 4	☹ 70¼	¼ A ¾
McDonald's® French fries	portion 2.47oz/70g	☺	☺ ☺	☹ 35½	☺ ☺
McDonald's® Hamburger	piece 3.53oz/100g	☺	3¾ 7¾	☹ 5	½ A 1
McDonald's® hot fudge sundae®	portion 6.32ozfl/179ml	¼ +¼ unit	☺+ ×7½ unit ☺+ ×3¾ unit	☹ 55¾	1¼ G 2½
McDonald's® hot mustard sauce	portion 0.71ozfl/20ml	☺	☺+ ×1¼ unit ☺+ ×½ unit	☺ ☺	☺ ☺
McDonald's® M & M's® McFlurry®	portion 8.05ozfl/228ml	☹² +0,18 unit	☺+ ×3½ unit ☺+ ×1¾ unit	☺ ☺	1 2¼
McDonald's® McCafe® shakes, chocolate flavors	portion 7.41ozfl/210ml	¼ +¼ unit	☺+ ×5¾ unit ☺+ ×2¾ unit	☹ 15¾	1½ 3¼
McDonald's® McCafe® shakes, vanilla or other flavors	portion 7.27ozfl/206ml	¼ +¼ unit	☺+ ×¼ unit ☺	☹ 12	1½ 3¼
McDonald's® McChicken®	piece 5.05oz/143g	☺	1½ 3	☹ 69¾	¼ A ¾
McDonald's® McDouble®	piece 5.33oz/151g	9¾ +8¼ unit	4¼ 8¾	☹ 4¼	¼ A ½
McDonald's® McRib®	piece 7.34oz/208g	☺	☺+ ×¾ unit ☺+ ×¼ unit	☹ 1¾	¼ A ½
McDonald's® Newman's Own® Creamy Caesar salad dressing	portion 1.06oz/30g	18¼ +15¼ unit	26¾ 53¾	☹ 7¼	☺ ☺
McDonald's® Newman's Own® Low Fat Balsamic Vinaigrette salad dressing	portion 1.06ozfl/30ml	☺	☺ ☺	☺ ☺	☺ ☺
McDonald's® orange juice	glass 8.4ozfl/240ml	☺	1½ 3¼	☹ ¼	☺ ☺
McDonald's® Quarter Pounder	piece 6.11oz/173g	☺	48 ☺	☹ 2½	¼ A ½
McDonald's® Sausage & EGG® McMuffin®	piece 5.79oz/164g	9¾ +8¼ unit	☺+ ×1 unit ☺+ ×½ unit	☺ ☺	¼ A ½

Keyword Index	Unit	Lactose [Level 1] + unit/[capsule]	Fructose* [Level 0] Fructose* [Level 1]	Sorbitol [Level 0] Sorbitol [Level 1]	FrucGalactans [Level 0] FrucGalactans [Level 1] [source]
McDonald's® side salad	portion 3.53oz/100g	☻	3¾ 7½	☹ 2½	☻ ☻
McDonald's® smoothies, all flavors	glass 8.4oz/240g	2¾ +2¼ unit	3¾ 7¾	☹ 1¼	15½ 31
McDonald's® Southwestern chipotle barbecue sauce	portion 1.1ozfl/31ml	☻	☻+ ×1¾ unit ☻+ ×¾ unit	☹ 2¾	☻ ☻
McDonald's® sweet and sour sauce	portion 1.06ozfl/30ml	☻	¼ ¾	☹ 41½	☻ ☻
Meat ravioli, with tomato sauce	portion 8.82oz/250g	☺	☻+ ×½ unit ☻+ ×¼ unit	☹ ½	¼ A ¾
Meatloaf, pork	portion 3oz/85g	2¼ +2 unit	☻+ ×¼ unit ☻	☹ 3½	☻ ☻
Meatloaf, tuna	portion 3oz/85g	5½ +4½ unit	☻ ☻	☹ 14½	☻ ☻
Melba Toast®, Classic (Old London®)	portion 0.53oz/15g	☻	☻+ ×¼ unit ☻	☹ ☺	½ A 1¼
Mentos®	piece 0.11oz/3g	☻	☻ ☻	☻ ☻	☻ ☻
Merlot, red	glass 8.4ozfl/240ml	☻	17¾ 35½	☹ ½	☻ ☻
Merlot, white	glass 8.4ozfl/240ml	☻	¾ 1¾	☻ ☻	☻ ☻
Milk chocolate bar, cereal	bar 4.77oz/135g	½ +½ unit	☻ ☻	☹ 40	¼ A ¾
Milk chocolate bar, cereal, sugar free	piece 0.43ozfl/12g	26½ +22 unit	80 ☺	☹ ☹	4½ A 9
Milk chocolate bar, sugar free	piece 0.43ozfl/12g	32½ +27 unit	80 ☺	☹ ☹	4½ 9
Milk Chocolate covered raisins	hand 1.06oz/30g	2¾ +2¼ unit	☻+ ×¼ unit ☺	☹ 3¼	3¼ G 6½
Milk, lactose reduced (Lactaid®), skim (fat free)	glass 8.4oz/240g	☻	☻+ ×10 unit ☻+ ×5 unit	☻ ☻	☻ ☻
Milk, lactose reduced (Lactaid®), whole	cup 5.2ozfl/150ml	☻	☻+ ×7½ unit ☻+ ×3¾ unit	☻ ☻	☻ ☻

[Level 0] *Level 0:* lactose measure ×½ + Unit/[capsule]: added tolerated amount of unit per strong lactase capsule
[Level 1] *Level 1:* fructose measure ×2 Fructose*: fructose, sorbitol adjusted

[Level 2] *Level 2:* fructose-/sorbitol measure ×4. the rest ×2
[Level 3] *Level 3:* sorbitol measure ×7. the rest ×3
[source]: source of fruc/galactans data

☻+ ×[Amount] unit: Per unit consumed you can additionally tolerate up to [amount] × fructose(*)-unit of another product.

☹: avoid; ☹¹: ¼ at TL 1; ☹²: ¼ at TL 2; ☹³: ¼ at TL 3; ☺: only contains traces; ☻: is free from it

KEYWORD INDEX	Unit	**Lactose** **+ unit/**	**Fructose*** **Fructose***	**Sorbitol** **Sorbitol**	**FrucGalactans** **FrucGalactans**
Milk, lactose reduced, skim (fat free), fortified with calcium (Lactaid®)	glass 8.4oz/240g	☺	☺+ ×10 unit ☺+ ×5 unit	☺ ☺	☺ ☺
Milk, unprepared dry powder, nonfat, instant	portion 0.78ozfl/22ml	¼ +0,21 unit	☺ ☺	☺ ☺	1¼ 2¾
Mineral Water	glass 8.4ozfl/240ml	☺	☺ ☺	☺ ☺	☺ ☺
Minestrone soup, condensed	portion 4.45oz/126g	☺	☺ ☺	☹ ¾	½ 1
Minestrone soup, homemade	portion 8.65oz/245g	☺	☺ ☺	☹ 1	¼ ½
Mint Julep	glass 8.4ozfl/240ml	☺	☺ ☺	☺ ☺	☺ ☺
Mocha, without flavored syrup	cup 5.2ozfl/150ml	½ +¼ unit	☺+ ×1¾ unit ☺+ ×¾ unit	☺ ☺	3 6
Mojito	glass 8.4ozfl/240ml	☺	☺ ☺	☺ ☺	☺ ☺
Molasses cookies, store bought	piece 0.53oz/15g	☺	☺ ☺	☺ ☺	3¼[A] 6¾
Molasses, dark	tbsp. 0.5ozfl/14.21ml	☺	3¾ 7½	☺ ☺	☺ ☺
Monster® Energy®	glass 8.4ozfl/240ml	☺	☺+ ×17½ unit ☺+ ×8¾ unit	☺ ☺	☺ ☺
Monster® Khaos	portion 8.47oz/240g	☺	☺+ ×9 unit ☺+ ×4¾ unit	☹ ¼	☺ ☺
Morel mushrooms, raw	tbsp. 0.5ozfl/14.21ml	☺	☺ ☺	☹ ¾	☺ ☺
Mortadella	portion 1.95oz/55g	☺	☺+ ×¼ unit ☺	☺ ☺	☺ ☺
Mountain Dew®	glass 8.4ozfl/240ml	☺	☹[1] ¼	☺ ☺	☺ ☺
Mountain Dew® Code Red	glass 8.4ozfl/240ml	☺	☹[1] ¼	☺ ☺	☺ ☺
Mozzarella cheese, fat free	portion 1.06oz/30g	½ +½ unit	☺ ☺	☺ ☺	3½ 7¼
Mozzarella cheese, whole milk	portion 1.06oz/30g	9¾ +8¼ unit	☺ ☺	☺ ☺	55 ☺
Mrs. Paul's® Calamari Rings	portion 3oz/85g	☺	☺ ☺	☺ ☺	2¼[A] 4½

KEYWORD INDEX	Unit	Lactose L1 + unit/capsule	Fructose* L0 Fructose* L1	Sorbitol L0 Sorbitol L1	FrucGalactans L0 FrucGalactans L1 📖
Muenster cheese, natural	portion 1.06oz/30g	8¾ +7¼ unit	☺ ☺	☺ ☺	49½ 🙂
Mueslix® (Kellogg's®)	portion 1.95oz/55g	☺	☺+ ×¾ unit ☺+ ×¼ unit	☹ 2¾	¼[A] ¾
Muffins, banana	piece 3.99oz/113g	2½ +2 unit	☺+ ×¼ unit ☺	☹ 29¼	¼[A] ¾
Muffins, blueberry, store bought	piece 3.99oz/113g	1½ +1¼ unit	☺ ☺	☺ ☺	¼[A] ¾
Muffins, carrot, homemade, with nuts	piece 3.99oz/113g	1½ +1¼ unit	☺ ☺	☹ 3¼	¼[A] ¾
Muffins, oat bran or oatmeal, store bought	piece 3.99oz/113g	1¼ +1 unit	☺+ ×¼ unit ☺	☺ ☺	½[A] 1
Muffins, pumpkin, store bought	piece 3.99oz/113g	1¾ +1¼ unit	☺+ ×¼ unit ☺	☹ 14½	¼[A] ¾
Mulberries	portion 4.94oz/140g	☺	½ 1¼	☺ ☺	☺ ☺
Mung beans, cooked from dried	portion 3.18oz/90g	☺	½ 1¼	☺ ☺	¾[A] 1¾
Murray® Sugar Free Oatmeal Cookies	piece 0.39oz/11g	☺	½ 1¼	☹ ☹[2]	4½[A] 9
Murray® Sugar Free Shortbread	piece 0.14oz/3.75g	☺	1½ 3¼	☹ ☹[2]	10½[A] 21¼
Muscatel	glass 8.4ozfl/240ml	☺	☹[2] ☹[2]	☹ ½	☺ ☺
Mushroom gravy, canned	tbsp. 0.5ozfl/14.21ml	75¼ +62¾ unit	☺ ☺	☹ 2¼	🙂 🙂
Mushrooms, batter dipped or breaded	portion 2.47oz/70g	☺	☺ ☺	☹ ¼	2½[B] 5¼
Muskmelon	portion 4.94oz/140g	☺	1¼ 2½	☺ ☺	1½[B] 3¼
Nabisco® 100 Calorie Packs, Honey Maid Cinnamon Roll Thin Crisps	piece 0.46oz/13g	☺	☺ ☺	☹ 42½	4¾[A] 9¾

L0 *Level 0:* lactose measure ×½ + Unit/capsule: added tolerated amount of unit per strong lactase capsule
L1 *Level 1:* fructose measure ×2 Fructose*: fructose, sorbitol adjusted

L2 *Level 2:* fructose-/sorbitol measure ×4. the rest ×2
L3 *Level 3:* sorbitol measure ×7. the rest ×3
📖: source of fruc/galactans data

☺+ ×[Amount] unit: Per unit consumed you can additionally tolerate up to [amount] × fructose(*)-unit of another product.

☹: avoid; ☹[1]: ¼ at TL 1; ☹[2]: ¼ at TL 2; ☹[3]: ¼ at TL 3; 🙂: only contains traces; ☺: is free from it

Keyword Index	Unit	Lactose + unit/	Fructose* Fructose*	Sorbitol Sorbitol	FrucGalactans FrucGalactans
Nectarine, fresh	tbsp. 0.5ozfl/14.21ml	☺	8¼ 16½	☹ 1	5½[B] 11¼
Nestea® 100% Tea, unsweetened, dry	glass 8.4ozfl/240ml	☺	☺+ ×22 unit ☺+ ×11 unit	☺ ☺	☺ ☺
Nestea® Iced Tea, Sugar Free, dry	glass 8.4ozfl/240ml	☺	☺+ ×11½ unit ☺+ ×5¾ unit	☺ ☺	☺ ☺
Nestea® Iced Tea, Sugar Free, prepared	glass 8.4ozfl/240ml	☺	☺ ☺	☺ ☺	☺ ☺
Nestea® Iced Tea, sweetened with sugar, dry	glass 8.4ozfl/240ml	☺	☺ ☺	☺ ☺	☺ ☺
Nestle® Hot Cocoa Dark Chocolate, prepared	cup 5.2ozfl/150ml	¼ +¼ unit	☺+ ×½ unit ☺+ ×¼ unit	☹ ☺	2[G] 4
Nestle® Hot Cocoa Rich Milk Chocolate, prepared	cup 5.2ozfl/150ml	¼ +¼ unit	☺ ☺	☺ ☺	2[G] 4
Newman's Own® Organic Pretzels, Spelt	slice 1.49oz/42g	☺	☺+ ×½ unit ☺+ ×¼ unit	☺ ☺	¾[A] 1½
Nilla Wafers® (Nabisco®)	piece 0.14oz/3.75g	32½ +27 unit	☺ ☺	☺ ☺	12¼[A] 24¾
No Fear®	glass 8.4ozfl/240ml	☺	☺+ ×6¼ unit ☺+ ×3 unit	☹ 50	☺ ☺
No Fear® Sugar Free	glass 8.4ozfl/240ml	☺	☺ ☺	☺ ☺	☺ ☺
Non-alcoholic wine	glass 8.4ozfl/240ml	☺	2¼ 4½	☹ 50	☺ ☺
Noodle soup mix, dry	portion 0.57oz/16g	☺	☺+ ×¼ unit ☺	☺ ☺	6¼[CB] 12½
Northland® Cranberry Juice, all flavors	glass 8.4ozfl/240ml	☺	☺+ ×7¼ unit ☺+ ×3½ unit	☹ 25	☺ ☺
Nougat	bar 4.77oz/135g	☺	☺+ ×18 unit ☺+ ×9 unit	☺ ☺	¼ ¾
Nutella® (filbert spread)	portion 1.31oz/37g	32¼ +27 unit	67½ ☺	☹ 20¾	1¼[G] 2¾
Nutter Butter® Cookies (Nabisco®)	portion 0.5oz/14g	☺	☺ ☺	☺ ☺	3½[A] 7¼
Oat milk	glass 8.4oz/240g	☺	☺ ☺	☺ ☺	¼[A] ¾

KEYWORD INDEX	Unit	Lactose [L1] + unit/capsule	Fructose* [L0] Fructose* [L1]	Sorbitol [L0] Sorbitol [L1]	FrucGalactans [L0] FrucGalactans [L1] 📖
Oatmeal cookies, store bought	piece 0.46oz/13g	45¾ +38 unit	☺ ☺	☺ ☺	3¾[A] 7½
Okra, raw	portion 3oz/85g	☺	2¼ 4½	☺ ☺	2[CB] 4¼
Old Dutch® Crunch Curls	hand 0.75oz/21g	4 +3¼ unit	☺ ☺	☹ ☺	7¼[A] 14½
Omelet, made with bacon	portion 3.89oz/110g	34¾ +29 unit	☺+ ×1¾ unit ☺+ ×¾ unit	☺ ☺	☺ ☺
Omelet, made with sausage, potatoes, onions, cheese	portion 3.89oz/110g	52¼ +43½ unit	☺+ ×1 unit ☺+ ×½ unit	☹ 6¾	¼[CB] ½
Onion, white, yellow or red, raw	tbsp. 0.5ozfl/14.21ml	☺	☺ ☺	☹ 6	1[CB] 2
Orange kiwi passion juice	glass 8.4ozfl/240ml	☺	☺ ☺	☹ ¾	☺[B] ☺
Orange peel	tbsp. 0.5ozfl/14.21ml	☺	3¼ 6½	☺ ☺	☺ ☺
Orange, fresh	portion 4.94oz/140g	☺	2¼ 4¾	☺ ☺	2¼[B] 4½
Oregano, dried	pinch 0.04oz/1g	☺	☺ ☺	☺ ☺	☺ ☺
Oreo® Brownie Cookies (Nabisco®)	piece 1.5oz/42.5g	☺	¼ ¾	☹ ☺	1[A] 2¼
Oreo® Cookies (Nabisco®)	piece 0.43oz/12g	☺	☺ ☺	☹ ☺	4¼[A] 8½
Oreo® Cookies, Sugar Free (Nabisco®)	piece 0.43oz/12g	☺	13¾ 27¾	☹ ☹	4¼[A] 8½
Ouzo	glass 8.4ozfl/240ml	☺	☺+ ×4½ unit ☺+ ×2½ unit	☹ ¼	☺ ☺
Oyster mushrooms, raw	portion 3oz/85g	☺	☺+ ×1¾ unit ☺+ ×¾ unit	☹ ¼	☺ ☺
Pad thai, without meat	portion 4.94oz/140g	☺	☺ ☺	☹ 3¾	☺[A] ☺

[L0] *Level 0:* lactose measure ×½
[L1] *Level 1:* fructose measure ×2
[L2] *Level 2:* fructose-/sorbitol measure ×4. the rest ×2
[L3] *Level 3:* sorbitol measure ×7. the rest ×3
📖: source of fruc/galactans data

+ Unit/capsule: added tolerated amount of unit per strong lactase capsule
Fructose*: fructose, sorbitol adjusted

☺+ ×[Amount] unit: Per unit consumed you can additionally tolerate up to [amount] × fructose(*)-unit of another product.

☹: avoid; ☹[1]: ¼ at TL 1; ☹[2]: ¼ at TL 2; ☹[3]: ¼ at TL 3; ☺: only contains traces; ☺: is free from it

Keyword Index	Unit	Lactose + unit/	Fructose* Fructose*	Sorbitol Sorbitol	FrucGalactans FrucGalactans
Paella	portion 8.47oz/240g	☺	2¼ 4½	☹ 2¼	1 2
Palm kernel oil	tbsp. 0.5ozfl/14.21ml	☺	☺ ☺	☺ ☺	☺ ☺
Pancake, buckwheat, from mix, add water only	piece 1.56oz/44g	☺	☺ ☺	☹ 3¾	1¼ [A] 2½
Pancake, whole wheat, homemade	piece 1.56oz/44g	2½ +2 unit	☺ ☺	☺ ☺	1 [A] 2¼
Papaya, fresh	portion 4.94oz/140g	☺	☺+ ×1 unit ☺+ ×½ unit	☺ ☺	☺ ☺
Parmesan cheese, dry (grated)	portion 0.18oz/5g	☺	☺ ☺	☺ ☺	☺ ☺
Parmesan cheese, dry (grated), nonfat	portion 0.18oz/5g	☺ +75¾ unit	☺ ☺	☺ ☺	☺ ☺
Parsley, fresh	pinch 0.04oz/1g	☺	☺ ☺	☹ ☺	☺ ☺
Parsnip, cooked	portion 3oz/85g	☺	☺+ ×¼ unit ☺	☺ ☺	☺ [C] ☺
Passion fruit (maracuya), fresh	portion 4.94oz/140g	☺	☺+ ×2½ unit ☺+ ×1¼ unit	☺ ☺	☺ ☺
Passion fruit juice	glass 8.4ozfl/240ml	☺	☺+ ×3¾ unit ☺+ ×1¾ unit	☺ ☺	☺ ☺
Pasta salad with vegetables, Italian dressing	portion 4.94oz/140g	☺	3¾ 7½	☹ 1½	1½ [A] 3¼
Peach juice	glass 8.4ozfl/240ml	☺	¾ 1½	☹ ¾	½ [B] 1¼
Peach pie, bottom crust only	piece 4.31oz/122g	☺	2¾ 5½	☹ 1	¼ [A] ¾
Peach, fresh	portion 4.94oz/140g	☺	☺+ ×½ unit ☺+ ×½ unit	☹ ¼	2¼ [B] 4½
Peanut butter, unsalted	portion 1.13oz/32g	☺	☺+ ×¼ unit ☺	☺ ☺	☺ [G] ☺
Peanut sauce, store bought	portion 1.24oz/35g	☺	☺ ☺	☹ 8¼	☺ [G] ☺
Peanuts, dry roasted, salted	hand 1.06oz/30g	☺	☺ ☺	☺ ☺	☺ [G] ☺
Pear juice	glass 8.4ozfl/240ml	☺	☹ [2] ☹ [2]	☹ ☹ [3]	1½ [C] 3
Pear, fresh	tbsp. 0.5ozfl/14.21ml	☺	½ 1	☹ ¼	☺ [B] ☺

Keyword Index	Unit	Lactose (Level 1) + unit/capsule	Fructose* (Level 0) Fructose* (Level 1)	Sorbitol (Level 0) Sorbitol (Level 1)	FrucGalactans (Level 0) FrucGalactans (Level 1)
Pecan praline	piece 1.95oz/55g	3½ +2¾ unit	☺+ ×1¼ unit ☺+ ×½ unit	☺ ☺	1¼[G] 2¾
Pepperidge Farm® Sweet & Simple, Soft Baked Sugar Cookies	piece 0.48oz/13.5g	☺	☹[1] ¼	☺ ☺	4¾[A] 9½
Pepperidge Farm® Turnover, Apple	piece 3.14oz/89g	9 +7½ unit	½ 1¼	☹ ¼	½[A] 1¼
Peppermint, fresh	pinch 0.04oz/1g	☺	☺ ☺	☺ ☺	☺ ☺
Pepsi®	glass 8.4ozfl/240ml	☺	½ 1¼	☺ ☺	☺ ☺
Pepsi® Max	glass 8.4ozfl/240ml	☺	☺ ☺	☺ ☺	☺ ☺
Pepsi® Twist	glass 8.4ozfl/240ml	☺	½ 1¼	☺ ☺	☺ ☺
Persimmon, fresh	piece 4.94oz/140g	☺	2¾ 5¾	☺ ☺	1[C] 2
Pesto sauce, store bought	portion 2.19oz/62g	☺	☺ ☺	☺ ☺	1¾[A] 3¾
Pho soup (Vietnamese noodle soup)	portion 8.65oz/245g	☺	☺ ☺	☹ 6¾	¾ 1¾
Pickled beef	portion 1.95oz/55g	☺	☺ ☺	☺ ☺	☺ ☺
Pickled beets	portion 1.06oz/30g	☺	☺ ☺	☹ 15	3[CB] 6
Pillsbury® Big Deluxe White Chunk Macadamia Nut Cookies	piece 1.35oz/38g	6¾ +5½ unit	☺ ☺	☺ ☺	½[A] 1¼
Pina colada	glass 8.4ozfl/240ml	☺	☺+ ×1¼ unit ☺+ ×½ unit	☹ 4	☺ ☺
Pine nuts, pignolias	hand 1.06oz/30g	☺	☺ ☺	☺ ☺	2¾[G] 5¾
Pineapple juice	glass 8.4ozfl/240ml	☺	☺+ ×3¼ unit ☺+ ×1½ unit	☹ 1¾	1½[CB] 3

Level 0: lactose measure ×½
Level 1: fructose measure ×2
Level 2: fructose-/sorbitol measure ×4. the rest ×2
Level 3: sorbitol measure ×7. the rest ×3
(book symbol): source of fruc/galactans data

+ Unit/capsule: added tolerated amount of unit per strong lactase capsule
Fructose*: fructose, sorbitol adjusted
☺+ ×[Amount] unit: Per unit consumed you can additionally tolerate up to [amount] × fructose(*)-unit of another product.

☹: avoid; ☹[1]: ¼ at TL 1; ☹[2]: ¼ at TL 2; ☹[3]: ¼ at TL 3; ☺: only contains traces; ☺: is free from it

KEYWORD INDEX	Unit	Lactose + unit/	Fructose* Fructose*	Sorbitol Sorbitol	FrucGalactans FrucGalactans
Pineapple orange drink	glass 8.4ozfl/240ml	☺	¾ 1½	☺ ☺	1½[CB] 3
Pineapple, dried	portion 1.42oz/40g	☺	½ 1¼	☹ ½	2[CB] 4
Pineapple, fresh	portion 4.94oz/140g	☺	¾ 1¾	☹ ¾	2¼[CB] 4½
Pistachio nuts, raw	hand 0.75oz/21g	☺	☺ ☺	☺ ☺	¼[G] ¾
Pizza Hut® cheese bread stick	piece 1.98oz/56g	61½ +51¼ unit	☺+ ×¼ unit ☺	☺ ☺	1¼[A] 2½
Pizza Hut® Pepperoni Lover's pizza, stuffed crust	portion 4.94oz/140g	30 +25 unit	☺ ☺	☹ 1	¾[A] 1½
Pizza Hut® Personal Pan, supreme	piece 9.03oz/256g	16¾ +14 unit	☺ ☺	☹ ¼	4¾[A] 9½
Pizza, homemade or restaurant, cheese, thin crust	piece 7.38oz/209g	12¼ +10¼ unit	☺+ ×¾ unit ☺+ ×¼ unit	☹ ¾	½[A] 1
Plain dumplings for stew, biscuit type	portion 1.95oz/55g	1¾ +1½ unit	☺ ☺	☺ ☺	½[A] 1
Plantains, green, boiled	piece 7.87oz/223g	☺	¾ 1¾	☺ ☺	¼[FB] ¾
Plum, fresh	tbsp. 0.5ozfl/14.21ml	☺	☺+ ×¼ unit ☺+ ×¼ unit	☹ ¾	21½[C] 43
Polenta	portion 8.47oz/240g	½ +½ unit	☺+ ×¼ unit ☺	☹ 20¾	3¼[B] 6¾
Pomegranate juice	glass 8.4ozfl/240ml	☺	¾ 1½	☹ ☹[2]	☺ ☺
Pomegranate, fresh (arils-seed/juice sacs)	tbsp. 0.5ozfl/14.21ml	☺	☺+ ×½ unit ☺+ ×¼ unit	☹ 2	☺ ☺
Poore Brothers® Potato Chips, Salt & Cracked Pepper	hand 0.75oz/21g	☺	54 ☺	☹ ☺	10¾[A] 21½
Popcorn, store bought (prepopped), "buttered"	portion 1.06oz/30g	36¾ +30¾ unit	☺ ☺	☺ ☺	☺[CB] ☺
Popsicle	piece 1.84oz/52g	☺	☺+ ×1¼ unit ☺+ ×½ unit	☺ ☺	☺ ☺
Popsicle, sugar free	piece 1.95oz/55g	☺	☺ ☺	☺ ☺	☺ ☺
Pork cutlet (sirloin cutlet), visible fat eaten	portion 3oz/85g	☺	☺ ☺	☺ ☺	1¼[A] 2¾
Port wine	glass 8.4ozfl/240ml	☺	☹[2] ☹[2]	☹ ½	☺ ☺

Keyword Index	Unit	Lactose [L1] + unit/capsule	Fructose* [L0] Fructose* [L1]	Sorbitol [L0] Sorbitol [L1]	FrucGalactans [L0] FrucGalactans [L1] [source]
Portabella mushrooms, cooked from fresh	tbsp. 0.5ozfl/14.21ml	☻	☻+ ×½ unit ☻+ ×¼ unit	☹ ½	12¼ [B] 24½
Potato bread	slice 1.2oz/34g	6¼ +5¼ unit	☻ ☻	☹ ☺	1½ [A] 3
Potato chips, salted	hand 0.75oz/21g	☻	41¾ 83½	☹ 79¼	10¾ [A] 21½
Potato dumpling (Kartoffel-kloesse)	portion 4.94oz/140g	45½ +37¾ unit	☻+ ×¼ unit ☻	☹ 35½	☺ [C] ☺
Potato gnocchi	portion 6.64oz/188g	2½ +2 unit	☻ ☻	☻ ☻	14 [A] 28¼
Potato pancakes	portion 2.47oz/70g	☻	☻+ ×½ unit ☻+ ×¼ unit	☹ 12¾	☻ [B] ☻
Potato salad, with egg, mayo dressing	portion 4.94oz/140g	☻	☻+ ×½ unit ☻+ ×¼ unit	☹ 2	1 [CB] 2
Potato soup with broccoli and cheese	portion 8.65oz/245g	29¾ +24¾ unit	☻ ☻	☹ 13½	½ [AC] 1
Potato sticks	hand 0.75oz/21g	☻	☻ ☻	☹ 79¼	10¾ [A] 21½
Potato, boiled, with skin	portion 3.89oz/110g	☻	☻ ☻	☹ 45¼	☻ [B] ☻
Potato, boiled, without skin	portion 3.89oz/110g	☻	☻ ☻	☹ 45¼	☻ [B] ☻
Power Bar® 20g Protein Plus, Chocolate Crisp	piece 2.16oz/61g	3 +2½ unit	☹[1] ¼	☹ ☹	4 [G] 8¼
Power Bar® 20g Protein Plus, Chocolate Peanut Butter	piece 2.16oz/61g	3 +2½ unit	☹[2] ☹[2]	☹ ☹	17 34¼
Power Bar® 30g Protein Plus, Chocolate Brownie	piece 2.47oz/70g	2 +1½ unit	☻+ ×1½ unit ☻+ ×¾ unit	☹ ☺	3¼ [G] 6½
Power Bar® Harvest Energy®, Double Chocolate Crisp	piece 2.3oz/65g	2¾ +2¼ unit	☻+ ×5¾ unit ☻+ ×2¾ unit	☹ 10¾	¼ [AG] ½
Power Bar® Performance Energy®, Banana	piece 2.3oz/65g	☻	¼ ¾	☹ ☺	10½ [A] 21

[L0] *Level 0:* lactose measure ×½
[L1] *Level 1:* fructose measure ×2
[L2] *Level 2:* fructose-/sorbitol measure ×4. the rest ×2
[L3] *Level 3:* sorbitol measure ×7. the rest ×3
[source]: source of fruc/galactans data

+ Unit/capsule: added tolerated amount of unit per strong lactase capsule
Fructose*: fructose, sorbitol adjusted

☻+ ×[Amount] unit: Per unit consumed you can additionally tolerate up to [amount] × fructose(*)-unit of another product.

☹: avoid; ☹[1]: ¼ at TL 1; ☹[2]: ¼ at TL 2; ☹[3]: ¼ at TL 3; ☺: only contains traces; ☻: is free from it

Keyword Index	Unit	Lactose + unit/	Fructose* Fructose*	Sorbitol Sorbitol	FrucGalactans FrucGalactans
Power Bar® Performance Energy®, Chocolate	piece 2.3oz/65g	☺	¼ ¾	☹ 76¾	3¼[AG] 6¾
Power Bar® Performance Energy®, Cookie Dough	piece 2.3oz/65g	☺	¼ ¾	☹ ☺	10½[A] 21
Power Bar® Performance Energy®, Mixed Berry Blast	piece 2.3oz/65g	☺	¼ ¾	☹ 19	10½[A] 21
Power Bar® Performance Energy®, Vanilla Crisp	piece 2.3oz/65g	☺	¼ ¾	☹ ☺	10½[A] 21
Powerade®, all flavors	glass 8.4oz/240g	7½ +6¼ unit	☺+ ×1¼ unit ☺+ ×½ unit	☺ ☺	41½ 83¼
Pretzels, hard, unsalted, sticks	hand 0.75oz/21g	☺	☺ ☺	☺ ☺	1½[A] 3¼
Pringles® Light Fat Free Potato Crisps, Barbecue	hand 0.75oz/21g	☺	37 74¼	☹ 79¼	10¾[A] 21½
Pringles® Potato Crisps, Loaded Baked Potato	hand 0.75oz/21g	☺	41¾ 83½	☹ 79¼	10¾[A] 21½
Pringles® Potato Crisps, Original	hand 0.75oz/21g	☺	76¾ ☺	☹ ☺	10¾[A] 21½
Pringles® Potato Crisps, Salt & Vinegar	hand 0.75oz/21g	☺	41¾ 83½	☹ 79¼	10¾[A] 21½
Pudding mix, other flavors, cooked type	portion 0.88oz/24.75g	☺	☺ ☺	☺ ☺	☺ ☺
Pumpernickel roll	slice 1.49oz/42g	☺	☺ ☺	☺ ☺	½[A] 1¼
Pumpkin or squash seeds, shelled, unsalted	hand 1.06oz/30g	☺	☺ ☺	☺ ☺	2¾[G] 5¾
Pumpkin seed oil	portion 0.46oz/13g	☺	☺ ☺	☺ ☺	☺ ☺
Purslane, raw	portion 3oz/85g	☺	58¾ ☺	☺ ☺	☺ ☺
Quince, fresh	tbsp. 0.5ozfl/14.21ml	☺	1¼ 2¾	☺ ☺	☺ ☺
Quinoa, cooked	portion 4.94oz/140g	☺	☺+ ×1¾ unit ☺+ ×¾ unit	☺ ☺	2½[A] 5
Radicchio, raw	portion 3oz/85g	☺	2¼ 4¾	☺ ☺	¾ 1½
Radish, raw	portion 3oz/85g	☺	☺+ ×½ unit ☺+ ×¼ unit	☹ 1	☺[C] ☺
Raisins, uncooked	portion 1.42oz/40g	☺	½ 1	☹ ½	2[B] 4

KEYWORD INDEX	Unit	Lactose (L1) + unit/capsule	Fructose* (L0) Fructose* (L1)	Sorbitol (L0) Sorbitol (L1)	FrucGalactans (L0) FrucGalactans (L1)
Rambutan, canned in syrup	portion 4.94oz/140g	☺	1¼ 2¾	☺ ☺	¾ CB 1¾
Raspberries, fresh, red	portion 4.94oz/140g	☺	½ 1¼	☹ 1½	1 B 2¼
Raspberry juice	glass 8.4ozfl/240ml	☺	☹[2] ☹[2]	☹ ☹[2]	¾ B 1½
Ratatouille	portion 3.89oz/110g	🙂	☺ ☺	☹ 1¼	4 B 8
Red beans and rice soup mix, dry	portion 1.8oz/51g	☺	¼ ¾	☹ ¼	1¼ AC 2¾
Red Bull® Energy Drink	glass 8.4ozfl/240ml	☺	☺+ ×7¾ unit ☺+ ×3¾ unit	☺ ☺	☺ ☺
Red Bull® Energy Drink Sugar Free	glass 8.4ozfl/240ml	☺	☺ ☺	☺ ☺	☺ ☺
Red pepper (cayenne), ground	pinch 0.04oz/1g	☺	51 🙂	☺ ☺	☺ ☺
Red wine vinegar	tbsp. 0.5ozfl/14.21ml	☺	🙂 🙂	☹ 20	☺ ☺
Rhubarb pie, bottom crust only	piece 4.31oz/122g	☺	☺ ☺	☺ ☺	¼ A ¾
Rhubarb, fresh	portion 4.94oz/140g	☺	☺ ☺	☺ ☺	☺ ☺
Ribs, beef, spare, visible fat eaten	portion 3oz/85g	☺	☺ ☺	☺ ☺	☺ ☺
Rice bread	slice 1.49oz/42g	☺	☺ ☺	☺ ☺	☺ A ☺
Rice cake	piece 0.32oz/9g	☺	☺ ☺	☺ ☺	☺ G ☺
Rice Krispies® (Kellogg's®)	portion 1.06oz/30g	☺	☺ ☺	☺ ☺	1½ A 3
Rice milk, plain or original, unsweetened, enriched	glass 8.4oz/240g	☺	☺+ ×¼ unit ☺	☺ ☺	☺ A ☺
Rice noodles, fried	portion 0.89oz/25g	☺	☺ ☺	☺ ☺	☺ A ☺

(L0) *Level 0:* lactose measure ×½ + Unit/capsule: added tolerated amount of unit per strong lactase capsule
(L1) *Level 1:* fructose measure ×2 Fructose*: fructose, sorbitol adjusted

(L2) *Level 2:* fructose-/sorbitol measure ×4. the rest ×2 ☺+ ×[Amount] unit: Per unit consumed you can additionally tolerate up to [amount] × fructose(*)-unit of another product.
(L3) *Level 3:* sorbitol measure ×7. the rest ×3
[book]: source of fruc/galactans data

☹: avoid; ☹[1]: ¼ at TL 1; ☹[2]: ¼ at TL 2; ☹[3]: ¼ at TL 3; 🙂: only contains traces; ☺: is free from it

Keyword Index	Unit	Lactose + unit/	Fructose* Fructose*	Sorbitol Sorbitol	FrucGalactans FrucGalactans
Rice pudding (arroz con leche), coconut, raisins	piece 7.06oz/200g	½ +¼ unit	27¾ 55½	☹ 1¼	3¼ 6½
Rice pudding (arroz con leche), plain	piece 7.06oz/200g	½ +¼ unit	☺+ ×½ unit ☺+ ×¼ unit	☺ ☺	2¾ 5¾
Rice pudding (arroz con leche), raisins	piece 7.06oz/200g	½ +¼ unit	3¾ 7½	☹ 1¼	3 6
Ricotta cheese, part skim milk	portion 1.95oz/55g	17½ +14½ unit	☺ ☺	☺ ☺	☺ ☺
Riesen®	piece 0.32oz/9g	12¾ +10½ unit	½ 1	☹ ☹[3]	71 ☺
Riesling	glass 8.4ozfl/240ml	☺	31¼ 62½	☹ ¾	☺ ☺
Ritz Cracker (Nabisco®)	portion 1.06oz/30g	☺	☺ ☺	☺ ☺	¼[A] ½
Rob Roy	glass 8.4ozfl/240ml	☺	¼ ½	☹ 2½	☺ ☺
Rocket (arugula), raw	portion 3oz/85g	☺	4¾ 9¾	☺ ☺	☺ ☺
Rockstar Original®	glass 8.4ozfl/240ml	☺	☺+ ×23¾ unit ☺+ ×11¾ unit	☹ 5	☺ ☺
Rockstar Original® Sugar Free	glass 8.4ozfl/240ml	☺	☺ ☺	☹ 5	☺ ☺
Rompope (eggnog with alcohol)	glass 8.4ozfl/240ml	¼ +¼ unit	☺ ☺	☺ ☺	2¾ 5½
Root beer	glass 8.4ozfl/240ml	☺	½ 1¼	☺ ☺	☺ ☺
Roquefort cheese	portion 1.06oz/30g	5 +4 unit	☺ ☺	☺ ☺	27¾ 55½
Rose hips	portion 4.94oz/140g	☺	☺+ ×½ unit ☺+ ×¼ unit	☺ ☺	☺ ☺
Rose wine, other types	glass 8.4ozfl/240ml	☺	¾ 1¾	☺ ☺	☺ ☺
Rosemary, dried	pinch 0.04oz/1g	☺	☺ ☺	☺ ☺	☺ ☺
Rum	glass 8.4ozfl/240ml	☺	☺ ☺	☺ ☺	☺ ☺
Rum and cola	glass 8.4ozfl/240ml	☺	1 2	☺ ☺	☺ ☺
Rusty nail	glass 8.4ozfl/240ml	☺	☺+ ×1¾ unit ☺+ ×1 unit	☹ ¾	☺ ☺

KEYWORD INDEX	Unit	Lactose (Level 1) + unit/capsule	Fructose* (Level 0) Fructose* (Level 1)	Sorbitol (Level 0) Sorbitol (Level 1)	FrucGalactans (Level 0) FrucGalactans (Level 1) (source)
Rutabaga, raw or blanched, marinated in oil mixture	portion 3oz/85g	☺	☺+ ×1 unit ☺+ ×½ unit	☺ ☺	☺ CB ☺
Rye bread	slice 1.49oz/42g	☺	☺ ☺	☺ ☺	¾ A 1¾
Rye flour,in recipes not containing yeast	portion 1.06oz/30g	☺	27¾ 55½	☺ ☺	1¼ A 2½
Rye roll	slice 1.49oz/42g	☺	☺ ☺	☺ ☺	¾ A 1¾
Safflower oil	portion 0.46oz/13g	☺	☺ ☺	☺ ☺	☺ ☺
Sake	glass 8.4ozfl/240ml	☺	☹² ☹²	☹ ½	☺ ☺
Salami, beer or beerwurst, beef	portion 1.95oz/55g	☺	☺+ ×1 unit ☺+ ×½ unit	☺ ☺	☺ ☺
Salmon, red (sockeye), smoked	portion 1.95oz/55g	☺	☺ ☺	☺ ☺	☺ ☺
Salsa, store bought	tbsp. 0.5ozfl/14.21ml	☺	6¼ 12½	☹ 6¾	5½ 11¼
Sambuca	glass 8.4ozfl/240ml	☺	☺+ ×4½ unit ☺+ ×2½ unit	☹ ¼	☺ ☺
Sandwich cookies, vanilla	piece 0.53oz/15g	9 +7½ unit	☺ ☺	☺ ☺	3 A 6¼
Sangria	glass 8.4ozfl/240ml	☺	7¾ 15½	☹ ¾	☺ ☺
Santa Claus melon	portion 4.94oz/140g	☺	1¼ 2½	☺ ☺	☺ ☺
Sapodilla, fresh	portion 4.94oz/140g	☺	☺+ ×3½ unit ☺+ ×1¾ unit	☺ ☺	☺ ☺
Sauerbraten	portion 5.61oz/159g	☺	34¾ 69¾	☺ ☺	☺ ☺
Sauerkraut	tbsp. 0.5ozfl/14.21ml	☺	☺ ☺	☹ ¾	7 B 14¼

Level 0: lactose measure ×½
Level 1: fructose measure ×2
+ Unit/capsule: added tolerated amount of unit per strong lactase capsule
Fructose*: fructose, sorbitol adjusted
Level 2: fructose-/sorbitol measure ×4. the rest ×2
Level 3: sorbitol measure ×7. the rest ×3
(book): source of fruc/galactans data
☺+ ×[Amount] unit: Per unit consumed you can additionally tolerate up to [amount] × fructose(*)-unit of another product.

☹: avoid; ☹¹: ¼ at TL 1; ☹²: ¼ at TL 2; ☹³: ¼ at TL 3; ☺: only contains traces; ☺: is free from it

KEYWORD INDEX	Unit	Lactose + unit/	Fructose* Fructose*	Sorbitol Sorbitol	FrucGalactans FrucGalactans
Scallions or spring onions, raw or blanched, tops and bulbs, marinated in oil	piece 0.56oz/15.7g	☺	☺+ ×¼ unit ☺	☹ 6	¼ G ¾
Scallop squash	portion 3oz/85g	☺	4 8¼	☺ ☺	☺ CB ☺
Scallops	portion 3oz/85g	☺	☺ ☺	☺ ☺	☺ ☺
Schnapps, all flavors	glass 8.4ozfl/240ml	☺	☺+ ×2¼ unit ☺+ ×1¼ unit	☹ ½	☺ ☺
Schweppes® Bitter Lemon	glass 8.4ozfl/240ml	☺	☹ 2 ☹ 2	☺ ☺	☺ ☺
Scotch and soda	glass 8.4ozfl/240ml	☺	☺ ☺	☺ ☺	☺ ☺
Scrambled egg with bacon	portion 3.89oz/110g	2¼ +1¾ unit	☺+ ×1¾ unit ☺+ ×¾ unit	☺ ☺	12½ 25¼
Screwdriver	glass 8.4ozfl/240ml	☺	2 4¼	☹ ¼	☺ ☺
Sea Pak® Seasoned Shrimp, Roasted Garlic	portion 3oz/85g	☺	☺ ☺	☺ ☺	☺ ☺
Sea Pak® Shrimp Scampi in Italian Parmesan Sauce	portion 3oz/85g	☺	☺ ☺	☺ ☺	☺ ☺
Seabreeze	glass 8.4ozfl/240ml	☺	☺+ ×5¼ unit ☺+ ×2½ unit	☹ 2½	☺ ☺
Semolina flour	portion 1.06oz/30g	☺	☺ ☺	☺ ☺	1¼ AD 2¾
Sesame chicken	portion 8.89oz/252g	☺	☺ ☺	☹ 3¾	☺ ☺
Sesame sticks	hand 0.75oz/21g	☺	☺ ☺	☹ ☺	1½ A 3¼
Shallot, raw	tbsp. 0.5ozfl/14.21ml	☺	☺ ☺	☺ ☺	¼ CB ½
Shiitake mushrooms, cooked	tbsp. 0.5ozfl/14.21ml	☺	☺+ ×1 unit ☺+ ×½ unit	☹ ½	☺ ☺
Singapore sling	glass 8.4ozfl/240ml	☺	☺+ ×¼ unit ☺	☹ 4½	☺ ☺
Slim-Fast® Easy to Digest, Vanilla, ready-to-drink can	glass 8.4oz/240g	2½ +2 unit	☺ ☺	☺ ☺	14¼ 28¾
Sloe gin	glass 8.4ozfl/240ml	☺	☺+ ×4½ unit ☺+ ×2½ unit	☹ ¼	☺ ☺

Keyword Index	Unit	Lactose 1 + unit/capsule	Fructose* 0 Fructose* 1	Sorbitol 0 Sorbitol 1	FrucGalactans 0 FrucGalactans 1 📖
Sloe gin fizz	glass 8.4ozfl/240ml	☻	☻+ ×¾ unit ☻+ ×¼ unit	☹ 1½	☻ ☻
Smart Balance® Light with Flax Oil Margarine, tub	portion 0.5oz/14g	32¼ +27 unit	☻ ☻	☻ ☻	☺ ☺
Smart Balance® Margarine	portion 0.5oz/14g	31 +25¾ unit	☻ ☻	☻ ☻	☺ ☺
Smarties®	hand 1.06oz/30g	☻	☻+ ×55 unit ☻+ ×27½ unit	☻ ☻	☻ ☻
Snickers®	piece 2.08oz/58.7g	1½ +1¼ unit	☻+ ×7 unit ☻+ ×3½ unit	☻ ☻	5¾ 11½
Snickers®, Almond	piece 1.77oz/49.9g	1¾ +1½ unit	☻+ ×8¾ unit ☻+ ×4¼ unit	☻ ☻	6½ G 13¼
Snow peas (edible pea pods), cooked from fresh	portion 3oz/85g	☻	☻+ ×3½ unit ☻+ ×1¾ unit	☻ ☻	¾ B 1¾
Sorbet, chocolate	portion 3.71oz/105g	☺	☻+ ×3¼ unit ☻+ ×1½ unit	☻ ☻	3 G 6¼
Sorbet, coconut	portion 3.74oz/106g	18¾ +15½ unit	☻+ ×5 unit ☻+ ×2½ unit	☻ ☻	3¼ 6½
Sorbet, fruit	portion 3.74oz/106g	☻	☻+ ×5½ unit ☻+ ×2¾ unit	☻ ☻	☻ ☻
Sorghum	portion 1.06oz/30g	☻	☻ ☻	☻ ☻	☻ ☻
Souffle, meat	portion 3.89oz/110g	1¼ +1 unit	☻+ ×½ unit ☻+ ×¼ unit	☹ ☺	1¾ B 3¾
Soup base	tbsp. 0.5ozfl/14.21ml	☻	64 ☺	☹ 74	☻ ☻
Sour cherries, fresh	tbsp. 0.5ozfl/14.21ml	☻	10 20	☹ ½	☻ ☻
Sour cream	portion 1.06oz/30g	3¼ +2¾ unit	☻ ☻	☻ ☻	19¼ 38½
Sour pickles	portion 1.06oz/30g	☻	☻+ ×¼ unit ☻	☹ 4¼	1 G 2¼

0 *Level 0:* lactose measure ×½
1 *Level 1:* fructose measure ×2
+ Unit/capsule: added tolerated amount of unit per strong lactase capsule
Fructose*: fructose, sorbitol adjusted

2 *Level 2*: fructose-/sorbitol measure ×4. the rest ×2
3 *Level 3:* sorbitol measure ×7. the rest ×3
📖: source of fruc/galactans data

☻+ ×[Amount] unit: Per unit consumed you can additionally tolerate up to [amount] × fructose(*)-unit of another product.

☹: avoid; ☹[1]: ¼ at TL 1; ☹[2]: ¼ at TL 2; ☹[3]: ¼ at TL 3; ☺: only contains traces; ☻: is free from it

Keyword Index	Unit	Lactose + unit/	Fructose* Fructose*	Sorbitol Sorbitol	FrucGalactans FrucGalactans
Sourdough bread	slice 1.49oz/42g	☺	☺ ☺	☺ ☺	¾[A] 1½
Soursop (guanabana), fresh	portion 4.94oz/140g	☺	1¼ 2¾	☺ ☺	☺ ☺
Southern Comfort®	glass 8.4ozfl/240ml	☺	☺ ☺	☺ ☺	☺ ☺
Soy bread	slice 1.49oz/42g	3½ +3 unit	11 22¼	☹ 2	1[A] 2
Soy chips	hand 0.75oz/21g	5¼ +4¼ unit	15 30	☹ 1	2[A] 4
Soy Kaas Fat Free, all flavors	portion 1.06oz/30g	9 +7½ unit	55½ ☺	☹ 18½	1¼[A] 2¾
Soy milk, chocolate, sweetened with sugar, not fortified	cup 5.2ozfl/150ml	☺	☺ ☺	☹ 4¼	¼[A] ½
Soy milk, plain or original, sweetened with artificial sweetener	glass 8.4oz/240g	☺	4¾ 9½	☹ 1½	☹[A] ¼
Soy milk, vanilla or other flavors, sweetened with sugar, fat free	glass 8.4oz/240g	☺	☺+ ×¾ unit ☺+ ×¼ unit	☹ 7	☹[A] ¼
Soy sauce	tbsp. 0.5ozfl/14.21ml	☺	☺ ☺	☹ 4½	3[A] 6
Soybean oil, unhydrogenated	tbsp. 0.5ozfl/14.21ml	☺	☺ ☺	☺ ☺	☺ ☺
Soybean sprouts, raw	portion 3oz/85g	☺	☺ ☺	☹ ½	3¾[CB] 7½
Soybeans, cooked from dried	tbsp. 0.5ozfl/14.21ml	☺	9 18	☹ 3	3[A] 6
Spaetzle (spatzen)	portion 4.94oz/140g	5¼ +4¼ unit	☺+ ×¼ unit ☺	☺ ☺	1[A] 2
Spaghetti squash	portion 3oz/85g	☺	☺+ ×¼ unit ☺	☺ ☺	☺[CB] ☺
Spaghetti, with carbonara sauce	portion 7.09oz/201g	13½ +11¼ unit	☺+ ×¾ unit ☺+ ×¼ unit	☹ 6	½[A] 1
Spearmint tea	glass 8.4ozfl/240ml	☺	☺ ☺	☺ ☺	☺[G] ☺
Special K® Blueberry cereal (Kellogg's®)	portion 1.06oz/30g	☺	☺+ ×½ unit ☺+ ×¼ unit	☹ 15	½[A] 1¼
Special K® Cinnamon Pecan cereal (Kellogg's®)	portion 1.06oz/30g	☺	☺ ☺	☺ ☺	½[A] 1¼

Keyword Index	Unit	Lactose + unit/	Fructose* Fructose*	Sorbitol Sorbitol	FrucGalactans FrucGalactans
Special K® Original cereal (Kellogg's®)	portion 1.06oz/30g	13 +10¾ unit	☺ ☺	☺ ☺	½[A] 1¼
Special K® Red Berries cereal (Kellogg's®)	portion 1.06oz/30g	☺	☺ ☺	☹ 41½	½[A] 1¼
Spelt flour	portion 1.06oz/30g	☺	☺+ ×¼ unit ☺	☺ ☺	☺[A] ☺
Spinach ravioli, with tomato sauce	portion 8.82oz/250g	5½ +4½ unit	☺+ ×¼ unit ☺	☹ ½	½[A] 1
Spinach, cooked from fresh	portion 3oz/85g	☺	☺ ☺	☹ 13	4[CB] 8¼
Splenda®	portion 0oz/0g	☺	☺ ☺	☺ ☺	☺ ☺
Split pea sprouts, cooked	tbsp. 0.5ozfl/14.21ml	☺	☺ ☺	☺ ☺	1¼[A] 2½
Spring roll	portion 4.94oz/140g	☺	21 42	☹ 2¾	¼ ½
Sprinkles Cookie Crisp® (General Mills®)	portion 1.06oz/30g	☺	☺+ ×¼ unit ☺	☹ ☺	¾[A] 1¾
Sprite®	glass 8.4ozfl/240ml	☺	☹ [2] ☹ [2]	☺ ☺	☺ ☺
Sprite® Zero	glass 8.4ozfl/240ml	☺	☺ ☺	☺ ☺	☺ ☺
Squash or pumpkin ravioli, with cream sauce	portion 8.82oz/250g	½ +½ unit	☺+ ×¼ unit ☺	☹ 40	½[A] 1
Starbucks® Hot Cocoa Double Chocolate, prepared	cup 5.2ozfl/150ml	¼ +¼ unit	37 74	☹ 66½	1[G] 2¼
Starbucks® Hot Cocoa Salted Caramel, prepared	cup 5.2ozfl/150ml	¼ +¼ unit	33¼ 66½	☹ 66½	2 4¼
Starburst®, Original	piece 0.18oz/5g	☺	☺+ ×½ unit ☺+ ×¼ unit	☹ 30¼	☺ ☺
Stewed green peas with sofrito	tbsp. 0.5oz.fl/14.8ml	☺ +2¾ unit	☺ ☺	☹ 5½	1¼[AB] 2½

Level 0: lactose measure ×½
Level 1: fructose measure ×2
+ Unit/: added tolerated amount of unit per strong lactase capsule
Fructose*: fructose, sorbitol adjusted

Level 2: fructose-/sorbitol measure ×4. the rest ×2
Level 3: sorbitol measure ×7. the rest ×3
: source of fruc/galactans data
☺+ ×[Amount] unit: Per unit consumed you can additionally tolerate up to [amount] × fructose(*)-unit of another product.

☹: avoid; ☹[1]: ¼ at TL 1; ☹[2]: ¼ at TL 2; ☹[3]: ¼ at TL 3; ☺: only contains traces; ☺: is free from it

Keyword Index	Unit	Lactose + unit/	Fructose* Fructose*	Sorbitol Sorbitol	FrucGalactans FrucGalactans
Sticky bun	piece 2.51oz/71g	8¾ +7¼ unit	☺+ ×¾ unit ☺+ ×¼ unit	☺ ☺	½[D] 1
Stonyfield® Oikos Greek Yogurt, Blueberry	piece 5.3oz/150g	¼ +¼ unit	☺+ ×1 unit ☺+ ×½ unit	☺ ☺	1¾ 3½
Stonyfield® Oikos Greek Yogurt, Caramel	piece 4.03oz/114g	½ +½ unit	☺+ ×½ unit ☺+ ×¼ unit	☺ ☺	4 8
Stonyfield® Oikos Greek Yogurt, Chocolate	piece 4.03oz/114g	½ +¼ unit	66½ ☺	☺ ☺	3 6¼
Stonyfield® Oikos Greek Yogurt, Strawberry	piece 5.3oz/150g	¼ +¼ unit	4 8¼	☹ 2	1¾ 3½
Straw mushrooms, canned, drained	portion 3oz/85g	☺	☺ ☺	☹ ¼	☺ ☺
Strawberries, fresh	portion 4.94oz/140g	☺	½ 1¼	☹ ¼	☺[C] ☺
Strawberry milk, plain, prepared	glass 8.4oz/240g	¼ +¼ unit	☺ ☺	☺ ☺	1¾ 3½
Strawberry pie, bottom crust only	piece 4.31oz/122g	☺	1¾ 3¾	☹ ¾	¼[A] ¾
Streusel topping, crumb	portion 0.68oz/19g	68¼ +57 unit	☺ ☺	☺ ☺	2¾[A] 5¾
Subway® 9-grain Wheat bread	piece 2.76oz/78g	☺	1 2	☺ ☺	¼[A] ¾
Subway® American cheese	portion 1.06oz/30g	4½ +3¾ unit	☺ ☺	☺ ☺	25¾ 51½
Subway® bacon	portion 0.53oz/15g	☺	☺ ☺	☺ ☺	☺ ☺
Subway® cheddar cheese	portion 1.06oz/30g	43¼ +36 unit	☺ ☺	☺ ☺	☺ ☺
Subway® chipotle southwest salad dressing	portion 1.06ozfl/30ml	7¼ +6 unit	☺ ☺	☺ ☺	40½ 81
Subway® chocolate chip cookie	piece 1.59oz/45g	☺	☺+ ×1 unit ☺+ ×½ unit	☹ ☺	½[A] 1
Subway® chocolate chunk cookie	piece 1.59oz/45g	☺	☺+ ×1 unit ☺+ ×½ unit	☹ ☺	½[A] 1
Subway® Ham Sandwich with Veggies, no mayo	piece 7.73oz/219g	12½ +10½ unit	¾ 1¾	☹ 1¼	¼[A] ½
Subway® honey mustard salad dressing	portion 1.06oz/30g	☺	4½ 9	☺ ☺	☺ ☺
Subway® honey mustard sauce, fat free	portion 0.99oz/28g	☺	4¾ 9½	☺ ☺	☺ ☺

Keyword Index	Unit	Lactose (Level 1) + unit/capsule	Fructose* (Level 0) Fructose* (Level 1)	Sorbitol (Level 0) Sorbitol (Level 1)	FrucGalactans (Level 0) FrucGalactans (Level 1) 🕮
Subway® Honey Oat bread	piece 3.14oz/89g	¾ +½ unit	2½ 5¼	☹ 6½	¼ ¾[A]
Subway® Italian BMT® Sandwich with Veggies, no mayo	piece 7.98oz/226g	12½ +10½ unit	¾ 1¾	☹ 1¼	¼[A] ½
Subway® M & M's® cookie	piece 1.59oz/45g	9 +7½ unit	☻+ ×½ unit ☻+ ×¼ unit	☹ ☺	½[A] 1
Subway® mustard	portion 0.18oz/5g	☻	☻ ☻	☻ ☻	☻ ☻
Subway® Oven Roasted Chicken Sandwich with Veggies, no mayo	piece 8.22oz/233g	12½ +10½ unit	1¾ 3¾	☹ 1¼	☹[A] ¼
Subway® Parmesan Oregano bread	piece 2.65oz/75g	☺	☻+ ×½ unit ☻+ ×¼ unit	☻ ☻	¾[A] 1½
Subway® ranch salad dressing	portion 1.06ozfl/30ml	☺	☻ ☻	☹ ☺	☺ ☺
Subway® Roast Beef Sandwich with Veggies, no mayo	piece 8.22oz/233g	12½ +10½ unit	¾ 1¾	☹ 1¼	☹[A] ¼
Subway® Spicy Italian Sandwich with Veggies, no meat	piece 7.84oz/222g	12½ +10½ unit	¾ 1¾	☹ 1¼	¼[A] ½
Subway® Steak & Cheese Sandwich with Veggies, no mayo	piece 8.65oz/245g	☺	1 2	☹ 1¼	☹[A] ¼
Subway® Sweet Onion Chicken Teriyaki Sandwich with Veggies, no mayo	piece 9.74oz/276g	12½ +10½ unit	22½ 45¼	☹ 1¼	☹[A] ¼
Subway® sweet onion salad dressing	portion 1.06ozfl/30ml	☻	☻+ ×1 unit ☻+ ×½ unit	☹ 55½	½ 1¼
Subway® Tuna Sandwich with Veggies, no mayo	piece 8.22oz/233g	12½ +10½ unit	¾ 1¾	☹ 1¼	☹[A] ¼
Subway® Turkey Breast & Ham Sandwich with Veggies, no mayo	piece 7.73oz/219g	12½ +10½ unit	¾ 1¾	☹ 1¼	¼[A] ½
Subway® Turkey Breast Sandwich with Veggies, no mayo	piece 7.73oz/219g	12½ +10½ unit	¾ 1¾	☹ 1¼	¼[A] ½

Level 0: lactose measure ×½
Level 1: fructose measure ×2
+ Unit/capsule: added tolerated amount of unit per strong lactase capsule
Fructose*: fructose, sorbitol adjusted

Level 2: fructose-/sorbitol measure ×4. the rest ×2
Level 3: sorbitol measure ×7. the rest ×3
🕮: source of fruc/galactans data
☻+ ×[Amount] unit: Per unit consumed you can additionally tolerate up to [amount] × fructose(*)-unit of another product.

☹: avoid; ☹[1]: ¼ at TL 1; ☹[2]: ¼ at TL 2; ☹[3]: ¼ at TL 3; ☺: only contains traces; ☻: is free from it

Keyword Index	Unit	Lactose + unit/	Fructose* Fructose*	Sorbitol Sorbitol	FrucGalactans FrucGalactans
Subway® Veggie Delite Salad, no dressing	portion 3.53oz/100g	34¼ +28½ unit	83¼ ☺	☹ 2¼	☺ ☺
Subway® Veggie Delite Sandwich, no mayo	piece 5.72oz/162g	12½ +10½ unit	¾ 1¾	☹ 1½	¼[A] ½
Subway® vinegar	portion 0.5ozfl/14ml	☺	☺ ☺	☹ 20¼	☺ ☺
Subway® white chip macadamia nut cookie	piece 1.59oz/45g	6¾ +5½ unit	☺ ☺	☺ ☺	½[A] 1
Subway® wrap bread	piece 3.64oz/103g	☺	☺ ☺	☺ ☺	½ 1[A]
Suckers®, sugar free	piece 0.5oz/14g	☺	☹ ☹	☹ ☹	☺ ☺
Sugar cookies, iced, store bought	piece 0.53oz/15g	☺	☺ ☺	☺ ☺	3¼[A] 6½
Sugar, white granulated	tbsp. 0.5ozfl/14.21ml	☺	☺ ☺	☺ ☺	☺ ☺
Summer squash, cooked from fresh	portion 3oz/85g	☺	2¼ 4¾	☺ ☺	2[CB] 4
Sunbelt Bakery® Chewy Granola Bar, Banana Harvest	piece 0.89oz/25g	49 +40¾ unit	☺+ ×½ unit ☺+ ×¼ unit	☹ ¾	¾[A] 1½
Sunbelt Bakery® Chewy Granola Bar, Blueberry Harvest	piece 0.89oz/25g	49 +40¾ unit	☺+ ×½ unit ☺+ ×¼ unit	☹ ¾	¾[A] 1½
Sunbelt Bakery® Chewy Granola Bar, Golden Almond	piece 0.99oz/28g	4 +3¼ unit	1½ 3¼	☹ ☹[2]	½[A] 1¼
Sunbelt Bakery® Chewy Granola Bar, Low Fat Oatmeal Raisin	piece 1.06oz/30g	11¾ +9¾ unit	½ 1	☹ ☹[2]	½[A] 1¼
Sunbelt Bakery® Chewy Granola Bar, Oats & Honey	piece 0.96oz/27g	17½ +14¾ unit	5¾ 11¾	☹ ☹[2]	½[A] 1¼
Sunbelt Bakery® Fudge Dipped Chewy Granola Bar, Coconut	piece 1.03oz/29g	17¼ +14½ unit	¾ 1½	☹ ☹[2]	½[A] 1¼
Sun-dried tomatoes, oil pack, drained	portion 1.06oz/30g	☺	¼ ½	☹ ¼	4½[B] 9¼
Sunflower oil	tbsp. 0.5ozfl/14.21ml	☺	☺ ☺	☺ ☺	☺ ☺
Sunflower seeds, raw	hand 1.06oz/30g	☺	☺ ☺	☺ ☺	2[G] 4
Sushi, with fish	portion 4.94oz/140g	☺	10½ 21	☹ 2½	☺ ☺

KEYWORD INDEX	Unit	Lactose (L1) + unit/capsule	Fructose* (L0) Fructose* (L1)	Sorbitol (L0) Sorbitol (L1)	FrucGalactans (L0) FrucGalactans (L1) [source]
Sushi, with fish and vegetables in seaweed	portion 4.94oz/140g	☻	☻ ☻	☹ 2	☻ ☻
Sushi, with vegetables in seaweed	portion 4.94oz/140g	☻	☻ ☻	☹ 1½	☻ ☻
Swedish Meatballs	portion 4.94oz/140g	1½ +1¼ unit	☻ ☻	☹ 71¼	9 18
Sweet and sour chicken	tbsp. 0.5ozfl/14.21ml	☻	2½ 5	☹ ☺	☻ ☻
Sweet and sour sauce, store bought	tbsp. 0.5ozfl/14.21ml	☻	½ 1¼	☹ 83¼	☻ ☻
Sweet cherries, fresh	tbsp. 0.5ozfl/14.21ml	☻	3¾ 7½	☹ ¼	☻ ☻
Sweet potato bread	slice 1.49oz/42g	☺	☻ ☻	☻ ☻	1½ A 3¼
Sweetened condensed milk	portion 1.35ozfl/38ml	½ +½ unit	☻ ☻	☻ ☻	3¾ 7½
Sweetened condensed milk, reduced fat	portion 1.38ozfl/39ml	½ +½ unit	☻ ☻	☻ ☻	3½ 7¼
Swiss cheese, natural	portion 1.06oz/30g	☺	☻+ ×¼ unit ☻	☻ ☻	☺ ☺
Swiss cheese, natural, low sodium	portion 1.06oz/30g	☺	☻+ ×¼ unit ☻	☻ ☻	☺ ☺
Sylvaner	glass 8.4ozfl/240ml	☻	31¼ 62½	☹ ¾	☻ ☻
Tabasco® sauce	tbsp. 0.5ozfl/14.21ml	☻	☻ ☻	☻ ☻	☻ ☻
Taco Bell® 7-Layer Burrito	portion 4.94oz/140g	25½ +21¼ unit	☻ ☻	☹ 5¾	¼ A ¾
Taco Bell® Crunchwrap Supreme	piece 8.65oz/245g	4¼ +3½ unit	☻ ☻	☹ 5	☹ A ¼
Taco Bell® Mexican Pizza	piece 7.52oz/213g	13¾ +11½ unit	23¼ 46¾	☹ 1	¼ A ¾

(L0) *Level 0:* lactose measure ×½
(L1) *Level 1:* fructose measure ×2
+ Unit/capsule: added tolerated amount of unit per strong lactase capsule
Fructose*: fructose, sorbitol adjusted

(L2) *Level 2*: fructose-/sorbitol measure ×4. the rest ×2
(L3) *Level 3:* sorbitol measure ×7. the rest ×3
[source]: source of fruc/galactans data
☻+ ×[Amount] unit: Per unit consumed you can additionally tolerate up to [amount] × fructose(*)-unit of another product.

☹: avoid; ☹[1]: ¼ at TL 1; ☹[2]: ¼ at TL 2; ☹[3]: ¼ at TL 3; ☺: only contains traces; ☻: is free from it

KEYWORD INDEX	Unit	Lactose + unit/	Fructose* Fructose*	Sorbitol Sorbitol	FrucGalactans FrucGalactans
Taco Bell® Nachos Supreme	portion 4.94oz/140g	6¼ +5¼ unit	☺ ☺	☹ 7¾	35¾[B] 71½
Taco John's® nachos	hand 0.75oz/21g	28 +23¼ unit	☺ ☺	☹ ☺	10[A] 20
Taco sauce, red	portion 1.13oz/32g	☺	2¾ 5¾	☹ 3	11 22
Taco, soft corn shell, with beans, cheese	portion 4,94 oz/140g	☺ +77 unit	12¾ 25½	☺ 4¼	¼ [A] ½
Taffy	piece 0.31oz/8.6g	☺	☺+ ×4¼ unit ☺+ ×2 unit	☺ ☺	☺ ☺
Tahini (sesame butter)	portion 1.06oz/30g	☺	☺ ☺	☺ ☺	1[G] 2¼
Tap water	glass 8.4ozfl/240ml	☺	☺ ☺	☺ ☺	☺ ☺
Tempeh	portion 3oz/85g	☺	3¼ 6¾	☹ ½	½[A] 1
Tequila	glass 8.4ozfl/240ml	☺	☺ ☺	☺ ☺	☺ ☺
Tequila sunrise	glass 8.4ozfl/240ml	☺	☺+ ×¼ unit ☺	☹ 3¼	☺ ☺
Thyme, dried	pinch 0.04oz/1g	☺	☺ ☺	☺ ☺	☺ ☺
Tic Tacs®	2 piece 0.05oz/1.15g	☺	☺ ☺	☺ ☺	☺ ☺
Tilsit cheese	portion 1.06oz/30g	5¼ +4¼ unit	☺ ☺	☺ ☺	29½ 59
Tiramisu	portion 1.95oz/55g	2½ +2 unit	☺ ☺	☺ ☺	12[A] 24
Toast, cinnamon and sugar, whole wheat bread	slice 1.49oz/42g	49½ +41¼ unit	1½ 3¼	☺ ☺	¾[A] 1¾
Toast, wheat bread, with butter	slice 1.49oz/42g	62½ +52 unit	1¾ 3¾	☺ ☺	1¼[A] 2½
Toblerone® Swiss Dark Chocolate with Honey & Almond Nougat	piece 0.89oz/25g	7¼ +6 unit	☺ ☺	☹ 40	1½ 3¼
Toblerone® Swiss Milk Chocolate with Honey & Almond Nougat	piece 0.89oz/25g	1½ +1¼ unit	☺ ☺	☺ ☺	1½ 3

KEYWORD INDEX	Unit	Lactose [Level 1] + unit/capsule	Fructose* [Level 0] Fructose* [Level 1]	Sorbitol [Level 0] Sorbitol [Level 1]	FrucGalactans [Level 0] FrucGalactans [Level 1] [source]
Toblerone® Swiss White Confection with Honey & Almond Nougat	piece 0.89oz/25g	1 +1 unit	☺ ☺	☺ ☺	6¾ 13½
Toffee	piece 0.25oz/7g	40¾ +34 unit	☺ ☺	☺ ☺	☺ ☺
Toffifay®	piece 0.29oz/8.2g	7½ +6¼ unit	½ 1	☹ ☹[2]	42¾ 85½
Tofu, raw (not silken), cooked, low fat	portion 3oz/85g	☺	2¼ 4¾	☹ ¾	½[A] 1
Tokaji Wine	glass 8.4ozfl/240ml	☺	☹[2] ☹[2]	☹ ½	☺ ☺
Tom Collins	glass 8.4ozfl/240ml	☺	31¼ 62½	☹ 16½	☺ ☺
Tomato juice	glass 8.4ozfl/240ml	☺	1¼ 2½	☹ ¼	2¾[B] 5½
Tomato relish	portion 0.53oz/15g	☺	☺ ☺	☹ 5¼	33 66¼
Tomato sauce	portion 2.12oz/60g	☺	☺+ ×¾ unit ☺+ ×¼ unit	☹ ¾	9¼[B] 18½
Tomato soup mix, dry	portion 1.2oz/34g	¼ +0,24 unit	13 26	☹ 2	1¼[B] 2¾
Tomato, cooked from fresh	portion 3oz/85g	☺	4¼ 8½	☹ ¾	6½[B] 13
Tonic water	glass 8.4ozfl/240ml	☺	☹[2] ☹[2]	☺ ☺	☺ ☺
Tonic water, diet	glass 8.4ozfl/240ml	☺	☺ ☺	☺ ☺	☺ ☺
Tootsie Pops®	piece 0.6oz/17g	☺	☺+ ×2½ unit ☺+ ×1¼ unit	☺ ☺	☺ ☺
Tortilla, white, store bought, fried	piece 2.05oz/58g	☺	☺ ☺	☺ ☺	¾[A] 1¾
Triple Sec	glass 8.4ozfl/240ml	☺	☺+ ×4½ unit ☺+ ×2½ unit	☹ ¼	☺ ☺

Level 0: lactose measure ×½
Level 1: fructose measure ×2
+ Unit/capsule: added tolerated amount of unit per strong lactase capsule
Fructose*: fructose, sorbitol adjusted
Level 2: fructose-/sorbitol measure ×4. the rest ×2
Level 3: sorbitol measure ×7. the rest ×3
[source]: source of fruc/galactans data
☺+ ×[Amount] unit: Per unit consumed you can additionally tolerate up to [amount] × fructose(*)-unit of another product.

☹: avoid; ☹[1]: ¼ at TL 1; ☹[2]: ¼ at TL 2; ☹[3]: ¼ at TL 3; ☺: only contains traces; ☺: is free from it

Keyword Index	Unit	Lactose + unit/	Fructose* Fructose*	Sorbitol Sorbitol	FrucGalactans FrucGalactans
Triticale bread	slice 1.49oz/42g	☺	2½ 5	☺ ☺	1 [A] 2
Tuna, canned, light, oil pack, not drained	portion 1.95oz/55g	☺	☺ ☺	☺ ☺	☺ ☺
Turnip, cooked	portion 3oz/85g	☺	☺+ ×½ unit ☺+ ×¼ unit	☹ 2½	☺ [CB] ☺
Twix®	piece 1.8oz/51g	2 +1¾ unit	☺+ ×1½ unit ☺+ ×¾ unit	☺ ☺	1¾ [A] 3½
Tzatziki sauce (yogurt and cucumber)	portion 1.06oz/30g	4½ +3¾ unit	38¾ 77½	☹ 9¼	11½ [FB] 23¼
V-8® 100% A-C-E Vitamin Rich Vegetable Juice	glass 8.4ozfl/240ml	☺	¼ ¾	☹ 3	2¾ [B] 5½
Vanilla Coke®	glass 8.4ozfl/240ml	☺	½ 1¼	☺ ☺	☺ ☺
Vanilla sauce	tbsp. 0.5ozfl/14.21ml	☺	☺ ☺	☺ ☺	☺ ☺
Vegetable soup, condensed	portion 4.45oz/126g	☺	☺+ ×¼ unit ☺	☹ 1	19¾ 39½
Venison or deer, stewed	portion 3oz/85g	☺	☺ ☺	☺ ☺	☺ ☺
Veryfine Cranberry Raspberry	glass 8.4ozfl/240ml	☺	☹ [1] ¼	☹ ☹ [2]	¾ [B] 1½
Vichyssoise soup	portion 8.65oz/245g	¾ +½ unit	☺+ ×¼ unit ☺	☹ 1¼	4¼ [AB] 8½
Vodka	glass 8.4ozfl/240ml	☺	☺ ☺	☺ ☺	☺ ☺
Waffles, bran	piece 3.36oz/95g	¾ +¾ unit	☺+ ×¼ unit ☺	☺ ☺	¼ [A] ¾
Waffles, whole wheat, from mix, add milk, fat and egg	piece 3.36oz/95g	1 +¾ unit	☺+ ×¼ unit ☺	☺ ☺	½ [A] 1
Walnut oil	tbsp. 0.5ozfl/14.21ml	☺	☺ ☺	☺ ☺	☺ ☺
Walnuts	hand 1.06oz/30g	☺	☺ ☺	☺ ☺	2¾ [G] 5¾
Watercress, raw	pinch 0.04oz/1g	☺	☺ ☺	☺ ☺	☺ ☺
Watermelon, fresh	tbsp. 0.5ozfl/14.21ml	☺	1¾ 3½	☹ ☺	10¼ [B] 20¾

Keyword Index	Unit	Lactose 1 / + unit/capsule	Fructose* 0 / Fructose* 1	Sorbitol 0 / Sorbitol 1	FrucGalactans 0 / FrucGalactans 1 (source)
Wax beans (yellow beans), canned, drained	portion 3oz/85g	☻	☻ ☻	☻ ☻	¼ A ¾
Weetabix® Organic Crispy Flakes & Fiber (Barbara's Bakery®)	portion 1.95oz/55g	☻	☻+ ×¾ unit ☻+ ×¾ unit	☻ ☻	¼ A ¾
Wendy's® Strawberry Shake	glass 8.4oz/240g	¼ +¼ unit	☻+ ×4¼ unit ☻+ ×2 unit	☹ 3¼	1¾ 3¾
Werther's® Original Caramel Coffee Hard Candies	piece 0.15oz/4g	17¾ +14¾ unit	☻+ ×½ unit ☻+ ×¼ unit	☻ ☻	☺ ☺
Wheat bran, unprocessed	tbsp. 0.5ozfl/14.21ml	☻	☻ ☻	☻ ☻	½ G 1
Wheaties® (General Mills®)	portion 1.06oz/30g	☻	83¼ ☺	☻ ☻	½ A 1¼
Whipped cream, aerosol	portion 0.25oz/7g	☺	☻ ☻	☻ ☻	☺ ☺
Whipped cream, aerosol, chocolate	portion 0.18oz/5g	9¾ +8 unit	☻ ☻	☹ ☺	54½ ☺
Whipped cream, aerosol, fat free	portion 0.18oz/5g	18¾ +15¾ unit	☻+ ×¼ unit ☻	☻ ☻	☺ ☺
Whiskey	glass 8.4ozfl/240ml	☻	☻ ☻	☻ ☻	☻ ☻
Whiskey sour	glass 8.4ozfl/240ml	☻	9½ 19	☹ 6¼	☻ ☻
whisky	glass 8ozfl/240mL	☻	☻ ☻	☻ ☻	☻ ☻
whisky sour	glass 8ozfl/240mL	☻	9½ 19	☹ 6¼	☻ ☻
White all-purpose flour, un-enriched	portion 1.06oz/30g	☻	☻ ☻	☻ ☻	1¼ A 2¾
White bean stew with sofrito	tbsp. 0.5ozfl/14.21ml	☻	☻ ☻	☹ ☺	3 AC 6
White bread, store bought	slice 1.49oz/42g	☺	1¼ 2¾	☻ ☻	1¼ A 2½

Level 0: lactose measure ×½ — + Unit/capsule: added tolerated amount of unit per strong lactase capsule
Level 1: fructose measure ×2 — Fructose*: fructose, sorbitol adjusted
Level 2: fructose-/sorbitol measure ×4. the rest ×2
Level 3: sorbitol measure ×7. the rest ×3
(book icon): source of fruc/galactans data
☻+ ×[Amount] unit: Per unit consumed you can additionally tolerate up to [amount] × fructose(*)-unit of another product.
☹: avoid; ☹1: ¼ at TL 1; ☹2: ¼ at TL 2; ☹3: ¼ at TL 3; ☺: only contains traces; ☻: is free from it

Keyword Index	Unit	Lactose + unit/	Fructose* Fructose*	Sorbitol Sorbitol	FrucGalactans FrucGalactans
White chocolate bar	piece 0.43ozfl/12g	2½ +2 unit	☺ ☺	☺ ☺	14 28¼
White Russian	glass 8.4ozfl/240ml	1½ +1¼ unit	☺ ☺	☹ 8¼	9 18¼
White sauce, store bought	tbsp. 0.5ozfl/14.21ml	4 +3¼ unit	☺ ☺	☺ ☺	22¼ 44½
White whole grain wheat bread	slice 1.49oz/42g	☺	¾ 1¾	☹ 26¼	¾[A] 1¾
White whole wheat flour	portion 1.06oz/30g	☺	33¼ 66½	☺ ☺	1¼[AD] 2¾
Whole wheat bread, store bought	slice 1.49oz/42g	☺	1¼ 2½	☺ ☺	1[A] 2¼
Wild 'n Fruity Gummi Bears (Brach's®)	hand 1.06oz/30g	☺	☺+ ×3½ unit ☺+ ×1¾ unit	☹ ☺	☺ ☺
Windmill cookies	piece 0.75oz/21g	☺	☺ ☺	☺ ☺	6¼[A] 12¾
Wine spritzer	glass 8.4ozfl/240ml	☺	27¾ 55½	☹ 1	☺ ☺
Winter (dark green or orange) squash, cooked	portion 4.59oz/130g	☺	1¾ 3¾	☺ ☺	☺[CB] ☺
Winter melon (waxgourd or chinese preserving melon)	portion 3oz/85g	☺	☺ ☺	☺ ☺	☺[CB] ☺
Wise Onion Flavored Rings	portion 1.06oz/30g	☺	☺ ☺	☹ ☺	10¼[AC] 20¾
Yams, sweet potato type, boiled	portion 3.89oz/110g	☺	☺ ☺	☺ ☺	☺[B] ☺
Yellow bell pepper, raw	portion 3oz/85g	☺	½ 1¼	☺ ☺	☺[CB] ☺
Yellow tomato, raw	portion 3oz/85g	☺	4½ 9¼	☹ 1	6½[B] 13
Yerba® Mate tea	glass 8.4ozfl/240ml	☺	☺ ☺	☺ ☺	☺ ☺
Yogurt, chocolate or coffee flavors, nonfat, sweetened with aspartame	tbsp. 0.5ozfl/14.21ml	4 +3¼ unit	☺ ☺	☺ ☺	22½ 45
Yogurt, chocolate or coffee flavors, whole milk, sweetened with sucralose	piece 6.04oz/171g	¼ +¼ unit	40 80	☺ ☺	1½ 3¼
Yogurt, fruited, whole milk	tbsp. 0.5ozfl/14.21ml	2¾ +2¼ unit	¾ 1½	☹ 60½	16 32¼

Keyword Index	Unit	Lactose 1 / + unit/💊	Fructose* 0 / Fructose* 1	Sorbitol 0 / Sorbitol 1	FrucGalactans 0 / FrucGalactans 1 📖
Zsweet®	portion 0.18ozfl/5ml	☺	☺ ☺	☹ ☹	☺ ☺

0 *Level 0:* lactose measure ×½
1 *Level 1:* fructose measure ×2
2 *Level 2*: fructose-/sorbitol measure ×4. the rest ×2
3 *Level 3:* sorbitol measure ×7. the rest ×3
📖: source of fruc/galactans data

+ Unit/💊: added tolerated amount of unit per strong lactase capsule
Fructose*: fructose, sorbitol adjusted

☺+ ×[Amount] unit: Per unit consumed you can additionally tolerate up to [amount] × fructose(*)-unit of another product.

☹: avoid; ☹[1]: ¼ at TL 1; ☹[2]: ¼ at TL 2; ☹[3]: ¼ at TL 3; ☺: only contains traces; ☺: is free from it

GLOSSARY

Abbreviation	Meaning
Brick dragon	Metaphor for discomfort induced by the presence of quickly fermentable carbohydrates in an "irritable bowel".
Bricks	Carbohydrates that are quickly fermented in the intestine. To this group belong oligosaccharides (Fructose, Fructans and Galactans, Lactose) and sugar alcohols.
BTL	Basic tolerance level, i.e. as long as you consume less of a problematic brick than the stated maximum amount for this level, you are likely to be untroubled by symptoms from it. It only applies in case of intolerance or certain testphases and then refers to the lowest allowable portion sizes and holds at least until a level test has been taken. Note that if you consume the maximum (B)TL portion size for a food at a meal, you cannot eat any other foods that contain the brick at that meal. To combine two foods that contain a certain brick you have to reduce the stated portion sizes accordingly, e.g. by dividing both by two.
BTLs	Basic tolerance levels.
EFSA	European Food Safety Authority.
FDA	Food and Drug Administration.
Fructans	Quickly fermentable carbohydrates that are contained in grain products for example. In this book only inulin, kestose and nystose are attributed to this group.
Fructose	Oligosaccharide that is primarily contained in fruit.
Galactans	Quickly fermentable carbohydrates that are contained in beans, cabbage, lentils and peas for example. In this book only raffinose and stachyose are attributed to this group.
Interception shield	Metaphor for the normal bodily resorbtion of bricks.

Abbreviation	Meaning
Irritable bowel	Definition of this book: An irritable bowel is one that reacts much more intensly to indigestions than it is commonly the case. These indigestions are often caused by the presence of "bricks" in the intestine.
Lactose	Oligosaccharide that is primarily contained in dairy products.
Meal	A meal is defined as one of three mainmeals of a given day. The first meal happen at about 7 am, the second one at about 1pm and the third one at about 7 pm. Hence, between each meal there has to be a gap of about six hours in order to avoid overloading your "interception shield". The tolerable portion sizes are based on this definition of a meal.
NCC	Nutrition Coordination Center of the University of Minnesota.
Sorbitol	Sugar alcohol that also limits the "interception" of fructose. Besides, see "sugar alcohols".
Sugar alcohols	These are contained in some fruit, like apples. Moreover, they are part of many diabetic, dietary and light products as well as chewing gums and mints. They are not contained in stevia. Part of the group of sugar alcohols besides sorbitol are erythritol, inositol, isomalt, lactitol, maltitol, mannitol, pinitol and xylitol.
TL	Tolerance level. These are employed to differentiate the portion sizes stated in the food tables according to the amount of the respective brick that is tolerated by you per meal. There are four tolerance levels for any brick. TL 0 being the BTL and TL 1 to TL 3 representing higher tolerable amounts of a brick and thus larger portion sizes of the foods that contain it. You can determine the level that applies to you by taking the level test that is described in chapter 21.4. Please also read the BTL definition.
TLs	Tolerance levels.

This page has been intentionally left blank.

SOURCES

Ali, M., Rellos, P., & Cox, T. M. (1998). Heriditary fructose intolerance. *Journal of Medical Genetics*, 35(5), 353-365.

Barrett, J. S., Gearry, R. B., Muir, J. G., Irving, P. M., Rose, R., Rosella, O., ... & Gibson, P. R. (2010). Dietary poorly absorbed, short-chain carbohydrates increase delivery of water and fermentable substrates to the proximal colon. *Alimentary Pharmacology & Therapeutics*, 31(8), 874-882.

Balasubramanya, N. N., Sarwar, & Narayanan, K. M. (1993). Effect of stage of lactation on oligosaccharides level in milk. *Indian Journal of Dairy & Biosciences*, 4, 58-60. Abstract Retrieved from http://www.cabdirect.com (Record Number 19950401205)

Belitz, H.-D., Grosch, W., & Schieberle, P. (2008). *Lehrbuch der Lebensmittelchemie* (6th ed.), Berlin Heidelberg: Springer.

Berekoven, L., Eckert, W., Ellenrieder, P. (2009). Marktforschung: *Methodische Grundlagen und praktische Anwendung* (12th ed.). Wiesbaden: Gabler.

Biesiekierski, J. R., Rosella, O., Rose, R., Liels, K., Barrett, J. S., Shepherd, S. J., ... & Muir, J. G. (2011). Quantification of fructans, galacto-oligosacharides and other short-chain carbohydrates in processed grains and cereals. *Journal of Human Nutrition and Dietetics*, 24(2), 154-176.

Binnendijk, K. H., & Rijkers, G. T. (2013). What is a health benefit? an evaluation of EFSA opinions on health benefits with reference to probiotics. *Beneficial Microbes*, 4(3), 223-230.

Blumenthal, M. (1998). *The Complete German Commission E Monographs; Therapeutic Guide to Herbal Medicine*. Boston, MA: Integrative Medicine Communications.

Boehm, G., & Stahl, B. (2007). Oligosaccharides from milk. *The Journal of Nutrition*, 137(3), 847S-849S.

Bowden, P. (2011). *Telling It Like It Is*. Paul Bowden.

Briançon, S., Boini, S., Bertrais, S., Guillemin, F., Galan, P., & Hercberg, S. (2011). Long-term antioxidant supplementation has no effect on health-related quality of life: The randomized, double-blind, placebo-controlled, primary prevention SU.VI.MAX trial. *International Journal of Epidemiology*, 40(6), 1605-1616.

Campbell, J. M., Fahey, G. C., & Wolf, B. W. (1997). Selected indigestible oligosaccharides affect large bowel mass, cecal and fecal short-chain fatty acids, pH and microflora in rats. *The Journal of Nutrition*, 127(1), 130-136.

Chi, W. J., Chang, Y. K., & Hong, S. K. (2012). Agar degradation by microorganisms and agar-degrading enzymes. *Applied Microbiology and Biotechnology*, 94(4), 917-930.

Choi, Y. K; Johlin Jr., F. C.; Summers, R.W., Jackson, M., & Rao, S. S. C. (2003). Fructose intolerance: an under-recognized problem. *The American Journal of Gastroenterology*, 98(6) 2003, S. 1348-1353.

CIAA (n. d.). *CIAA agreed reference values for GDAs* [Table]. Retrieved from http://gda.fooddrinkeurope.eu/asp2/gdas_portions_rationale.asp?doc_id=127.

Connor, W. E. (2000). Importance of n– 3 fatty acids in health and disease. *The American journal of clinical nutrition, 71*(1), 171S-175S.

Coraggio, L. (1990). *Deleterious Effects of Intermittent Interruptions on the Task Performance of Knowledge Workers: A Laboratory Investigation* (Doctoral Dissertation). Retrieved from http://arizona.openrepository.com.

Corazza, G. R., Strocchi, A., Rossi, R., Sirola, D., & Fasbarrini, G. (1988). Sorbitol malabsorption in normal volunteers and in patients with celiac disease. *Gut*, 29(1), 44-48.

Cummings, J. H. (1981). Short chain fatty acids in the human colon. *Gut*, 22(9), 763-779.

Cummings, J. H., & Macfarlane, G. T. (1997). Role of intestinal bacteria in nutrient metabolism. *Journal of Parental and Enteral Nutrition*, 21(6), 357-365.

DGE (2013). Vollwertig essen und trinken nach den 10 Regeln der DGE. 9th Edition, Bonn.

Diamond, J. (2005). *Collapse – How Societies Choose to Fail or to Survive*. New York: Viking Penguin.

Donker, G. A., Foets, M., & Spreeuwenberg, P. (1999). Patients with irritable bowel syndrome: health status and use of healthcare services. *British Journal of General Practice*, 49(447), 787-792.

Drossman, D. A., Li, Z., Andruzzi, E., Temple, R. D., Talley, N. J., Thompson, W. G. …Corazziari, E. et al., (1993). US householder survey of functional gastrointestinal disorders: prevalence, sociodemography, and health impact. *Digestive Diseases and Sciences*, 38(9), 1569-1580.

Dukas, L., Willett, W. C., & Giovannucci, E. L. (2003). Association between physical activity, fiber intake, and other lifestyle variables and constipation in a study of women. *The American Journal of Gastroenterology*, 98(8), 1790-1796.

EFSA (2007). Opinion of the Scientific Panel on Dietetic Products, Nutrition and Allergies on a request from the Commission related to a notification from EPA on lactitol pursuant to Article 6, paragraph 11 of Directive 2000/13/EC- for permanent exemption from labeling. *The EFSA Journal*, 5(10), 565-570.

EFSA (2012a). Scientific Opinion on Dietary Reference Values for protein. *The EFSA Journal*, 10(2), 2557-2622.

EFSA (2012b). Scientific Opinion on the substantiation of health claims related to Lactobacillus casei DG CNCM I-1572 and decreasing potentially pathogenic gastro-intestinal microorganisms (ID 2949, 3061, further assessment) pursuant to Article 13(1) of Regulation (EC) No 1924/2006. *The EFSA Journal*, 10(6), 2723-2637.

EFSA (2012c). Scientific opinion on the tolerable upper intake level of eicosapentaenoic acid (epa), docosahexaenoic acid (dha) and docosapentaenoic acid (dpa). *The EFSA Journal*, 10(7), 2815-2862.

EFSA (2013). Scientific Opinion on the substantiation of a health claim related to Bimuno® GOS and reducing gastro-intestinal discomfort pursuant to Article 13(5) of Regulation (EC) No 1924/2006. *The EFSA Journal*, 11(6), 3259-3268.

Eisenführ, F., Weber, M., & Langer, T. (2010): *Rational Decision Making*, Heidelberg, Berlin: Springer.

Erdman, K., Tunnicliffe, J., Lun, V. M., & Reimer, R. A. (2013). Eating Patterns and Composition of Meals and Snacks in Elite Canadian Athletes. *International Journal Of Sport Nutrition & Exercise Metabolism*, 23(3), 210-219.

Falony, G., Verschaeren, A. De Bruycker, F., De Preter, V., Verbecke, F. L., & De Vuyst L. (2009b). In vitro kinetics of prebiotic inulin-type fructan fermentation by butyrate-producing colon bacteria: implementation of online gas chromatography for quantitative analysis of carbon dioxide and hydrogen gas production. *Applied Environmental Microbiology*, 75(18), 5884-5892.

FAO (2008). Fats and fatty acids in human nutrition. *FAO Food and Nutrition Paper*, 91, 9-20.

Farquhar, P. H., & Keller, L. R. (1989). Preference intensity measurement. *Annals of Operations Research*, 19(1), 205-217.

Farshchi, H. R., Taylor, M. A., & Macdonald, I. A. (2004). Regular meal frequency creates more appropriate insulin sensitivity and lipid profiles compared with irregular meal frequency in healthy lean women. *European Journal Of Clinical Nutrition*, 58(7), 1071-1077.

Fass, R., Fullerton, S., Naliboff, B., Hirsh, T., & Mayer, E. A. (1998). Sexual dysfunction in patients with irritable bowel syndrom and non-ulcer dyspepsia. *Digestion*, 59(1), 79-85.

Fernández-Bañares, F., Esteve-Pardo, M., de Leon, R., Humbert, P., Cabré, E., Llovet, J. M., & Gassull, M. A. (1993). Sugar malabsorption in functional bowel disease: clinical implications. *American Journal of Gastroenterology*, 88(12), 2044-2050.

Fox, K. (2013). N. t.. In Wells, V., Wyness, L., & Coe, S. (Eds.). The British Nutrition Foundation's 45th Anniversary Conference: Behaviour change in relation to healthier lifestyles. *Nutrition Bulletin*, 38(1), 100-107.

Gaby, A. R. (2005). Adverse effects of dietary fructose. *Alternative medicine review*, 10(4).

Gay-Crosier, F., Schreiber, G., & Hauser, C. (2000). Anaphylaxis from inulin in vegetables and processed food. *The New England Journal of Medicine*, 342(18), 1372.

German, J., Freeman, S., Lebrilla, C., & Mills, D. (2008). Human milk oligosaccharides: evolution, structures and bioselectivity as substrates for intestinal bacteria, *Nestlé Nutrition Workshop, Pediatric Program*, 62, 205-222.

Gibson, P. R., Newnham, E., Barrett, J. S., Shepherd, S. J., & Muir, J. G. (2007). Review article: Fructose malabsorption and the bigger picture. *Alimentary pharmacology & therapeutics*, 25(4), 349-363.

Gibson, P. R., & Shepherd, S. J. (2010). Evidence-based dietary management of functional gastrointestinal symptoms: the fodmap approach. Journal of *Gastroenterology and Hepatology*, 25(2), 252-258.

Gilbert, P. (2013). N. t.. In Wells, V., Wyness, L., & Coe, S. (Eds.). The British Nutrition Foundation's 45th Anniversary Conference: Behaviour change in relation to healthier lifestyles. *Nutrition Bulletin*, 38(1), 100-107.

Goldstein, R., Braverman, D., & Stankiewicz, H. (2000). Carbohydrate malabsorption and the effect of dietary restriction on symptoms of irritable bowel syndrome and functional bowel complaints. *Israel Medical Association Journal*, 2(8), 583-587.

Gralnek, I. M., Hays, R. D., Kilbourne, A., Naliboff, B., & Mayer, E. A. (2000). The impact of irritable bowel syndrome on health-related quality of life. *Gastroenterology*, 119(3), 654-660.

Hahn, B. A., Kirchdoerfer, L. J., Fullerton, S., & Mayer, S. (1997). Patient perceived severity of irritable bowel syndrome in relation to symptoms, health resource utilization and quality of life. *Alimentary Pharmacology and Therapeutics*, 11(3), 553-559.

Hawthorne, B., Lambert, S., Scott, D., & Scott, B. (1991). Food intolerance and the irritable bowel syndrome. *Journal of Human Nutrition and Dietetics,* 4(1), 19-23.

Hawking, S. (n. d.). Publications. Retrieved from http://www.hawking.org.uk/publications.html.

Hillson, M. (2013). N. t.. In Wells, V., Wyness, L., & Coe, S. (Eds.). The British Nutrition Foundation's 45th Anniversary Conference: Behaviour change in relation to healthier lifestyles. *Nutrition Bulletin,* 38(1), 100-107.

Hoekstra, J. H., van Kempen, A. A. M. W., & Kneepkens, C. M. F. (1993). Apple juice malabsorption: Fructose or sorbitol?. *Journal of Pediatric Gastroenterology and Nutrition,* 16(1), 39-42.

Huether, G. (Lecturer). (2014). Interview mit Prof. Dr. Gerald Hüther zu Angst & Berufung. Retrieved from http://www.coach-your-self.tv/Startseite/TV/InterviewmitProfDrH%C3%BCtherzu AngstBerufung/tabid/1341/Default.aspx

Hyams, J. S. (1983). Sorbitol intolerance: an unappreciated cause of functional gastrointestinal complaints. *Gastroenterology,* 84(1)1, 30-33.

Hyams, J. S., Etienne, N. L., Leichtner, A. M., & Theuer, R. C. (1988). Carbohydrate Malabsorption Following Fruit Juice Ingestion in Young Children. *Pediatrics,* 82(1), 64-68.

Jensen, R. G., Blanc, B., & Patton, S. (1995). Particulate Constituents in Human and Bovine Milks. In Jensen, R. G. (Ed.), *Handbook of Milk Composition* (pp. 51-62). San Diego: Academic Press.

Kennedy, E. (2004). Dietary diversity, diet quality, and body weight regulation. *Nutrition reviews,* 62(s2), S78-S81.

Kneepkens, C. M. F., Vonk, R. J., & Fernandes, J. (1984). Incomplete intestinal absorption of fructose. *Archives of Disease in Childhood,* 59(8), 735-738.

Kneepkens, C. M. F., Jakobs, C., & Douwes, A. C. (1989): Apple juice, fructose, and chronic nonspecific diarrhoea. *Pediatrics,* 148(6), 571-573.

Knudsen, B. K., & Hessov, I. (1995). Recovery of inulin from Jerusalem artichoke (Helianthus tuberosus L.) in the small intestine of man. *British Journal of Nutrition,* 74(01), 101-113.

Komericki, P., Akkilic-Materna, M., Strimitzer, T., Weyermair, K., Hammer, H. F., & Aberer, W. (2012). Oral xylose isomerase decreases breath hydrogen excretion and improves gastrointestinal symptoms in fructose malabsorption – a double-blind, placebo-controlled study. *Alimentary Pharmacology & Therapeutics,* 36(10), 980-987.

Kuhn, R., & Gauhe, A. (1965). Bestimmung der Bindungsstelle von Sialinsäureresten in Oligosacchariden mit Hilfe von Perjodat. *Chemische Berichte*, 98(2), 395-314.

Ladas, S. D., Grammenos, I., Tassios, P. S., & Raptis, S. A. (2000). Coincidental malabsorption of lactose, fructose, and sorbitol ingested at low doses is not common in normal adults. *Digestive Diseases and Sciences*, 45(12), 2357-2362.

Langkilde, A. M., Andersson, H., Schweizer, T. F., & Würsch, P. (1994). Digestion and absorption of sorbitol, maltitol and isomalt from the small bowel. A study in ileostomy subjects. *European Journal of Clinical Nutrition*, 48(11), 768-775.

Latulippe, M. E., & Skoog, S. M. (2011). Fructose malabsorption and intolerance: effects of fructose with and without simultaneous glucose ingestion. *Critical Reviews in Food Science and Nutrition*, 51(7), 583-592.

Le, A. S., & Mulderrig, K. B. (2001). *Sorbitol and mannitol*. Nabors, O'B. (Ed.). New York, NY: Marcel Dekker.

Ledochowski, M., Widner, B., Sperner-Unterweger, B., Probst, T., Vogel, W., & Fuchs, D. (2000). Carbohydrate malabsobtion syndromes and early signs of mental depression in females. *Digestive Diseases and Sciences*, 45(12), 1255-1259.

Ledochowski, M., Sperner-Unterweger, B., Widner, B., & Fuchs, D. (1998a). Fructose malabsorption is associated with early signs of mentral depression. *European Journal of Medical Research*, 3(6), 295-298.

Ledochowski, M., Sperner-Unterweger, B., & Fuchs, D. (1998b). Lactose malabsorption is associated with early signs of mental depression in females – a preliminary report. *Digestive Diseases and Sciences*, 43(11), 2513-2517.

Ledochowski, M., Überall, F., Propst, T., & Fuchs, D. (1999). Fructose malabsorption is associated with lower plasma folic acid concentrations in middle-aged subjects. *Clinical Chemistry*, 45(11), 2013-2014.

Ledochowski, M., Widner, B., Bair, H., Probst, T., & Fuchs, D. (2000a). Fructose-and sorbitol-reduced diet improves mood and gastrointestinal disturbances in fructose malabsorbers. *Scandinavian Journal of Gastroenterology*, 35(10), 1048-1052.

Ledochowski, M., Widner, B., Sperner-Unterweger, B., Probst, T., Vogel, W., & Fuchs, D. (2000b). Carbohydrate malabsobtion syndromes and early signs of mental depression in females. *Digestive Diseases and Sciences*, 45(12), 1255-1259.

Leinoel (n. d.). *Leinöl(Leinsamen)*. Retrieved from http://www.vitalstoff-journal.de/vitalstoff-lexikon/l/leinoel-leinsamen/

Lewis, S. J., & Heaton, K. W. (1997). Stool form scale as a useful guide to intestinal transit time. *Scandinavian Journal of Gastroenterology*, 32(9), 920-924.

Lifschitz, C. H. (2000). Carbohydrate absorption from fruit juices in infants. *Pediatrics*, 105(1), e4.

Lombardi, D. A., Jin, K., Courtney, T. K., Arlinghaus, A., Folkard, S., Liang, Y., & Perry, M. J. (2014). The effects of rest breaks, work shift start time, and sleep on the onset of severe injury among workers in the People's Republic of China. *Scandinavian Journal of Work, Environment & Health*, 40(2), 146-155.

Lomer, M. C. E., Parkes, G. C., & Sanderson, J. D. (2008). Review article: Lactose intolerance in clinical practice – myths and realities. *Alimentary Pharmacology & Therapeutics*, 27(2), 93-103.

Longstreth, G. F., Thompson, W. G., Chey, W. D., Houghton, L. A., Mearin, F., & Spiller, R. C. (2006). Functional bowel disorders. *Gastroenterology*, 130(5), 1480-1491.

Maintz, L., & Novak, N. (2007). Histamine and histamine intolerance. *The American Journal of Clinical Nutrition*, 85(5), 1185-1196.

Makras, L., Van Acker, G., & De Vuyst, L. (2005). Lactobacillus paracasei subsp. paracasei 8700: 2 degrades inulin-type fructans exhibiting different degrees of polymerization. *Applied and Environmental Microbiology*, 71(11), 6531-6537.

McCoubrey, H., Parkes, G. C., Sanderson, J. D., & Lomer, M. C. E. (2008). Nutritional intakes in irritable bowel syndrome. *Journal of Human Nutrition and Dietetics*, 21(4), 396-397.

McKenzie, Y. A., Alder, A., Anderson, W. Goddard, L, Gulia, P., Jankovich, E. ...Lomer, M. C. E. (2012). British Dietic Association evidence-based guidelines for the dietary management of irritable bowel syndrome in adults. *Journal of Human Nutrition and Dietics*, 25(3), 260-274.

Meyrand, M., Dallas, D. C., Caillat, H., Bouvier, F., Martin, P., & Barile, D. (2013). Comparison of milk oligosaccharides between goats with and without the genetic ability to synthesize αs1-casein. *Small Ruminant Research*, 113(2), 411-420.

Michel, G., Nyval-Collen, P., Barbeyron, T., Czjzek, M., & Helbert, W. (2006). Bioconversion of red seaweed galactans: a focus on bacterial agarases and carrageenases. *Applied Microbiology and Biotechnology*, 71(1), 23-33.

Michie, S. (2013). N. t.. In Wells, V., Wyness, L., & Coe, S. (Eds.). The British Nutrition Foundation's 45th Anniversary Conference: Behaviour change in relation to healthier lifestyles. *Nutrition Bulletin*, 38(1), 100-107.

Mishkin, D., Sablauskas, L., Yalovsky, M., & Mishkin, S. (1997). Fructose and sorbitol malabsorption in ambulatory patients with functional dyspepsia: comparison with lactose maldigestion/malabsorption. *Digestive Diseases and Sciences*, 42(12), 2591-2598.

Montalto, M., Curigliano, V., Santoro, L., Vastola, M., Cammarota, G., Manna, R., ... & Gasbarrini, G. (2006). Management and treatment of lactose malabsorption. *World Journal of Gastroenterology*, 12(2), 187.

Molis, C., Flourié, B., Ouarne, F., Gailing, M. F., Lartigue, S., Guibert, A., Bornet, F., & Galmiche, F. P. (1996). Digestion, excretion, and energy value of fructooligosaccharides in healthy humans.*The American Society for Clinical Nutrition*, 64(3), 324-328.

Mosby's Medical Dictionary (8th ed.). St. Louis, MO: Mosby.

Monash University (2014). The Monash University Low Foodmap Diet [Software]. Available from http://www.med.monash.edu/cecs/gastro/fodmap/education.html

Moshfegh, A. J., James, E. F., Goldman, J. P., & Ahuja, J. L. C. (1999). Presence of inulin and oligofructose in the diets of Americans. *The Journal of Nutrition*, 129(7), 1407S-1411S.

Mount Sinai (n. d.). *Fiber Chart*. Retrieved from https://www.wehealny.org/healthinfo/dietaryfiber/fibercontentchart.html.

Mozaffarian, D., & Wu, J. H. (2011). Omega-3 fatty acids and cardiovascular disease effects on risk factors, molecular pathways, and clinical events. *Journal of the American College of Cardiology*, 58(20), 2047-2067.

Muir, J. G., Shepherd, S. J., Rosella, O., Rose, R., Barrett, J. S., & Gibson, P. R. (2007). Fructan and free fructose content of common Australian vegetables and fruit. *Journal of Agricultural and Food Chemistry*, 55(16), 6619-6627.

Muir, J. G., Rose, R., Rosella, O., Liels, K., Barrett, J. S., Shepherd, S. J., & Gibson, P. R. (2009). Measurement of short-chain carbohydrates in common Australian vegetables and fruits by high-performance liquid chromatography (HPLC). *Journal of Agricultural and Food Chemistry*, 57(2), 554-565.

Nanda, R., James, R., Smith, H., Dudley, C. R. K., & Jewell, D. P. (1989). Food intolerance and the irritable bowel syndrome. *Gut*, 30(8), 1099-1104.

Necas, J., Bartosikova, L. (2013). Carageenan: a review. *Veterinarni Medicina*, 58(4), 187-205.

Nelis, G. F., Vermeeren, M. A., & Jansen, W. (1990). Role of fructose-sorbitol malabsorbtion in the irritable bowel syndrome. *Gastroenterology*, 99(4), 10156-1020.

Newburg, D. S. & Neubauer, S. H. (1995). Carbohydrates in Milks: Analysis, Quantities, and Significance. In Jensen, R. G. (Ed.), *Handbook of Milk Composition* (pp. 273-349). San Diego: Academic Press.

NICNAS (2008). Multiple chemical sensitivity: identifying key research needs. *Scientific review report.*

Nucera, G., Gabrielli, M., Lupascu, A., Lauritano, E. C., Santoliquido, A., Cremonini, F., …Gasbarrini, A. (2005). Abnormal breath tests to lactose, fructose and sorbitol in irritable bowel syndrome may be explained by small intestinal bacterial overgrowth. *Alimentary Pharmacology & Therapeutics,* 21(11), 1391-1395.

O'Connell, S., & Walsh, G. (2006). Physicochemical characteristics of commercial lactases relevant to their application in the alleviation of lactose intolerance. *Applied Biochemistry and Biotechnology,* 134(2), 179-191.

Ong, D., Mitchell, S., Barrett, J., Shepherd, S., Irving, P., Biesiekierski, J., & ... Muir, J. (2010). Manipulation of dietary short chain carbohydrates alters the pattern of gas production and genesis of symptoms in irritable bowel syndrome. *Journal of Gastroenterology & Hepatology,* 25(8), 1366-1373.

Park, Y. K., & Yetley, E. A. (1993). Intakes and food sources of fructose in the United States. *The American Journal of Clinical Nutrition,* 58(5), 737S-747S.

Parker, T. J., Naylor, S. J., Riordan, A. M., & Hunter, J. O. (1995). Management of patients with food intolerance in irritable

bowel syndrome. The development and use of an exclusion diet. *Journal of Human Nutrition and Dietetics,* 8(3), 159-166.

Petitpierre, M., Gumowski, P., & Girard, J. P. (1985). Irritable bowel syndrome and hypersensitivity to food. *Annals of Allergy, Asthma & Immunology,* 54(6), 538-540.

Quigley, E., Fried, M., Gwee, K. A., Olano, C., Guarner, F., Khalif, I., ... & Le Mair, A. W. (2009). Irritable bowel syndrome: a global perspective. *WGO Practice Guideline.*

Quigley, E., M., M., Hunt, R. H., Emmanuel, A., & Hungin, A. P. S. (2013). Irritable Bowel Syndrome (IBS): What is it, what causes it and can I do anything about it? Retrieved from http://client.blueskybroadcast.com/WGO/indeux.html

Raithel, M., Weidenhiller, M., Hagel, A.-F.-K., Hetterich, U., Neurath, M. F., & Konturek, P. C. (2013). The malabsorption of commonly occurring mono and disaccharides: levels of investigation and differential diagnoses. *Dtsch Arztebl Int,* 110(46), 775-782.

Riby, J. E., Fujisawa, T., & Kretchmer, N. (1993). Fructose absorption. *The American Journal of Clinical Nutrition,* 58(5), 748S-753S.

Ross, A. C., Manson, J. E., Abrams, S. A., Aloia, J. F., Brannon, P. M., Clinton, S. K., ... & Shapses, S. A. (2011). The 2011 report on dietary reference intakes for calcium and vitamin D from the Institute of Medicine: what clinicians need to know. *Journal of Clinical Endocrinology & Metabolism*, 96(1), 53-58.

Rumessen, J. J., & Gudmand-Høyer, E. (1986). Absorption capacity of fructose in healthy adults. Comparison with sucrose and its constituent monosaccharides. *Gut*, 27(10), 1161-1168.

Rumessen, J. J., & Gudmand-Høyer, E., (1987). Malabsoption of Fructose-sorbitol mixtures. Interactions causing abdominal distress. *Scandinavian Journal of Gastroenterology*, 22(4), 431-436.

Rumessen, J. J. (1992). Fructose and related food carbohydrates. sources, intake, absorbtion, and clinical implications. *Scandinavian Journal of Gastroenterology*, 27(10), 819-828.

Ruppin, H., Bar-Meir, S., Soergel, K. H., Wood, C. M., & Schmitt Jr, M. G. (1980). Absorption of short-chain fatty acids by the colon. *Gastroenterology*, 78(6), 1500-1507.

Rycroft, C. E., Jones, M. R., Gibson, G. R., & Rastall, R. A. (2001). A comparative in vitro evaluation of the fermentation properties of prebiotic oligosaccharides. *Journal of Applied Microbiology*, 91(5), 878-887.

Scientific Community on Food (2000). Opinion of the Scientific Committee on Food on the Tolerable Upper Intake Level of Folate.

Shepherd, S. J., & Gibson, P. R. (2006). Fructose malabsorption and symptoms of irritable bowel syndrome: guidelines for effective dietary management. *Journal of the American Dietetic Association*, 106(10), 1631-1639.

Shepherd, S. J., Parker, F. C., Muir, J. G., & Gibson, P. R. (2008). Dietary triggers of abdominal symptoms in patients with irritable bowel syndrome: randomized placebo-controlled evidence. *Clinical Gastroenterology and Hepatology*, 6(7), 765-771.

Silk, D. B. A., Davis, A., Vulevic, J., Tzortzis, G., & Gibson, G. R. (2009). Clinical trial: the effects of a trans-galactooligosaccharide prebiotic on faecal microbiota and symptoms in irritable bowel syndrome. *Alimentary pharmacology & therapeutics*, 29(5), 508-518.

Simopoulos, A. P. (1999). Essential fatty acids in health and chronic disease. *The American Journal of Clinical Nutrition*, 70(3), 560s-569s.

Speier, C., Vessey, I., & Valacich, J. S. (2003). The Effects of Interruptions, Task Complexity, and Information Presentation on Computer-Supported Decision-Making Performance. *Decision Sciences*, 34(4), 771-797.

Stefanini, G. F., Saggioro, A., Alvisi, V., Angelini, G., Capurso, L., Di, L. G., ...Melzi, G. (1995). Oral cromolyn sodium in comparison with elimination diet in the irritable bowel syndrome, diarrheic type. Multicenter study of 428 patients. *Scandinavian Journal of Gastroenterology*, 30(6), 535–541.

Stockwell, M. (n. d.). *Awards/Events*. Retrieved from http://www.melissastockwell.com/Melissa_Stockwell/Awards.html.

Stubbs, J. (2013). N. t.. In Wells, V., Wyness, L., & Coe, S. (Eds.). The British Nutrition Foundation's 45th Anniversary Conference: Behaviour change in relation to healthier lifestyles. *Nutrition Bulletin*, 38(1), 100-107.

Suarez, F. L., Savaiano, D. A., & Levitt, M. D. (1995). A comparison of symptoms after the consumption of milk or lactose-hydrolyzed milk by people with self-reported severe lactose intolerance. *New England Journal of Medicine*, 333(1), 1-4.

Suarez, F. L., Springfield, J., Furne, J. K., Lohrmann, T. T., Kerr, P. S., & Levitt, M. D. (1999). Gas production in humans ingesting a soybean flour derived from beans naturally low in oligosaccharides. *The American Journal of Clinical Nutrition*, 69(1), 135-139.

Tarpila, S., Tarpila, A., Grohn, P., Silvennoinen, T., & Lindberg, L. (2004). Efficacy of ground flaxseed on constipation in patients with irritable bowel syndrome. *Current Topics in Nutraceutical Research*, 2(2), 119–125.

Test (2008). Schneller, schöner, stärker. *test – Journal Gesundheit*, 43(02), 88-92.

Teuri, U., Vapaatalo, H., & Korpela, R. (1999). Fructooligosaccharides and lactulose cause more symptoms in lactose maldigesters and subjects with pseudohypolactasia than in control lactose digesters. *The American Journal of Clinical Nutrition*, 69(5), 973-979.

Thompson, Kyle (2006). Bristol Stool Chart [Graphical illustration]. Retrieved from http://commons.wikimedia.org/wiki/File:Bristol_Stool_Chart.png

Nanda, R., Shu, L. H., & Thomas, J. R. (2012). A fodmap diet update: craze or credible. *Practical Gastroenterology*, 10(12), 37-46.

Toschke, A. M., Thorsteinsdottir, K. H., & von Kries, R. (2009). Meal frequency, breakfast consumption and childhood obesity. *International Journal Of Pediatric Obesity*, 4(4), 242-248.

Tou, J. C., Chen, J., & Thompson, L. U. (1998). Flaxseed and its lignan precursor, secoisolariciresinol diglycoside, affect pregnancy outcome and reproductive development in rats. *The Journal of nutrition*, 128(11), 1861-1868.

Truswell, A. S., Seach, J. M., & Thorburn, A. W. (1988). Incomplete absorption of pure Fructose in healthy subjects and the facilitating effect of glucose. *The American Journal of Clinical Nutrition*, 48(6), 1424-1430.

U. S. Department of Agriculture and U. S. Department of Health and Human Services (2010). *Dietary Guidelines for Americans* (7th ed.). Washington, DC: U. S. Government Printing Office.

U. S. Department of Agriculture, Agricultural Research Service (2013). USDA National Nutrient Database for Standard Reference, Release 26. Nutrient Data Laboratory HomePage, http://www.ars.usda.gov/ba/bhnrc/ndl.

van Loo, J., Coussement, P., De Leenheer, L., Hoebregs, H., & Smits, G. (1995). On the presence of inulin and oligoFructose as natural ingredients in the western diet. *Critical Reviews in Food Science and Nutrition*, 35(6), 525–552.

Varea, V., de Carpi, J. M., Puig, C., Alda, J. A., Camacho, E., Ormazabal, A., ... & Gómez, L. (2005). Malabsorption of carbohydrates and depression in children and adolescents. *Journal of pediatric gastroenterology and nutrition*, 40(5), 561-565.

Verhoef, P., Stampfer, M. J., Buring, J. F., Gaziano, J. M., Allen, R. H., Stabler, S. P., ... & Willett, W. C. (1996). Homocysteine metabolism and risk of myocardial infarction: relation with vitamins B6, B12, and folate. *American Journal of Epidemiology*, 143(9), 845-859.

Vernia, P., Ricciardi, M. R., Frandina, C., Bilotta, T., & Frieri, G. (1995). Lactose malabsorption and irritable bowel syndrome. Effect of a long-term lactose-free diet. *The Italian Journal of Gastroenterology*, 27(3), 117-121.

Vesa, T. H., Korpela, R. A., & Sahi, T. (1996). Tolerance to small amounts of lactose in lactose maldigesters. *The American journal of clinical nutrition*, 64(2), 197-20.

Virtanen, S. M., Räsänen, L., Mäenpää, J., & Åkerblom, H. K. (1987). Dietary Survey of Finnish Adolescent Diabetics and Non-Diabetic Controls. *Acta Paediatrica*, 76(5), 801-808.

Vos, M. B., Kimmons, J. E., Gillespie, C., Welsh, J., & Blanck, H. M. (2008). Dietary Fructose consumption among US children and adults: the Third National Health and Nutrition Examination Survey. *The Medscape Journal of Medicine*, 10(7), 160.

Watson, B. D. (2008). Public health and carrageenan regulation : a review and analysis. *Journal of Applied Phycology*, 20(5), 505-513.

Webb, F. S., & Whitney, E. N. (2008). *Nutrition: Concepts and controversies* (11th ed.). Belmont, CA: Thomson/ Wadsworth.

Wells, N. E. J., Hahn, B. A., & Whorwell, P. J. (1997). Clinical economics review: irritable bowel syndrome. *Allimentary Pharmacology and Therapeutics*, 11, 1019-1030.

Winterfeldt, D. von, & Edwards, W. (1986). *Decision analysis and behavioral research*. Cambridge: Cambridge University Press.

--

Sources regarding the prevalence of IBS:

England

Jones, R., & Lydeard, S. (1992). Irritable bowel syndrom in the general population. *British Medical Journal*, 304(6819), 87-90.

Japan and the Netherlands

Schlemper, R. J., van der Werf, S. D. J., Vandenbroucke, J. P., Blemond, I., & Lamers, C. B. H. W. (1993). Peptic ulcer, non-ulcer dysepsia and irritable bowel syndrom in the Netherlands and Japan. *Scandinavian Journal of Gastroenterology*, 28(200), 33-41.

Nigeria

Olubuykle, I. O., Olawuyl, F., & Fasanmade, A. A. (1995). A study of irritable bowel syndrom diagnosed by manning criteria in an african population. *Digestive Diseases and Sciences*, 40(5), 983-985.

USA

Longstreth, G. F., & Wolde-Tsadik, G. (1993). Irritable bowel-type symptoms in hmo examinees. *Digestive Diseases and Sciences*, 38(9), 1581-1589.

Talley, N. J., Zinsmeister, A. R., van Dyke, C., & Melton, L. J. (1991). Epidemiology of colonic symptoms and the irritable bowel syndrome. *Gastroenterology*, 101(4), 927-934.

O'Keefe, E. A., Talley, N. J., Zinsmeister, A. R., & Jacobsen, S. J. (1995). Bowel disorders impair functional status and quality of life in the elerdly: a population-based study. *Journal of Gastroenterology*, 50A, M184-M189.

--

Wilder-Smith, C. H., Materna, A., Wermelinger, C., & Schuler, J. (2013). Fruktose and Laktose intolerance and malabsorption testing: the relationship with symptoms in functional gastrointestinal disorders. *Alimentary Pharmacology and Therapeutics*, 37(11), 1074-1083.

Winterfeldt, D. von, & Edwards, W. (1986). *Decision analysis and behavioral research*. Cambridge: Cambridge University Press.

Zohar, D. (1999). When things go wrong: The effect of daily work hassles on effort, exertion and negative mood. *Journal of Occupational and Organizational Psychology*, 72(3), 265-283.

www.ingramcontent.com/pod-product-compliance
Ingram Content Group UK Ltd.
Pitfield, Milton Keynes, MK11 3LW, UK
UKHW051450290926
15471UKWH00008B/1114

9 781941 978245